The Role of Telemedicine in Transforming Healthcare Delivery—Capabilities and Barriers

The Role of Telemedicine in Transforming Healthcare Delivery—Capabilities and Barriers

Guest Editor

Motti Haimi

MDPI

Basel • Beijing • Wuhan • Barcelona • Belgrade • Novi Sad • Cluj • Manchester

Guest Editor
Motti Haimi
Health Systems Management
Department
Yezreel Valley College
Yezreel Valley
Israel

Editorial Office
MDPI AG
Grosspeteranlage 5
4052 Basel, Switzerland

This is a reprint of the Special Issue, published open access by the journal *Healthcare* (ISSN 2227-9032), freely accessible at: https://www.mdpi.com/journal/healthcare/special_issues/SRI81W939S.

For citation purposes, cite each article independently as indicated on the article page online and as indicated below:

Lastname, A.A.; Lastname, B.B. Article Title. *Journal Name* **Year**, *Volume Number*, Page Range.

ISBN 978-3-7258-6346-4 (Hbk)
ISBN 978-3-7258-6347-1 (PDF)
https://doi.org/10.3390/books978-3-7258-6347-1

Contents

About the Editor vii

Preface ix

Motti Haimi
Editorial: The Role of Telemedicine in Transforming Healthcare Delivery—Capabilities and Barriers
Reprinted from: *Healthcare* **2025**, *13*, 2927, https://doi.org/10.3390/healthcare13222927 1

Gillie Gabay, Hana Ornoy, Attila Gere and Howard Moskowitz
Personalizing Communication of Clinicians with Chronically Ill Elders in Digital Encounters—A Patient-Centered View
Reprinted from: *Healthcare* **2024**, *12*, 434, https://doi.org/10.3390/healthcare12040434 9

Nancy Chen, Jen-Hung Wang and Cheng-Jen Chiu
Satisfaction with Teleophthalmology Services: Insights from Remote Areas of Taiwan
Reprinted from: *Healthcare* **2024**, *12*, 818, https://doi.org/10.3390/healthcare12080818 21

Motti Haimi and Aaron Lerner
Utilizing Telemedicine Applications in Celiac Disease and Other Gluten-Free-Diet-Dependent Conditions: Insights from the COVID-19 Pandemic
Reprinted from: *Healthcare* **2024**, *12*, 1132, https://doi.org/10.3390/healthcare12111132 34

Abigaela Bîlbîie, Andreea-Ionela Puiu, Viorel Mihăilă and Marin Burcea
Investigating Physicians' Adoption of Telemedicine in Romania Using Technology Acceptance Model (TAM)
Reprinted from: *Healthcare* **2024**, *12*, 1531, https://doi.org/10.3390/healthcare12151531 47

Emily Johnson, Ryan Kruis, Rosaura Orengo-Aguayo, Rebecca Verdin, Kathryn King, Dee Ford and Regan Stewart
Telehealth Outreach Program for Child Traumatic Stress: Strategies for Long-Term Sustainability
Reprinted from: *Healthcare* **2024**, *12*, 2110, https://doi.org/10.3390/healthcare12212110 68

Sharon Cobb, Attallah Dillard, Ehsan Yaghmaei, Mohsen Bazargan and Shervin Assari
Telehealth Perceived Benefits and Self-Efficacy Do Not Mediate the Effects of Demographic, Health, and Social Determinants on Telehealth Use of Low-Income African American and Latino Residents of Public Housing in Los Angeles
Reprinted from: *Healthcare* **2025**, *13*, 286, https://doi.org/10.3390/healthcare13030286 87

Chiara Bernuzzi, Maria Adele Piccardo and Chiara Guglielmetti
Mapping Research Trends on the Implications of Telemedicine for Healthcare Professionals: A Comprehensive Bibliometric Analysis
Reprinted from: *Healthcare* **2025**, *13*, 1149, https://doi.org/10.3390/healthcare13101149 101

Sinaa Al-Aqeel, Alaa Mutlaq, Njood Alkhalifa, Deem Alnassar, Rashed Alghanim, Wafa Algarni and Sultanah Alshammari
Pharmacists' Interventions in Virtual Diabetes Clinics: Cost-Effectiveness Feasibility Study
Reprinted from: *Healthcare* **2025**, *13*, 2130, https://doi.org/10.3390/healthcare13172130 121

Angelica Gherman, Codrina Mihaela Levai, Ovidiu Alin Haţegan, Călin Marius Popoiu, Emil Robert Stoicescu and Anca Laura Maghiari
Telemedicine-Supported Intervention Versus Standard Care for Managing Cardiovascular Risk Factors in a Socially Deprived Urban Population: A Prospective Study
Reprinted from: *Healthcare* **2025**, *13*, 2202, https://doi.org/10.3390/healthcare13172202 133

Rafael Pizarro-Mena, Elena S. Rotarou, Hendrik Adrián Baracaldo-Campo, Samuel Duran-Aguero, Solange Parra-Soto, Felipe Retamal-Walter, et al.
Implementation of Telehealth Among Older People: A Challenge and Opportunity for Latin America and the Caribbean—A Literature Review
Reprinted from: *Healthcare* **2025**, *13*, 2680, https://doi.org/10.3390/healthcare13212680 . . . . . **146**

About the Editor

Motti Haimi

Motti Haimi is an experienced pediatrician, pediatric onco-hematologist, and Medical Director. He has demonstrated a history of working in the hospital and healthcare industry. He is skilled in clinical research, medical education, epidemiology, pediatrics, hematology, telehealth, and anti-healthcare disparities activism.

He is a Senior Clinical Lecturer at the Rappaport Faculty of Medicine, Technion; a senior lecturer at the Max Stern Yezreel Valey Academic College; and a telemedicine lecturer and researcher. Haimi is a strong healthcare services professional with an MD degree from the medical school of the Hebrew University in Jerusalem. He also received his Ph.D. degree and master's degree (Cum Laude) in Health Administration, focusing on healthcare management, from the School of Public Health at Haifa University.

In 2019, he received a Travel Fellowship from the Daniel Turnberg UK/Middle East Travel Fellowships program (Academy of Medical Sciences) to support a visit to Oxford University.

His areas of research and interest include pediatric hematology; dysmorphology and familial genetic syndromes in children; genetics, cancer, and hereditary predispositions for cancer; infections in immune-suppressed children; gastroenterology and nutrition in children; micronutrient deficiencies in the pediatric age group; and the decision-making of primary care doctors in telemedicine.

In recent years, he has become especially interested in the fields of telehealth, telemedicine, health informatics, and pediatric telemedicine services and is especially interested in finding telehealth solutions for the elderly population and for other populations who may experience difficulties in accessing digital solutions (the digital divide).

He is part of the Healthcare Disparities and Digital Health working group of the International Society for Telemedicine and e-Health.

Preface

The rapid evolution of digital health has fundamentally reshaped global healthcare, with telemedicine becoming a cornerstone of modern patient care. Accelerated dramatically by the COVID-19 pandemic, this transformation has highlighted both the immense potential and persistent challenges of remote healthcare delivery.

This Special Issue of *Healthcare* compiles a diverse collection of research and review articles exploring telemedicine's multifaceted role in transforming healthcare across various populations, clinical settings, and geographical contexts. The ten featured contributions collectively address critical implementation dimensions, including technological adoption, provider acceptance, patient satisfaction, cost-effectiveness, and equity considerations. These studies cover diverse domains, such as chronic disease management, mental health, specialty care, and geriatric medicine, and examine populations from socioeconomically disadvantaged urban areas to remote rural regions globally. Understanding these diverse applications is essential as telemedicine moves from an emergency measure to an integral component of sustainable healthcare systems.

Motti Haimi
Guest Editor

healthcare MDPI

Editorial

Editorial: The Role of Telemedicine in Transforming Healthcare Delivery—Capabilities and Barriers

Motti Haimi [1,2,3]

[1] Health Systems Management Department, The Max Stern Yezreel Valley Academic College, D.N Emek Yezreel 1930600, Israel; mottih@yvc.ac.il
[2] Rappaport Faculty of Medicine, Technion—Israel Institute of Technology, Haifa 3109601, Israel
[3] Meuhedet Healthcare Services, North District, Haifa 3109601, Israel

1. Introduction

The rapid evolution of digital health technologies has fundamentally reshaped healthcare delivery worldwide, with telemedicine emerging as a cornerstone of modern patient care. This transformation, dramatically accelerated by the COVID-19 pandemic, has revealed both the immense potential and persistent challenges inherent in delivering healthcare services remotely [1,2]. This Special Issue of *Healthcare* brings together a diverse collection of research and review articles that explore telemedicine's multifaceted role in transforming healthcare delivery across various populations, clinical settings, and geographical contexts.

The ten contributions featured in this Special Issue collectively address critical dimensions of telemedicine and its implementation: from technological adoption and provider acceptance to patient satisfaction, cost-effectiveness, and equity considerations. These studies span diverse healthcare domains, including chronic disease management, mental health services, specialty care, and geriatric medicine, while examining populations ranging from socioeconomically disadvantaged urban communities to remote rural areas across multiple continents. Understanding these diverse applications is essential as telemedicine evolves from an emergency response measure to an integral component of sustainable healthcare delivery systems [3].

2. Provider Adoption and Acceptance

Understanding the factors that influence healthcare providers' adoption of telemedicine is fundamental to successful implementation. Bîlbîie et al. (Contribution 1) [4] investigate the acceptance that Romanian physicians practiced for telemedicine through the Technology Acceptance Model (TAM), analyzing 1093 nationwide survey responses. Their findings reveal that perceived usefulness emerges as a stronger predictor of adoption compared to perceived ease of use, while subjective norms, perceived incentives, and accessibility to medical records significantly influence behavioral intention to use telemedicine. This study underscores that successful telemedicine implementation requires addressing not only technological barriers but also systemic factors, including regulatory frameworks and financial incentives. These findings align with broader research demonstrating that organizational support and clear reimbursement policies are critical enablers of telemedicine adoption [5,6].

The human dimension of healthcare delivery in digital settings is explored by Gabay et al. (Contribution 2) [7], who examine communication between clinicians and chronically ill elderly patients during digital encounters. Their patient-centered analysis reveals that personalized communication strategies can help preserve therapeutic relationships in virtual settings, addressing concerns about losing personal connections that are particularly acute among elderly populations. This work emphasizes that technology alone cannot ensure quality care; rather, clinicians must adapt their communication approaches to maintain empathy and connection in digital environments. The importance of the quality of communication in telemedicine has been increasingly recognized as a determinant of patient satisfaction and treatment adherence [8].

3. Disease-Specific Applications and Clinical Effectiveness

Several contributions demonstrate telemedicine's efficacy in managing specific conditions and populations. Gherman et al. (Contribution 3) [9] present a prospective controlled study examining telemedicine-supported interventions versus standard care for cardiovascular risk factor management in a socially deprived urban population in Romania. Their six-month intervention, incorporating regular phone calls focused on adherence to medication, self-monitoring, and lifestyle modifications, demonstrates telemedicine's potential to address healthcare disparities in underserved communities where traditional healthcare access remains limited. These findings contribute to growing evidence that telemedicine interventions can effectively reduce cardiovascular risk factors when integrated with patient education and remote monitoring [10,11].

Al-Aqeel et al. (Contribution 4) [12] contribute valuable evidence on the cost-effectiveness of pharmacist-led virtual diabetes clinics. Their feasibility study characterizes pharmacists' interventions in telepharmacy settings, demonstrating improved diabetes-related outcomes while enhancing access to specialized pharmaceutical care. This work illustrates how telemedicine can expand the roles of various healthcare professionals beyond traditional boundaries, optimizing resource utilization in the management of diabetes. The integration of telepharmacy into chronic disease management represents a promising avenue for healthcare system optimization, particularly given the global shortage of healthcare professionals [13].

Haimi and Lerner (Contribution 5) [14] provide a comprehensive narrative review of telemedicine applications in celiac disease and gluten-free diet-dependent conditions, drawing insights from the COVID-19 pandemic experience. Their analysis reveals how telehealth facilitated essential dietary counseling during lockdowns and suggests sustained benefits for ongoing disease management. This review demonstrates telemedicine's value in conditions requiring long-term nutritional support and monitoring, particularly in regions with limited access to specialized dietitians. The role of telemedicine in nutritional counseling and dietary management remains an underexplored area, warranting further investigation [15].

The application of telemedicine to specialized care is exemplified by Chen et al. (Contribution 6) [16], who assessed satisfaction with teleophthalmology services in remote areas of Taiwan. Their study validates the efficacy of an integrated real-time videoconferencing system incorporating ophthalmic instruments, demonstrating that specialty telemedicine services can effectively reach geographically isolated populations while maintaining high patient satisfaction levels. Teleophthalmology has emerged as one of the most successful applications of telemedicine, with its effectiveness demonstrated in diabetic retinopathy screening and glaucoma management [17,18].

4. Mental Health and Pediatric Applications

Johnson et al. (Contribution 7) [19] address a critical gap in mental health services by examining a telehealth outreach program for traumatic stress in children. Their study on Trauma-Focused Cognitive Behavioral Therapy (TF-CBT) delivery via telehealth identifies strategies for long-term sustainability, which is particularly important given documented disparities in access to mental health services for racial and ethnic minority youths and rural communities. This contribution highlights telemedicine's potential to democratize access to evidence-based mental health interventions for vulnerable pediatric populations. The expansion of telepsychiatry and tele-mental health services was one of the most significant developments during the pandemic, with evidence suggesting comparable outcomes to in-person care for many conditions [20,21].

5. Health Equity and Socioeconomic Determinants

A crucial theme emerging from this Special Issue concerns health equity and the digital divide. Cobb et al. (Contribution 8) [22] present sobering findings on telehealth use among low-income African American and Latino residents of public housing in Los Angeles. Notably, their research reveals that perceived benefits and self-efficacy do not mediate the effects of demographic, health, and social determinants on telehealth utilization. These findings challenge assumptions that simply improving attitudes toward telemedicine will overcome structural barriers, emphasizing instead the need for comprehensive interventions addressing internet access, digital literacy, and systemic inequities. The persistence of digital health disparities represents one of the most pressing challenges for the implementation of telemedicine, requiring policy interventions that extend beyond healthcare systems to address broader social determinants of health [23,24].

6. Synthesis of Systematic Evidence

Two comprehensive review articles provide broader perspectives on telemedicine's evolving landscape. Bernuzzi et al. (Contribution 9) [25] offer a bibliometric analysis that maps research trends on telemedicine's implications for healthcare professionals. Their systematic analysis of 160 articles reveals that successful telemedicine implementation requires more than technological readiness—healthcare professionals' wellbeing must also be considered a strategic priority, as this directly impacts sustainability and quality of care. This framework reframes telemedicine as a complex organizational transformation rather than a merely technological intervention. The impact of telemedicine on healthcare workforce dynamics, including potential burnout prevention through increased flexibility and concerns about professional isolation, requires ongoing monitoring and research [26].

Pizarro-Mena et al. (Contribution 10) [27] conduct an extensive literature review on the implementation of telehealth among older people in Latin America and the Caribbean. While the COVID-19 pandemic accelerated the adoption of telehealth in gerontology and geriatrics, their analysis identifies persistent challenges, including digital literacy barriers, limited infrastructure, and cultural factors that must be addressed to ensure equitable access for aging populations in resource-limited settings. The unique needs of elderly populations in the adoption of telemedicine, including age-related sensory and cognitive changes, unfamiliarity with technology, and preference for in-person care, make tailored implementation strategies necessary [28,29].

7. Future Directions

Collectively, these contributions paint a nuanced picture of telemedicine's transformation of healthcare delivery. The evidence demonstrates clear benefits: improved access to care for geographically isolated and underserved populations, enhanced chronic disease management, cost-effectiveness in specific applications, and consistent patient satisfaction across diverse clinical contexts. Telemedicine has proven particularly valuable for follow-up care, chronic disease monitoring, mental health services, and specialty consultations. However, the research also reveals significant barriers that threaten the equitable implementation of telehealth.

Infrastructure limitations, particularly inadequate broadband access in rural and low-income areas, remain fundamental obstacles [30]. The digital divide extends beyond connectivity to encompass digital literacy, device availability, and technological comfort, particularly among the elderly and socioeconomically disadvantaged populations. Provider-related barriers include concerns about reimbursement, uncertainty regarding regulation, and the need for training in telemedicine-specific communication skills [31]. System-level challenges involve interoperability, data security, and the integration of telemedicine platforms with existing healthcare infrastructure.

8. Critical Research Gaps and Future Priorities

While this Special Issue advances our understanding of telemedicine's implementation, several critical research gaps warrant attention. First, longitudinal outcome studies are needed to assess the long-term effectiveness of telemedicine interventions across various clinical conditions. Most existing studies, including several in this collection, focus on short-to-medium term outcomes. Research examining 5–10-year outcomes, including clinical endpoints, healthcare utilization patterns, and patient satisfaction trajectories, would provide crucial evidence for sustainable telemedicine integration [32].

Second, comparative effectiveness research must expand beyond simple telemedicine-versus-usual-care designs to examine optimal modalities for specific conditions and populations. Which patients benefit most from synchronous video consultations versus asynchronous store-and-forward approaches? When are hybrid models superior to purely virtual or in-person care? Understanding these nuances will enable precise implementation tailored to patient needs and healthcare contexts [33].

Third, the economic evaluation of telemedicine remains incomplete. While studies like Al-Aqeel et al. [12] provide valuable feasibility data, comprehensive health economic analyses incorporating societal costs, productivity gains, patient time savings, and long-term cost trajectories are essential for policy decision-making. Standardized frameworks for telemedicine's cost-effectiveness assessment across different healthcare systems would facilitate evidence synthesis and policy translation [34].

Fourth, the implementation of science research must identify effective strategies for scaling telemedicine in diverse settings. The contributions by Johnson et al. [19] and Pizarro-Mena et al. [27] highlight sustainability challenges, but more research is needed on organizational factors, workflow integration, payment models, and training programs that enable successful large-scale implementation. Comparative implementation studies across different healthcare systems could identify transferable success factors [35].

Fifth, research on the integration of artificial intelligence with telemedicine represents an area for development. While not extensively covered in this Special Issue, AI-assisted triage, diagnostic support, and automated monitoring have the potential to enhance telemedicine capabilities while raising new questions about clinical validation, liability, and the preservation of human connection in care delivery [36,37]. Studies examining optimal human–AI collaboration in telemedicine settings are urgently needed.

Sixth, research on patient preference and satisfaction must move beyond simple satisfaction scores to understand the factors driving patient choices between telemedicine and in-person care. What clinical scenarios do patients prefer to receive through virtual care? How do preferences vary by demographic characteristics, health literacy, prior technology experience, and clinical condition? Understanding patient decision-making will inform the design of patient-centered hybrid care models [38].

Finally, health equity research must examine not only disparities in access but also disparities in quality for the delivery of care through telemedicine. Do outcomes differ by race, ethnicity, socioeconomic status, or language proficiency when care is delivered via telemedicine? Are certain populations receiving lower-quality virtual care due to communication barriers, technological limitations, or implicit biases? As Cobb et al. [22] demonstrate, structural interventions beyond changes in attitude are necessary to achieve health equity in digital healthcare delivery [39,40].

9. Implications for Policy and Practice

Moving forward, several priority areas emerge from this body of work. First, policies must address structural barriers to access, including universal broadband infrastructure, device provision programs, and digital literacy initiatives targeted at vulnerable populations. Telemedicine cannot achieve its potential for equity without fundamental investments in digital infrastructure as a social determinant of health [41,42].

Second, reimbursement models must evolve to fairly compensate telemedicine services while incentivizing quality care. Payment parity between virtual and in-person visits, when clinically appropriate, should be accompanied by quality metrics ensuring that telemedicine maintains high standards of care delivery. Value-based payment models may better capture telemedicine's contributions to access, convenience, and prevention than traditional fee-for-service approaches [43].

Third, provider training programs should incorporate telemedicine-specific competencies, including digital communication skills, cultural sensitivity in virtual care delivery, and proficiency with various telemedicine platforms and technologies. Medical education must evolve to prepare future healthcare professionals for hybrid practice environments where telemedicine is integrated seamlessly with in-person care [44].

Fourth, regulatory frameworks must balance innovation with patient safety. Licensure portability, privacy protections, prescribing regulations, and liability standards need modernization to support telemedicine expansion while safeguarding patients. International collaboration on telemedicine standards and regulations could facilitate cross-border care delivery where appropriate [45].

10. Conclusions

The pandemic served as an unprecedented catalyst for the adoption of telemedicine, demonstrating both its potential and its limitations. As healthcare systems transition to post-pandemic normalcy, the challenge lies in preserving telemedicine's benefits while addressing its shortcomings. Hybrid care models that thoughtfully integrate virtual and in-person services may offer the most promising path forward, allowing personalized care delivery that leverages technology's strengths while maintaining essential aspects of traditional healthcare relationships.

This Special Issue contributes valuable evidence to guide the continued evolution of telemedicine. By examining its implementation across diverse populations, healthcare systems, and clinical applications, these studies provide actionable insights for policymakers, healthcare administrators, clinicians, and researchers working to ensure that telemedicine fulfills its promise of becoming more accessible, efficient, and equitable healthcare for all. The research gaps identified here represent opportunities for the scientific community to advance knowledge and improve practice, ultimately enhancing patient care in an increasingly digital healthcare landscape.

Conflicts of Interest: The authors declare no conflicts of interest.

List of Contributions

1. Bîlbîie, A.; Puiu, A.-I.; Mihăilă, V.; Burcea, M. Investigating Physicians' Adoption of Telemedicine in Romania Using Technology Acceptance Model (TAM). *Healthcare* **2024**, *12*, 1531.
2. Gabay, G.; Ornoy, H.; Gere, A.; Moskowitz, H. Personalizing Communication of Clinicians with Chronically Ill Elders in Digital Encounters—A Patient-Centered View. *Healthcare* **2024**, *12*, 434.
3. Gherman, A.; Levai, C.M.; Haţegan, O.A.; Popoiu, C.M.; Stoicescu, E.R.; Maghiari, A.L. Telemedicine-Supported Intervention Versus Standard Care for Managing Cardiovascular Risk Factors in a Socially Deprived Urban Population: A Prospective Study. *Healthcare* **2025**, *13*, 2202.
4. Al-Aqeel, S.; Mutlaq, A.; Alkhalifa, N.; Alnassar, D.; Alghanim, R.; Algarni, W.; Alshammari, S. Pharmacists' Interventions in Virtual Diabetes Clinics: Cost-Effectiveness Feasibility Study. *Healthcare* **2025**, *13*, 2130.
5. Haimi, M.; Lerner, A. Utilizing Telemedicine Applications in Celiac Disease and Other Gluten-Free-Diet-Dependent Conditions: Insights from the COVID-19 Pandemic. *Healthcare* **2024**, *12*, 1132.
6. Chen, N.; Wang, J.-H.; Chiu, C.-J. Satisfaction with Teleophthalmology Services: Insights from Remote Areas of Taiwan. *Healthcare* **2024**, *12*, 818.
7. Johnson, E.; Kruis, R.; Orengo-Aguayo, R.; Verdin, R.; King, K.; Ford, D.; Stewart, R. Telehealth Outreach Program for Child Traumatic Stress: Strategies for Long-Term Sustainability. *Healthcare* **2024**, *12*, 2110.
8. Cobb, S.; Dillard, A.; Yaghmaei, E.; Bazargan, M.; Assari, S. Telehealth Perceived Benefits and Self-Efficacy Do Not Mediate the Effects of Demographic, Health, and Social Determinants on Telehealth Use of Low-Income African American and Latino Residents of Public Housing in Los Angeles. *Healthcare* **2025**, *13*, 286.
9. Bernuzzi, C.; Piccardo, M.A.; Guglielmetti, C. Mapping Research Trends on the Implications of Telemedicine for Healthcare Professionals: A Comprehensive Bibliometric Analysis. *Healthcare* **2025**, *13*, 1149.
10. Pizarro-Mena, R.; Rotarou, E.S.; Baracaldo-Campo, H.A.; et al. Implementation of Telehealth Among Older People: A Challenge and Opportunity for Latin America and the Caribbean—A Literature Review. *Healthcare* **2025**, *13*, 2680.

References

1. Hollander, J.E.; Carr, B.G. Virtually Perfect? Telemedicine for COVID-19. *N. Engl. J. Med.* **2020**, *382*, 1679–1681. [CrossRef]
2. Wosik, J.; Fudim, M.; Cameron, B.; Gellad, Z.F.; Cho, A.; Phinney, D.; Curtis, S.; Roman, M.; Poon, E.G.; Ferranti, J.; et al. Telehealth Transformation: COVID-19 and the Rise of Virtual Care. *J. Am. Med. Inform. Assoc.* **2020**, *27*, 957–962. [CrossRef] [PubMed]
3. Kichloo, A.; Albosta, M.; Dettloff, K.; Wani, F.; El-Amir, Z.; Singh, J.; Aljadah, M.; Chakinala, R.C.; Kanugula, A.K.; Solanki, S.; et al. Telemedicine, the Current COVID-19 Pandemic and the Future: A Narrative Review and Perspectives Moving Forward in the USA. *Fam. Med. Community Health* **2020**, *8*, e000530. [CrossRef] [PubMed]
4. Bîlbîie, A.; Puiu, A.-I.; Mihăilă, V.; Burcea, M. Investigating Physicians' Adoption of Telemedicine in Romania Using Technology Acceptance Model (TAM). *Healthcare* **2024**, *12*, 1531. [CrossRef] [PubMed]
5. Jacob, C.; Sanchez-Vazquez, A.; Ivory, C. Social, Organizational, and Technological Factors Impacting Clinicians' Adoption of Mobile Health Tools: Systematic Literature Review. *JMIR Mhealth Uhealth* **2020**, *8*, e15935 [CrossRef]; Erratum in *JMIR Mhealth Uhealth* **2022**, *10*, e37747. [CrossRef] [PubMed] [PubMed Central]
6. Kruse, C.S.; Karem, P.; Shifflett, K.; Vegi, L.; Ravi, K.; Brooks, M. Evaluating barriers to adopting telemedicine worldwide: A systematic review. *J. Telemed. Telecare* **2018**, *24*, 4–12. [CrossRef] [PubMed] [PubMed Central]
7. Gabay, G.; Ornoy, H.; Gere, A.; Moskowitz, H. Personalizing Communication of Clinicians with Chronically Ill Elders in Digital Encounters—A Patient-Centered View. *Healthcare* **2024**, *12*, 434. [CrossRef]
8. Rho, M.J.; Kim, S.R.; Kim, H.-S.; Cho, J.-H.; Yoon, K.-H.; Mun, S.K.; Choi, I.Y. Exploring the Relationship Among User Satisfaction, Compliance, and Clinical Outcomes of Telemedicine Services for Glucose Control. *Telemed. e-Health* **2014**, *20*, 712–720. [CrossRef]

9. Gherman, A.; Levai, C.M.; Haţegan, O.A.; Popoiu, C.M.; Stoicescu, E.R.; Maghiari, A.L. Telemedicine-Supported Intervention Versus Standard Care for Managing Cardiovascular Risk Factors in a Socially Deprived Urban Population: A Prospective Study. *Healthcare* **2025**, *13*, 2202. [CrossRef]
10. Omboni, S.; Caserini, M.; Coronetti, C. Telemedicine and M-Health in Hypertension Management: Technologies, Applications and Clinical Evidence. *High Blood Press Cardiovasc. Prev.* **2016**, *23*, 187–196. [CrossRef] [PubMed]
11. Kario, K.; Harada, N.; Okura, A. Digital Therapeutics for Essential Hypertension Using a Smartphone Application: A Randomized, Open-Label, Multicenter Pilot Study. *J. Clin. Hypertens.* **2021**, *23*, 923–934. [CrossRef]
12. Al-Aqeel, S.; Mutlaq, A.; Alkhalifa, N.; Alnassar, D.; Alghanim, R.; Algarni, W.; Alshammari, S. Pharmacists' Interventions in Virtual Diabetes Clinics: Cost-Effectiveness Feasibility Study. *Healthcare* **2025**, *13*, 2130. [CrossRef] [PubMed]
13. Hussain, A.; Bowen, A.M. Exploring Pharmacist Roles in Telepharmacy for Chronic Disease Management in New York State: A Qualitative Inquiry into Improving Implementation, Patient Communication, and Healthcare Technology Support. *Cureus* **2024**, *16*, e62982. [CrossRef] [PubMed] [PubMed Central]
14. Haimi, M.; Lerner, A. Utilizing Telemedicine Applications in Celiac Disease and Other Gluten-Free-Diet-Dependent Conditions: Insights from the COVID-19 Pandemic. *Healthcare* **2024**, *12*, 1132. [CrossRef] [PubMed]
15. Calcaterra, V.; Verduci, E.; Vandoni, M.; Rossi, V.; Di Profio, E.; Carnevale Pellino, V.; Tranfaglia, V.; Pascuzzi, M.C.; Borsani, B.; Bosetti, A.; et al. Telehealth: A Useful Tool for the Management of Nutrition and Exercise Programs in Pediatric Obesity in the COVID-19 Era. *Nutrients* **2021**, *13*, 3689. [CrossRef] [PubMed] [PubMed Central]
16. Chen, N.; Wang, J.-H.; Chiu, C.-J. Satisfaction with Teleophthalmology Services: Insights from Remote Areas of Taiwan. *Healthcare* **2024**, *12*, 818. [CrossRef]
17. Rathi, S.; Tsui, E.; Mehta, N.; Zahid, S.; Schuman, J.S. The Current State of Teleophthalmology in the United States. *Ophthalmology* **2017**, *124*, 1729–1734. [CrossRef]
18. Sim, D.A.; Mitry, D.; Alexander, P.; Mapani, A.; Goverdhan, S.; Aslam, T.; Bunce, C.; Keane, P.A.; Hamilton, R.; Welch, S.; et al. The Evolution of Teleophthalmology Programs in the United Kingdom: Beyond Diabetic Retinopathy Screening. *J. Diabetes Sci. Technol.* **2016**, *10*, 308–317. [CrossRef]
19. Johnson, E.; Kruis, R.; Orengo-Aguayo, R.; Verdin, R.; King, K.; Ford, D.; Stewart, R. Telehealth Outreach Program for Child Traumatic Stress: Strategies for Long-Term Sustainability. *Healthcare* **2024**, *12*, 2110. [CrossRef]
20. Hubley, S.; Lynch, S.B.; Schneck, C.; Thomas, M.; Shore, J. Review of Key Telepsychiatry Outcomes. *World J. Psychiatry* **2016**, *6*, 269–282. [CrossRef]
21. Hilty, D.M.; Ferrer, D.C.; Parish, M.B.; Johnston, B.; Callahan, E.J.; Yellowlees, P.M. The effectiveness of telemental health: A 2013 review. *Telemed. e-Health* **2013**, *19*, 444–454. [CrossRef] [PubMed] [PubMed Central]
22. Cobb, S.; Dillard, A.; Yaghmaei, E.; Bazargan, M.; Assari, S. Telehealth Perceived Benefits and Self-Efficacy Do Not Mediate the Effects of Demographic, Health, and Social Determinants on Telehealth Use of Low-Income African American and Latino Residents of Public Housing in Los Angeles. *Healthcare* **2025**, *13*, 286. [CrossRef]
23. Crawford, A.; Serhal, E. Digital Health Equity and COVID-19: The Innovation Curve Cannot Reinforce the Social Gradient of Health. *J. Med. Internet Res.* **2020**, *22*, e19361. [CrossRef]
24. Rodriguez, J.A.; Clark, C.R.; Bates, D.W. Digital Health Equity as a Necessity in the 21st Century Cures Act Era. *JAMA* **2020**, *323*, 2381–2382. [CrossRef] [PubMed]
25. Bernuzzi, C.; Piccardo, M.A.; Guglielmetti, C. Mapping Research Trends on the Implications of Telemedicine for Healthcare Professionals: A Comprehensive Bibliometric Analysis. *Healthcare* **2025**, *13*, 1149. [CrossRef] [PubMed]
26. Chereka, A.A.; Mekonnen, G.B.; Yirsaw, A.N.; Mengistie, B.A.; Getachew, E.; Lakew, G.; Shibabaw, A.A.; Kitil, G.W. Attitudes towards Telemedicine Services and Associated Factors among health professionals in Ethiopia: A systematic review and meta-analysis. *BMC Health Serv. Res.* **2024**, *24*, 1505. [CrossRef] [PubMed] [PubMed Central]
27. Pizarro-Mena, R.; Rotarou, E.S.; Baracaldo-Campo, H.A.; Duran-Aguero, S.; Parra-Soto, S.; Retamal-Walter, F.; Wachholz, P.A.; Maranzano, S.; Tirro, V.; Aguilar-Navarro, S.; et al. Implementation of Telehealth Among Older People: A Challenge and Opportunity for Latin America and the Caribbean—A Literature Review. *Healthcare* **2025**, *13*, 2680. [CrossRef]
28. Wildenbos, G.A.; Peute, L.; Jaspers, M. Aging Barriers Influencing Mobile Health Usability for Older Adults: A Literature Based Framework. *Int. J. Med. Inform.* **2018**, *114*, 66–75. [CrossRef]
29. Haimi, M.; Goren, U.; Grossman, Z. Barriers and challenges to telemedicine usage among the elderly population in Israel in light of the COVID-19 era: A qualitative study. *Digit. Health* **2024**, *10*, 20552076241240235. [CrossRef] [PubMed] [PubMed Central]
30. Nouri, S.; Khoong, E.C.; Lyles, C.R.; Karliner, L. Addressing Equity in Telemedicine for Chronic Disease Management During the COVID-19 Pandemic. *NEJM Catal. Innov. Care Deliv.* **2020**, *1*, 220728183.
31. Gajarawala, S.N.; Pelkowski, J.N. Telehealth Benefits and Barriers. *J. Nurse Pract.* **2021**, *17*, 218–221. [CrossRef]
32. Ezeamii, V.C.; Okobi, O.E.; Wambai-Sani, H.; Perera, G.S.; Zaynieva, S.; Okonkwo, C.C.; Ohaiba, M.M.; William-Enemali, P.C.; Obodo, O.R.; Obiefuna, N.G. Revolutionizing Healthcare: How Telemedicine Is Improving Patient Outcomes and Expanding Access to Care. *Cureus* **2024**, *16*, e63881. [CrossRef] [PubMed] [PubMed Central]

33. Moulaei, K.; Sheikhtaheri, A.; Fatehi, F.; Shanbehzadeh, M.; Bahaadinbeigy, K. Patients' perspectives and preferences toward telemedicine versus in-person visits: A mixed-methods study on 1226 patients. *BMC Med. Inform. Decis. Mak.* **2023**, *23*, 261. [CrossRef] [PubMed] [PubMed Central]
34. Santos, A.R.; Sampaio, F.; Londral, A.R.; Perelman, J. Mapping methodologies for economic assessment of digital health technologies: A scoping review protocol. *BMJ Open* **2025**, *15*, e099933. [CrossRef] [PubMed] [PubMed Central]
35. Hadian, M.; Jelodar, Z.K.; Khanbebin, M.J.; Atafimanesh, P.; Asiabar, A.S.; Dehagani, S.M.H. Challenges of Implementing Telemedicine Technology: A systematized Review. *Int. J. Prev. Med.* **2024**, *15*, 8. [CrossRef] [PubMed] [PubMed Central]
36. Rossi, M.; Rehman, S. Integrating Artificial Intelligence Into Telemedicine: Evidence, Challenges, and Future Directions. *Cureus* **2025**, *17*, e90829. [CrossRef] [PubMed] [PubMed Central]
37. Topol, E.J. High-Performance Medicine: The Convergence of Human and Artificial Intelligence. *Nat. Med.* **2019**, *25*, 44–56. [CrossRef] [PubMed]
38. Donelan, K.; Barreto, E.A.; Sossong, S.; Michael, C.; Estrada, J.J.; Cohen, A.B.; Wozniak, J.; Schwamm, L.H. Patient and Clinician Experiences with Telehealth for Patient Follow-up Care. *Am. J. Manag. Care* **2019**, *25*, 40–44.
39. Perzynski, A.T.; Roach, M.J.; Shick, S.; Callahan, B.; Gunzler, D.; Cebul, R.; Kaelber, D.C.; Huml, A.; Thornton, J.D.; Einstadter, D. Patient Portals and Broadband Internet Inequality. *J. Am. Med. Inform. Assoc.* **2017**, *24*, 927–932. [CrossRef]
40. Richardson, S.; Lawrence, K.; Schoenthaler, A.M.; Mann, D. A framework for digital health equity. *npj Digit. Med.* **2022**, *5*, 119. [CrossRef]
41. Nouri, S.S.; Avila-Garcia, P.; Cemballi, A.G.; Sarkar, U.; Aguilera, A.; Lyles, C.R. Assessing Mobile Phone Digital Literacy and Engagement in User-Centered Design in a Diverse, Safety-Net Population: Mixed Methods Study. *JMIR Mhealth Uhealth* **2019**, *7*, e14250. [CrossRef]
42. Rabbani, M.G.; Alam, A.; Prybutok, V.R. Telehealth as a Sociotechnical System: A Systems Analysis of Adoption and Efficacy Among Older Adults Post-COVID-19. *Systems* **2025**, *13*, 843. [CrossRef]
43. Ellimoottil, C.; An, L.; Moyer, M.; Sossong, S.; Hollander, J.E. Challenges and Opportunities Faced by Large Health Systems Implementing Telehealth. *Health Aff.* **2018**, *37*, 1955–1959. [CrossRef]
44. Jumreornvong, O.; Yang, E.; Race, J.; Appel, J. Telemedicine and Medical Education in the Age of COVID-19. *Acad. Med.* **2020**, *95*, 1838–1843. [CrossRef]
45. Mehrotra, A.; Bhatia, R.S.; Snoswell, C.L. Paying for Telemedicine After the Pandemic. *JAMA* **2021**, *325*, 431–432. [CrossRef]

healthcare

MDPI

Article

Personalizing Communication of Clinicians with Chronically Ill Elders in Digital Encounters—A Patient-Centered View

Gillie Gabay [1,*], Hana Ornoy [2], Attila Gere [3] and Howard Moskowitz [4]

1 Faculty of Social Sciences, Achva Academic College, Arugot 7980400, Israel
2 Faculty of Business, Ono Academic College, Kiryat Ono 5545173, Israel; hana.or@ono.ac.il
3 Institute of Food Science and Technology, Hungarian University of Agriculture and Life Sciences, 1118 Budapest, Hungary; gere.attila@uni-mate.hu
4 Mind-Genomics Associates, White Plains, NY 10605, USA; mjihrm@gmail.com
* Correspondence: gillie.gabay@gmail.com

Abstract: Background: Chronically ill elderly patients are concerned about losing the personal connection with clinicians in digital encounters and clinicians are concerned about missing nonverbal cues that are important for the diagnosis, thus jeopardizing quality of care. Aims: This study validated the expectations and preferences of chronically ill elderly patients regarding specific communication messages for communication with clinicians in telemedicine. Methods: The sample comprised 600 elderly chronically ill patients who use telehealth. We used a conjoint-based experimental design to test numerous messages. The outcome variable is elder patient expectations from communication with clinicians in telemedicine. The independent variables were known categories of patient–clinician communication. Respondents rated each of the 24 vignettes of messages. Results: Mathematical clustering yielded three mindsets, with statistically significant differences among them. Members of mindset 1 were most concerned with non-verbal communication, members of mindset 2 prefer communication that enhances the internal locus of control, and members of mindset 3 have an external locus of control and strongly oppose any dialogue about their expectations from communication. Conclusions: The use of the predictive algorithm that we developed enables clinicians to identify the belonging of each chronically ill elderly patient in the clinic to a sample mindset, and to accordingly personalize the communication in the digital encounters while structuring the encounter with greater specificity, therefore enhancing patient-centered care.

Keywords: communication; digital medical encounters; elderly chronically ill patients; experimental design; health expectations; mindsets; patient-centered care

1. Introduction

The Institute of Medicine defines patient-centered care (PCC) as respectful care that responds to the preferences, needs, and values of each patient [1,2]. Evidence suggests that PCC results in higher patient trust, lower costs of care, shorter hospital stays, higher patient self-efficacy, better self-management of illness, lower stress among clinicians, higher adherence, lower re-admissions to the hospital, improved clinical outcomes, and higher patient satisfaction [2–6]. PCC entails the beliefs and needs of the patient and a partnership is established between patients and clinicians [7–9]. Studies on PCC highlight the formation of personhood as an activity that requires interaction with others so that the clinician as a partner has a crucial role in supporting personal communication with vulnerable patients [10–12]. This approach to care calls for a therapeutic alliance that encompasses effective patient–provider communication [13]. Although PCC is the advocated approach to care, health systems are still far from obtaining it [14]. Furthermore, the degree to which PCC is delivered at the clinician level and the individual patient level is not characterized [1,9]. Health systems have established platforms for digital medical encounters (telemedicine) for patients, including for chronically ill elders.

Telemedicine, i.e., providing a wide range of medical care and information from a distance mediated by technology, has been globally expanding since the outbreak of the COVID-19 pandemic [15–18]. Telemedicine is being integrated into practice in value-based health systems, increasing accessibility to health services and delivery of care [19–21]. Telemedicine visits conveniently connect clinicians to patients in their own homes as well as connect clinicians to each other, enhancing coordination of care [22]. Health systems aspire to utilize telemedicine platforms across 51 chronic illnesses and patients living in rural distant cities [23–26]. However, telemedicine alters the face-to-face encounter, negatively affecting personalization in patient–provider communication [27]. Adopting the lack of face-to-face interaction that characterizes telemedicine may fail to satisfy the emotional needs of elderly patients while also decreasing their engagement [28].

Patient-tailored communication in telemedicine was found to improve clinical outcomes, but barriers of depersonalization decrease patient satisfaction and involvement in telemedicine, jeopardizing effective communication [29–31]. Also, with elders, communication itself is a barrier to innovative mobile health solutions [32]. As for clinicians, they feel that without the personal encounter, assessing patients' emotional states and attending to their needs as individuals is challenging [31]. Clinicians acknowledged that their assumptions about their patients' needs may be mistaken, impairing quality care [29]. Although both patients and clinicians articulate some unease about the lack of face-to-face interaction, clinicians stress the importance of understanding their patients' expectations and preferences [29]. While patients focused on issues of non-verbal communication and the lack of personal "connection", clinicians focused on the potential for "missing something" medically important when delivering care to elder patients [29].

The dearth of original research on telemedicine in primary care suggests limited evidence on utility and quality [33]. Provider–patient communication in telemedicine must enable chronically ill patients and clinicians to gain a higher sense of control in the encounter while supporting a holistic view of care [19,34,35]. Previous studies tested provider–patient interaction frequency [36], interactional unfairness [37], communication competencies [38], and engagement in the interaction [39]. One study demonstrated that telemedicine may be adequate for the empathetic connection of clinicians with patients, allaying patients' concerns, offering emotional and informational support, and enhancing patient cooperation [40]. Furthermore, multiple studies tested self-disclosure, social support, and patient–provider trust in telemedicine [41–43].

Based on the PCC view, patient-tailored communication may enhance the engagement of elderly chronically ill patients in telemedicine encounters, contributing to clinical outcomes [30,44,45]. Research on specific communication messages that patients prefer in communication with clinicians, which may guide them to better customize telemedicine communication with elderly chronically ill patients, is scant. More insight is essential to remove current barriers among elderly patients in telemedicine [46]. Previous studies called to illuminate how clinicians may personalize communication in telemedicine to provide elderly chronically ill patients with PCC and optimize the quality of care in telemedicine [29,30,33,43,46,47]. This study validates the expectations and preferences of chronically ill elderly patients regarding specific communication messages for communication with clinicians in telemedicine, testing the following questions: What messages do elderly chronically ill patients prefer in communication in telemedicine? Do different subgroups of chronically ill patients differ in their preferences for telemedicine communication with clinicians? To the best of our knowledge, this is the first study to validate communication preferences in the elderly.

2. Materials and Methods

2.1. Ethics

The institutional board of ethics at the academic college in which the second author is affiliated granted ethical approval for this study, in accordance with the 1964 Declaration of Helsinki.

2.2. Sample

The sample comprised 600 chronically ill elderly patients who received medical care through digital encounters since the outbreak of the COVID-19 pandemic and accords with the suggested number of respondents in studies that aim at stable utilities [48]. The inclusion criteria were chronic illnesses such as cardiovascular diseases, neurological diseases, diabetes, metabolic disorders, lung disease, chronic back pain, and osteoporosis. Exclusion criteria were mental illness and cancer, which differ in their constructs. Six hundred undergraduate students in business administration programs at one of four campuses of the academic institution with which the second author is affiliated interviewed patients. A total of 90 interviewers are from the first campus, 100 interviewers are from a second campus, 350 interviewers are from the third campus, and 60 interviewers are from a fourth campus. The data were obtained as part of the students' research obligations in a research laboratory course. Each student was asked to interview one elderly chronically ill patient in the age group of 65 and over from a nursing home. The students were trained by the second author. They read the questions to the patient and entered their responses on the online questionnaire. This study was active between 15 June 2021–16 November 2021 as part of a series of testing expectations of patients from communication in telemedicine.

2.3. Procedure

This study is part of a series. The first study in this series focused on the expectations of young patients from doctors in telemedicine [17]. This study focuses on the expectations of chronically ill elders from communication with clinicians in telemedicine. For all papers in this series, we applied a conjoint-based experimental design. Typical of such designs, participants are allocated into groups which all respond to repeated measures, under the same conditions [49]. The respondents were asked to rate vignettes of messages relating to their expectations from communication with clinicians in telehealth. Using a computerized program, the order of the vignettes was alternated. Compared with observational studies, this alteration reduced potential bias by increasing the variation, randomization, co-variance analysis, and control [48]. Simulating the complexity in reality, where multiple stimuli may operate together, we tested numerous communication messages with no limitation of degrees of freedom through the Mind Genomics conjoint experimental design methodology [50]. Responses to the vignettes of messages were statistically analyzed [48,50,51]. Conjoint-based experimental designs require the setting of categories and elements. We set four categories determined by a thorough literature review to identify independent variables and four elements to be used as communication messages under each category representing patient expectations regarding communication with clinicians [50,51]. Each respondent evaluated a unique set of 24 combinations of messages, constituting a full experimental design [51].

2.4. Instrument

After reading the orientation page of the study and signing the informed consent for participation and publication, respondents answered three demographic questions and consequently rated 24 vignettes of messages. The outcome variable was elders' expectations of communication with clinicians in telemedicine. The rating question was: "How important are these communication messages when communicating with clinicians in telemedicine?" The rating scale ranges from 1 (not at all important to me) to 9 (extremely important to me). The independent variables were four acknowledged patient expectations of clinician–patient communication: locus of control [44], education and health literacy [52,53], and attentive listening [17]. The sixteen messages were arranged into 24 vignettes, with each category consisting of two to four messages, for a total of 24 vignettes that each respondent rated. The respondents were asked to rate the vignettes as a unit rather than relate to each message separately [50,51].

A conjoint-based software organized the random order of the vignettes ensuring statistical independence of the independent variables for subsequent regression analyses at both the individual level and the group level [50,51]. Table 1 presents categories and the messages regarding expectations in each.

Table 1. Categories and the messages regarding expectations in each.

	Category 1—Locus of Control
A1	The clinician walks me through a process of change to maintain my health.
A2	The clinician initiates a dialogue about my expectations.
A3	The clinician explains the treatment plan.
A4	The clinician navigates me to take responsibility for my health.
	Category 2—Health Literacy
B1	The clinician provides me with specific information for my conditions, not just general info.
B2	The clinician recommends an accredited site for information to learn about my condition.
B3	The clinician ensures that I understood the information.
B4	The clinician encourages me to ask questions.
	Category 3—Attentive Listening
C1	The clinician invests all the time that I need.
C2	The clinician cares about my feelings.
C3	The clinician enables me to express myself without interrupting me.
C4	The clinician invests more time if I need it.
	Category 4—Non-verbal Communication
D1	The clinician respects my time.
D2	The clinician does not maintain direct eye contact with me.
D3	The clinician is short and succinct and even sends me the prescription.
D4	Upon entry to the telehealth visit, the clinician greets me warmly.

2.5. Data Analysis

Ordinary least regression was performed on an individual level for each message [50]. Ordinary least regression was performed for the whole sample by gender and age group to test the contribution of each message to the importance of the vignette of messages. Next, k-means clustering analysis was performed to uncover the response patterns of respondents to each message with 1-Pearsons's R distance measure [48,50,51]. This group-level analysis of response patterns yielded subgroups (mindsets). ANOVA and Tukey post hoc tests were performed to test if differences among mindsets were significant [52–54]. The high coefficients in each mindset guided the characterization of what is most important to members of each mindset. To connect the insights from this study to practice, we developed a predictive algorithm to easily assign a chronically ill elder patient in the population to a sample mindset.

3. Results

3.1. Preliminary Analysis

We used split halves to test reliability by testing internal consistency between the data for the whole sample and the data for half of the sample (0.70; 0.76). Sixty-one percent were females (367), and thirty-nine percent (233) were males. The age ranged from 65 to 92 years. The age distribution amongst the four age groups was as follows: 377 respondents, age group 65–70; 140 respondents, age group 71–79; 59 respondents, age group 80–87; and 24 respondents, age group 88–95.

3.2. Secondary Analysis

Data analysis was conducted using R-project (version R-3.6.0) and lm.beta package (R Core Team, Vienna, Austria, 2020). The additive constant is the intercept in the linear regression equation and presents the likelihood that respondents will agree with a vignette of messages. High additive constants (60+) represent groups who strongly agreed with the vignettes and low additive constants (<35) represent groups whose agreement with the vignettes was low. The additive constant was 0.53 for the whole sample and 0.55 for the age group of 65–70, reflecting the high importance of the subject. To crystalize the results of the importance of each message, this outcome variable was recoded as a categorical variable. Ratings of 1–6 were recoded as zero and ratings of 7–9 were recoded as 100.

The regression analysis yielded coefficients for the 16 messages. The higher the coefficients, the higher the importance of the message. In conjoint analysis, coefficients of 6 and higher are statistically significant indicating a high importance of the message. Coefficients that are lower than 6, or negative coefficients, indicate a lack of agreement with the message. The regression analysis was performed for the whole sample by gender and age testing the contribution of each message to the importance of the whole vignette of messages [50]. With 600 respondents and 24 vignettes rated by each respondent, there were 600 (14,000) different observations for the regression analysis (Systat Software Inc., San Jose, CA, USA, SYSTAT v13.2. 2020. www.sigmaplot.com). Regression coefficients for the total sample were not significant, indicating that there were no significant differences in the importance of messages in communication via telemedicine.

Likewise, no significant differences were found between the coefficients of males and females across age groups. Looking into differences among age groups, the strongest expectation of respondents in the age group of 80–87 was "Upon entry to the telehealth visit, the clinician greets me warmly" (beta = 10). The strongest expectations of respondents in the age groups of 88–95 were: "The clinician provides me with specific information for my conditions, not just general info" (beta = 11) and "The clinician walks me through a process of change to maintain my health" (beta = 12).

Next, using k-means mathematical clustering, we analyzed response patterns to each message with 1-Pearsons's R distance measure [48,50,51]. Commonalities in response patterns to each message uncovered groups of participants with similar responses to messages [52]. The clustering analysis yielded three subgroups (mindsets). ANOVA and Tukey post hoc tests showed indices that indicated that the differences among mindsets were significant [54]. The three mindsets are based on mathematical clustering, from which the commonalities in patterns of response to each message facilitated the assignment of each participant into mindsets presenting distinct expectations of elder patients from communication with clinicians in telemedicine. The mindsets reflect various ways of thinking about communication with clinicians. In each mindset, the highest coefficients guided the characterization of the expectations of members in that mindset [55,56]. Table 2 presents mindset segmentation. Figure 1 illustrates the mathematical clustering of messages by importance.

Members of mindset 1, comprising 36% of the sample, were most concerned with non-verbal communication; they sought a warm greeting and eye contact. The growing elderly population and the immense benefits of telemedicine call upon clinicians to address the needs of chronically ill patients in telemedicine communication and optimize its utilization [55]. Members of mindset 2, comprising 32% of the sample, are interested in communication that enhances internal locus of control. They would like to talk about their expectations and for the clinician to guide them through a change process to take responsibility and maintain their health. They would like relevant specific information about their condition rather than general information about the disease. The strongest messages for this mindset were "The clinician walks me through a change process to maintain my health" (beta = 12); "The clinician talks to me about my expectations" (beta = 12); and "The clinician helps me take responsibility for my health" (beta = 9). They expect clinicians to use messages that empower and navigate them to better manage their illness leading to higher resilience [57–59]. Members of mindset 3, comprising 31% of the sample, have an external locus of control and strongly oppose a change process guided by the clinician to maintain their health (beta = −12), to help them take responsibility for their health (beta = −13), or dialogue about their communication expectations (beta = −14).

Table 2. The results of segmentation by mindset (MS) and Tukey post hoc tests.

	Group (Binary Ratings) Total		**MS1**	**MS2**	**MS3**
	Base Size	600	217	194	189
	Additive Constant	53	54	53	51
	Category A: Internal Locus of Control				
A1	The clinician walks me through a process of change to maintain my health.	1	6 [b]	**9 [b]**	**−12 [a]**
A2	The clinician initiates a dialogue about my expectations.	1	6 [b]	**12 [b]**	**−14 [a]**
A3	The clinician explains the treatment plan.	1	7 [b]	**9 [b]**	**−13 [a]**
A4	The clinician navigates me to take responsibility for my health.	2	6 [b]	8 [b]	−9 [a]
	Category B: Health Literacy				
B1	The clinician provides me with specific information for my conditions, not just general info.	−1	−4 [a]	2 [b]	0 [b]
B2	The clinician recommends an accredited site to learn about my disease.	0	−3 [a]	1 [b]	2 [b]
B3	The clinician ensures that I understood the information.	0	−3 [a]	0 [b]	3 [b]
B4	The clinician encourages me to ask questions.	−1	−4 [a]	−3 [ab]	4 [b]
	Category C: Attentive Listening				
C1	The clinician invests all the time that I need.	0	−9 [a]	5 [b]	5 [b]
C2	The clinician cares about my feelings.	−1	−7 [a]	1 [b]	5 [c]
C3	The clinician enables me to express myself without interrupting.	1	−6 [a]	3 [b]	6 [b]
C4	The clinician invests more time if I need it.	1	−7 [a]	5 [b]	5 [b]
	Category D: Non-verbal Communication				
D1	The clinician respects my time.	2	**10 [c]**	−10 [a]	4 [b]
D2	The clinician does not maintain direct eye contact with me.	1	**9 [c]**	−13 [a]	4 [b]
D3	The clinician is short and succinct.	−1	7 [c]	−12 [a]	2 [b]
D4	Upon entry to the telehealth visit, the clinician greets me warmly.	2	**11 [c]**	−12 [a]	6 [b]

Letters indicate the homogenous subgroups created by Tukey post hoc tests after running an analysis of variance on the individual regression coefficients.

To connect the insights from this study to practice, we developed a predictive algorithm. To develop the algorithm, we considered a total of sixty-four potential response patterns to each message and the messages that strongly distinguished among the three mindsets. Based on six messages that distinguished among the mindsets, we employed a mathematical Monte Carlo simulation and developed the predictive algorithm [55]. The predictive algorithm enables clinicians to easily assign a chronically ill elder patient in the clinic to one of the study mindsets and choose to communicate by mindset-tailored communication messages. Since respondents are distributed across age groups and genders in the population, we created a predictive algorithm to quickly assign elderly patients to mindsets and accord communication to meet the expectations of members of each mindset. Figure 2 presents the predictive algorithm available at https://www.pvi360.com/TypingToolPage.aspx?projectid=2312&userid=2008 (accessed on 19 July 2022).

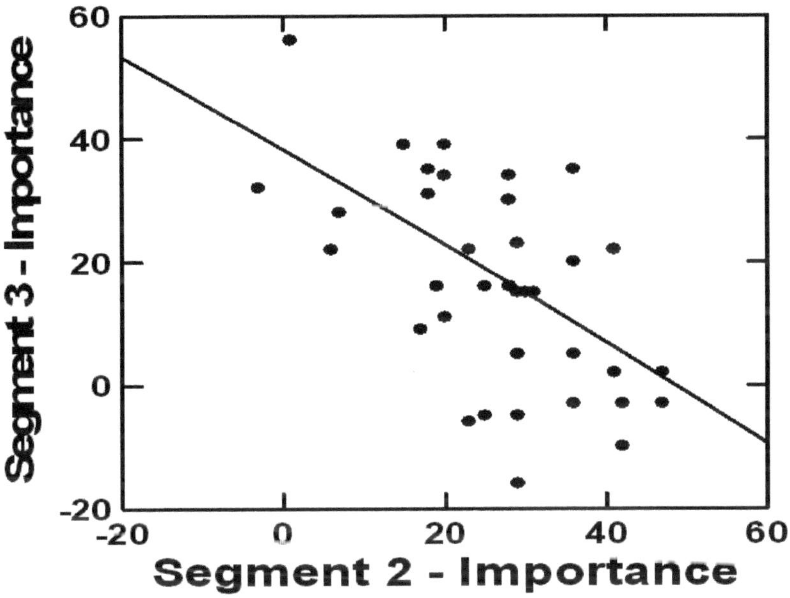

Figure 1. An example of mathematical clustering to identify commonalities by the perceived importance of messages.

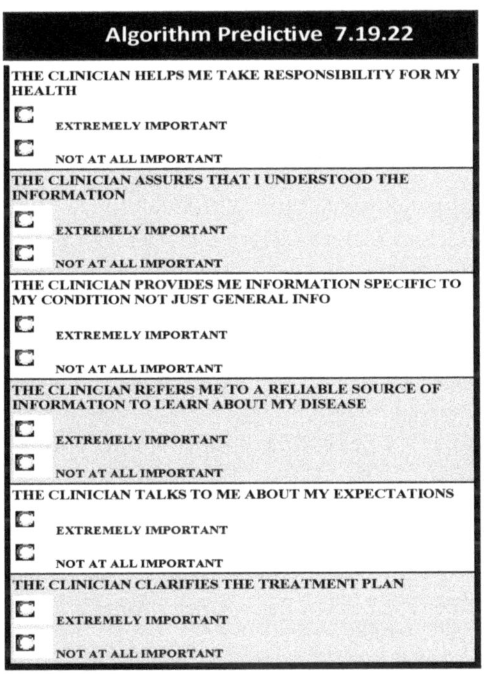

Algorithm Predictive 7.19.22

THE CLINICIAN HELPS ME TAKE RESPONSIBILITY FOR MY HEALTH
- EXTREMELY IMPORTANT
- NOT AT ALL IMPORTANT

THE CLINICIAN ASSURES THAT I UNDERSTOOD THE INFORMATION
- EXTREMELY IMPORTANT
- NOT AT ALL IMPORTANT

THE CLINICIAN PROVIDES ME INFORMATION SPECIFIC TO MY CONDITION NOT JUST GENERAL INFO
- EXTREMELY IMPORTANT
- NOT AT ALL IMPORTANT

THE CLINICIAN REFERS ME TO A RELIABLE SOURCE OF INFORMATION TO LEARN ABOUT MY DISEASE
- EXTREMELY IMPORTANT
- NOT AT ALL IMPORTANT

THE CLINICIAN TALKS TO ME ABOUT MY EXPECTATIONS
- EXTREMELY IMPORTANT
- NOT AT ALL IMPORTANT

THE CLINICIAN CLARIFIES THE TREATMENT PLAN
- EXTREMELY IMPORTANT
- NOT AT ALL IMPORTANT

Figure 2. The predictive algorithm listing the six most discriminating elements with binary answers needed to predict the mindset membership of new participants.

4. Discussion

This study tested expectations of elderly chronically ill patients based on communication messages in telemedicine, presenting a novel strategy of testing patterns of thinking and expectations of elders from communication in telemedicine, creating a predictive algorithm for detecting patient mindset and using mindset-tailored communication with clinicians. The identified mindsets contradict previous findings, which viewed patient expectations from telehealth services as varying by services provided and respondent demographics [60]. This study filled several gaps in the knowledge. First, this study identified what elders with chronic illness expect and perceive as important in communication with clinicians in telemedicine and how they are segmented in their expectations. Methodologically, this study conducted a conjoint-based experimental design that reduces biases of typical observational studies while testing a great many messages with no limitations of degrees of freedom.

This work allowed us to answer the following research questions:

(a) What messages do elderly chronically ill patients prefer in communication in telemedicine? Surprisingly, no significant differences were found between male and female chronically ill elders across age groups. The strongest expectation of elders ages 80–87 was that the clinicians will greet them warmly upon the beginning of the virtual encounter. The strongest expectations of elders ages 88–95 were that the clinicians will provide them with information that is specific to their conditions, rather than general information, and that clinicians will guide them through a process to maintain their health.

(b) Do different subgroups of chronically ill patients differ in their preferences for telemedicine communication with clinicians? Three mindsets, which are similar in size, represent subgroups of chronically ill patients and the expectations of members of one mindset are significantly distinct from expectations of members of other mindsets. Thus, expectations of members of one mindset are irrelevant to members of other mindsets. Members of mindset 1 expect a warm greeting and eye contact. Members of mindset 2 expect communication that enhances their internal locus of control, a dialogue concerning their expectations, and for clinicians to guide them through a change process to maintain their health. These elders expect specific information about their condition and for the clinician to help them take responsibility for their health, empower them, and navigate them to better manage their illness, leading to higher resilience. Members of mindset 3 have an external locus of control and oppose dialogue and a change process guided by clinicians.

Although the COVID-19 pandemic brought about rapid adaptation to telemedicine to complement "in-person" primary care, it also highlighted challenges [33]. Telemedicine is indeed a key response in primary care to support public health. Patient experience in telemedicine, however, entails barriers for clinicians and patients that decrease utility and quality of care [33]. This study begins to validate the removal of barriers to both patients and clinicians in communication in telemedicine with elderly chronically ill patients [61]. While regression on the total sample indicated no significant differences among chronically ill patients by expectations from communication, mathematical clustering yielded three distinct mindsets. Thus, offerings of communication in telemedicine should not be tailored to different demographic groups but rather to mindsets. These findings echo previous studies that suggested that patients should be segmented by their expectations from clinicians based on their mindset-belonging description rather than on demographics, driving patient satisfaction and health behaviors and enabling clinicians to use mindset-tailored communication to meet patient expectations and enhance the quality of care [57–59,62–64].

The novel strategy we presented to test communication expectations of chronically ill elders in telemedicine is not without limitations. First, the generalizability of this study. While the presented novel statistical strategy itself is replicable and generalizable across health settings and countries and is expected to yield distinct mindsets of patients, communication has cultural roots, which reduces the generalizability of the communication messages based on mindsets. First, attitudes toward the elderly differ between Western and Eastern cultures; in the latter, the elderly are highly respected, and all their needs must be fulfilled affecting patient–clinician communication in telemedicine. Second, there are cultural differences in attitudes and perceptions of authority figures that may affect the involvement of elders in communication with clinicians as authority figures, regardless of whether the clinician will use mindset-tailored communication messages. Third, our global landscape is becoming rich in immigrant diversity and elderly immigrants may not be fully versed in the dominant local language. Another limitation is that we did not test elder patient expectations by diseases included in this study, which may yield different mindset-belonging description results and varying importance levels of the messages in each mindset. Along with the patient-centered care framework, future studies may test the expectations of chronically ill patients from clinicians, by disease and by culture. Also, future studies may test the effect of implementing mindset-tailored messages with chronically ill elder patients on their satisfaction with interactions with clinicians in telemedicine.

5. Relevance to Clinical Practice

Telemedicine is developing, expanding, and creating new opportunities to meet patient expectations, improve the quality and delivery of care by personalizing care, and closing the chasm between aspiring for PCC and obtaining PCC. To meet patients' expectations and to put patients into focus, clinicians are advised to support communication with patients using mindset-tailored messages, which are considered the most important emphases for members of each mindset. The use of the predictive algorithm developed for this study detects the mindset-belonging description of each elder patient at the clinic linking it to a sample mindset, enabling personalized communication while delivering care via telemedicine. Understanding the expectations of patients regarding communication with clinicians based on mindset can structure the telehealth visit more effectively, thus enhancing patient-centered care and quality of care. Moreover, greater personalization will remove a major barrier for patients regarding telemedicine. Since personalized communication was proven to establish higher patient trust in clinicians, it may yield trust in clinicians in telemedicine as well. Trust was proven to enhance medication adherence and self-management of diseases [65]. Hence, it is possible that using mindset-tailored communication with chronically ill elder patients will contribute to optimal self-management of chronic diseases, creating an added value to telemedicine and enhancing the quality of care [66–71]. Greater utilization of telemedicine by patients and greater patient involvement may increase if clinicians meet patient expectations in communication with clinicians, which may improve health behaviors and overall clinical outcomes [27,68].

6. Conclusions

In terms of practice implications, the insights developed from this study enable clinicians to employ our predictive algorithm, or develop one, to easily assign elder patients with chronic illnesses (excluding mental illness) in telemedicine into mindsets from the sample. Detecting the mindset to which a patient belongs and understanding the strongest expectations of members in that mindset will provide clinicians with the choice to communicate with the patient through personalized, mindset-tailored messages.

Author Contributions: Conceptualization, G.G. and H.O.; methodology, G.G. and A.G.; software, H.M.; validation, G.G. and H.O.; formal analysis, A.G.; investigation, G.G. and A.G.; resources, H.M.; data curation, H.O.; writing—original draft preparation G.G. and A.G.; writing—review and editing, G.G., H.O. and H.M.; visualization, G.G.; supervision, G.G.; project administration, G.G. and A.G.; funding acquisition, G.G. and H.O. All authors have read and agreed to the published version of the manuscript.

Funding: This research received no external funding.

Institutional Review Board Statement: The ethics review board at the Ono Academic Center granted ethical approval for this study (IRB # 2021ono) on 15 June 2021. This study was conducted in accordance with the approval granted and with the 1964 Declaration of Helsinki.

Informed Consent Statement: Informed consent was obtained from all subjects involved in this study.

Data Availability Statement: All relevant data is included in the paper.

Acknowledgments: A.G. thanks the National Research, Development, and Innovation Office of Hungary (OTKA, contract no. FK 137577).

Conflicts of Interest: Author Howard Moskowitz was employed by the company Mind-Genomics Associates. The remaining authors declare that the research was conducted in the absence of any commercial or financial relationships that could be construed as a potential conflict of interest.

References

1. Babione, J.; Panjwani, D.; Murphy, S.; Kelly, J.; Van Dyke, J.; Santana, M.; Kaufman, J.; Sargious, P.; Rabi, D. Alignment of patient-centredness definitions with real-life patient and clinician experiences: A qualitative study. *Health Expect.* **2023**, *26*, 419–428. [CrossRef]
2. American Geriatrics Society Expert Panel on Person-Centered Care; Brummel-Smith, K.; Butler, D.; Frieder, M.; Gibbs, N.; Henry, M.; Koons, E.; Loggers, E.; Porock, D.; Reuben, D.B.; et al. Person-Centered Care: A Definition and Essential Elements. *J. Am. Geriatr. Soc.* **2016**, *64*, 15–18. [CrossRef]
3. Edvardsson, D.; Sandman, P.O.; Borell, L. Implementing national guidelines for person-centered care of people with dementia in residential aged care: Effects on perceived person-centeredness, staff strain, and stress of conscience. *Int. Psychogeriatr.* **2014**, *26*, 1171–1179. [CrossRef]
4. Fors, A.; Ekman, I.; Taft, C.; Björkelund, C.; Frid, K.; Larsson, M.E.; Thorn, J.; Ulin, K.; Wolf, A.; Swedberg, K. Person-centred care after acute coronary syndrome, from hospital to primary care—A randomised controlled trial. *Int. J. Cardiol.* **2015**, *187*, 693–699. [CrossRef] [PubMed]
5. Kim, S.K.; Park, M. Effectiveness of person-centered care on people with dementia: A systematic review and meta-analysis. *Clin. Interv. Aging* **2017**, *12*, 381–397. [CrossRef] [PubMed]
6. Hansson, E.; Ekman, I.; Swedberg, K.; Wolf, A.; Dudas, K.; Ehlers, L.; Olsson, L.-E. Person-centred care for patients with chronic heart failure—A cost-utility analysis. *Eur. J. Cardiovasc. Nurs.* **2016**, *15*, 276–284. [CrossRef] [PubMed]
7. Britten, N.; Ekman, I.; Naldemirci, Ö.; Javinger, M.; Hedman, H.; Wolf, A. Learning from Gothenburg model of person centred healthcare. *BMJ* **2020**, *370*, m2738. [CrossRef] [PubMed]
8. Ekman, I.; Swedberg, K.; Taft, C.; Lindseth, A.; Norberg, A.; Brink, E.; Carlsson, J.; Dahlin-Ivanoff, S.; Johansson, I.-L.; Kjellgren, K.; et al. Person-centered care—Ready for prime time. *Eur. J. Cardiovasc. Nurs.* **2011**, *10*, 248–251. [CrossRef] [PubMed]
9. Forsgren, E.; Saldert, C. Implementation of communication routines facilitating person-centred care in long-term residential care: A pilot study. *Health Expect.* **2022**, *25*, 2982–2991. [CrossRef]
10. Kagan, A.; Black, S.E.; Duchan, F.J.; Simmons-Mackie, N.; Square, P. Training volunteers as conversation partners using "Supported Conversation for Adults with Aphasia" (SCA): A controlled trial. *J. Speech Lang. Hear. Res.* **2001**, *44*, 624–638. [CrossRef] [PubMed]
11. Simmons, S.; Sharp, B.; Fowler, J.; Fowkes, H.; Paz-Arabo, P.; Dilt-Skaggs, M.K.; Singal, B.; Carter, T. Mind the (knowledge) gap: The effect of a communication instrument on emergency department patients' comprehension of and satisfaction with care. *Patient Educ. Couns.* **2015**, *98*, 257–262. [CrossRef] [PubMed]
12. Savundranayagam, M.Y.; Ryan, E.B.; Anas, A.P.; Orange, J.B. Communication and dementia: Staff perceptions of conversational strategies. *Clin. Gerontol.* **2007**, *31*, 47–63. [CrossRef]
13. Dong, K.; Jameel, B.; Gagliardi, A.R. How is patient-centred care conceptualized in obstetrical health? comparison of themes from concept analyses in obstetrical health- and patient-centred care. *Health Expect.* **2022**, *25*, 823–839. [CrossRef] [PubMed]
14. Tomaselli, G.; Buttigieg, S.C.; Rosano, A.; Cassar, M.; Grima, G. Person-Centered Care From a Relational Ethics Perspective for the Delivery of High Quality and Safe Healthcare: A Scoping Review. *Front. Public Health* **2020**, *8*, 44. [CrossRef] [PubMed]
15. Calton, B.; Abedini, N.; Fratkin, M. Telemedicine in the Time of Coronavirus. *J. Pain Symptom Manag.* **2020**, *60*, e12–e14. [CrossRef] [PubMed]
16. Contreras, C.M.; Metzger, G.A.; Beane, J.D.; Dedhia, P.H.; Ejaz, A.; Pawlik, T.M. Telemedicine: Patient-Provider Clinical Engagement During the COVID-19 Pandemic and Beyond. *J. Gastrointest. Surg.* **2020**, *24*, 1692–1697. [CrossRef]
17. Gabay, G.; Ornoy, H.; Moskowitz, H. Patient-centered care in telemedicine—An experimental-design study. *Int. J. Med. Inform.* **2022**, *159*, 104672. [CrossRef]
18. Tan, A.J.; Rusli, K.D.; McKenna, L.; Tan, L.L.; Liaw, S.Y. Telemedicine experiences and perspectives of healthcare providers in long-term care: A scoping review. *J. Telemed. Telecare* **2024**, *30*, 230–249. [CrossRef]
19. Caffery, L.J.; Bradford, N.K.; Smith, A.C.; Langbecker, D. How telehealth facilitates the provision of culturally appropriate healthcare for Indigenous Australians. *J. Telemed. Telecare* **2018**, *24*, 676–682. [CrossRef] [PubMed]

20. Chen, S.; Guo, X.; Wu, T.; Ju, X. Exploring the Online Doctor-Patient Interaction on Patient Satisfaction Based on Text Mining and Empirical Analysis. *Inf. Process. Manag.* **2020**, *57*, 102253. [CrossRef]
21. Emmett, A.; Kent, B.; James, A.; March-McDonald, J. Experiences of health professionals towards using mobile electrocardiogram (ECG) technology: A qualitative systematic review. *J. Clin. Nurs.* **2022**, *32*, 3205–3218. [CrossRef]
22. Frey, M.B.; Chiu, S.-H. Considerations When Using Telemedicine As the Advanced Practice Registered Nurse. *J. Nurse Pract.* **2021**, *17*, 289–292. [CrossRef] [PubMed]
23. Fatehi, F.; Wootton, R. Telemedicine, telehealth or e-health? A bibliometric analysis of the trends in the use of these terms. *J. Telemed. Telecare* **2012**, *18*, 460–464. [CrossRef]
24. Hennemann-Krause, L.; Lopes, A.J.; Araújo, J.A.; Petersen, E.M.; Nunes, R.A. The assessment of telemedicine to support outpatient palliative care in advanced cancer. *Palliat. Support. Care* **2015**, *13*, 1025–1030. [CrossRef] [PubMed]
25. Hanna, G.M.; Fishman, I.; Edwards, D.A.; Shen, S.; Kram, C.; Liu, X.; Shotwell, M.; Gilligan, C. Development and Patient Satisfaction of a New Telemedicine Service for Pain Management at Massachusetts General Hospital to the Island of Martha's Vineyard. *Pain Med.* **2016**, *17*, 1658–1663. [CrossRef] [PubMed]
26. Pahl, C.; Zare, M.; Ahmad, A.; Detschew, V. Identification of quality parameters for an e-health platform in the federal state of thuringia in germany. *J. Soft Comput. Decis. Support Syst.* **2014**, *1*, 17–23.
27. Barberio, J.A.; Jenkins, M.L. Transitioning to Telehealth: Today's Guidelines for Future Sustainability. *J. Nurse Pract.* **2021**, *17*, 795–798. [CrossRef]
28. EFORTT. Ethical Frameworks for Telecare Technologies for Older People at Home. Available online: http://www.lancs.ac.uk/efortt (accessed on 15 March 2022).
29. Hiratsuka, V.; Delafield, R.; Starks, H.; Ambrose, A.J.; Mau, M.M. Patient and provider perspectives on using telemedicine for chronic disease management among Native Hawaiian and Alaska Native people. *Int. J. Circumpolar Health* **2013**, *72*. [CrossRef]
30. Mohr, D.C.; Burns, M.N.; Schueller, S.M.; Clarke, G.; Klinkman, M. Behavioral Intervention Technologies: Evidence review and recommendations for future research in mental health. *Gen. Hosp. Psychiatry* **2013**, *35*, 332–338. [CrossRef]
31. Rubeis, G.; Schochow, M.; Steger, F. Patient Autonomy and Quality of Care in Telehealthcare. *Sci. Eng. Ethics* **2018**, *24*, 93–107. [CrossRef]
32. Kruse, C.S.; Mileski, M.; Moreno, J. Mobile health solutions for the aging population: A systematic narrative analysis. *J. Telemed. Telecare* **2017**, *23*, 439–451. [CrossRef]
33. Jonnagaddala, J.; Godinho, M.A.; Liaw, S.-T. From telehealth to virtual primary care in Australia? A Rapid scoping review. *Int. J. Med. Inform.* **2021**, *151*, 104470. [CrossRef]
34. Nemetz, E.T.A.; Urbach, D.R.; Devon, K.M. The Art of Surgery: Balancing Compassionate with Virtual Care. *J. Med. Internet Res.* **2020**, *22*, e22417. [CrossRef] [PubMed]
35. Vassilev, I.; Rowsell, A.; Pope, C.; Kennedy, A.; O'Cathain, A.; Salisbury, C.; Rogers, A. Assessing the implementability of telehealth interventions for self-management support: A realist review. *Implement. Sci.* **2015**, *10*, 59. [CrossRef] [PubMed]
36. Yang, H.; Guo, X.; Wu, T. Exploring the Influence of the Online Physician Service Delivery Process on Patient Satisfaction. *Decis. Support Syst.* **2015**, *78*, 113–121. [CrossRef]
37. Zhang, X.; Guo, X.; Lai, K.; Yi, W. How does online interactional unfairness matter for patient–doctor relationship quality in online health consultation? The contingencies of professional seniority and disease severity. *Eur. J. Inf. Syst.* **2019**, *28*, 336–354. [CrossRef]
38. Vaz de Almeida, C.; Belim, C. Health Professionals' Communication Competences as a Light on the Patient Pathway: The Assertiveness, Clarity, and Positivity (ACP) Model. *Int. J. Appl. Res. Public Heal. Manag.* **2021**, *6*, 14–29. [CrossRef]
39. Zhao, Y.; Da, J.; Yan, J. Detecting health misinformation in online health communities: Incorporating behavioral features into machine learning based approaches. *Inf. Process. Manag.* **2021**, *58*, 102390. [CrossRef]
40. Hobson, E.V.; Baird, W.O.; Cooper, C.L.; Mawson, S.; Shaw, P.J.; Mcdermott, C.J. Using technology to improve access to specialist care in amyotrophic lateral sclerosis: A systematic review. *Amyotroph. Lateral Scler. Frontotemporal Degener.* **2016**, *17*, 313–324. [CrossRef]
41. Guo, Y.; Goh, D.H.-L. "I Have AIDS": Content analysis of postings in HIV/AIDS support group on a Chinese microblog. *Comput. Hum. Behav.* **2014**, *34*, 219–226. [CrossRef]
42. Huang, H.-Y. Examining the beneficial effects of individual's self-disclosure on the social network site. *Comput. Hum. Behav.* **2016**, *57*, 122–132. [CrossRef]
43. Zhang, R. The stress-buffering effect of self-disclosure on Facebook: An examination of stressful life events, social support, and mental health among college students. *Comput. Hum. Behav.* **2017**, *75*, 527–537. [CrossRef]
44. Gabay, G. Perceived control over health, communication and patient-physician trust. *Patient Educ. Couns.* **2015**, *98*, 1550–1557. [CrossRef]
45. Liu, J.; He, J.; He, S.; Li, C.; Yu, C.; Li, Q. Patients' Self-Disclosure Positively Influences the Establishment of Patients' Trust in Physicians: An Empirical Study of Computer-Mediated Communication in an Online Health Community. *Front. Public Health* **2022**, *10*, 823692. [CrossRef]
46. Wildenbos, G.A.; Peute, L.; Jaspers, M. Aging barriers influencing mobile health usability for older adults: A literature based framework (MOLD-US). *Int. J. Med. Inform.* **2018**, *114*, 66–75. [CrossRef] [PubMed]

47. Rush, K.L.; Howlett, L.; Munro, A.; Burton, L. Videoconference compared to telephone in healthcare delivery: A systematic review. *Int. J. Med. Inform.* **2018**, *118*, 44–53. [CrossRef] [PubMed]
48. Cattin, P.; Wittink, D.R. Commercial Use of Conjoint Analysis: A Survey. *J. Mark.* **1982**, *46*, 44–53. [CrossRef]
49. Kirk, R.E. Experimental Design. In *Handbook of Psychology*; Weiner, I.B., Schinka, J.A., Velicer, W.F., Eds.; Wiley: New York, NY, USA, 2012; pp. 23–46. ISBN 978-0-470-89064-6.
50. Moskowitz, H.R. "Mind genomics": The experimental, inductive science of the ordinary, and its application to aspects of food and feeding. *Physiol. Behav.* **2012**, *107*, 606–613. [CrossRef] [PubMed]
51. Porretta, S.; Gere, A.; Radványi, D.; Moskowitz, H. Mind Genomics (Conjoint Analysis): The new concept research in the analysis of consumer behaviour and choice. *Trends Food Sci. Technol.* **2019**, *84*, 29–33. [CrossRef]
52. Zandbelt, L.C.; Smets, E.M.; Oort, F.J.; Godfried, M.H.; de Haes, H.C. Patient participation in the medical specialist encounter: Does physicians' patient-centered communication matter? *Patient Educ. Couns.* **2007**, *65*, 396–406. [CrossRef] [PubMed]
53. Paterick, T.E.; Patel, N.; Tajik, A.J.; Chandrasekaran, K. Improving health outcomes through patient education and partnerships with patients. *Baylor Univ. Med. Center Proc.* **2017**, *30*, 112–113. [CrossRef]
54. Milutinovic, V.; Salom, J. *Mind Genomics. A Guide to Data-Driven Marketing Strategy*; Springer International Publishing: Berlin, Germany, 2016; ISBN 978-3-319-39733-7.
55. Wildenbos, G.A.; Jaspers, M.W.M.; Schijven, M.P.; Dusseljee-Peute, L.W. Mobile health for older adult patients: Using an aging barriers framework to classify usability problems. *Int. J. Med. Inform.* **2019**, *124*, 68–77. [CrossRef]
56. Provencher, C. Towards A Better Understanding of Cognitive Polyphasia. *J. Theory Soc. Behav.* **2011**, *41*, 377–395. [CrossRef]
57. Gabay, G.; Gere, A.; Zemel, G.; Moskowitz, H.R. Personalized Communication with Patients at the Emergency Department. *J. Personal. Med.* **2022**, *12*, 1542. [CrossRef]
58. Gabay, G.; Gere, A.; Moskowitz, H. Communication Preferences of Obese Female Adolescents with Clinicians, Archives of Women Health, and Care. 2023. Available online: https://researchopenworld.com/category/archives-of-women-health-and-care (accessed on 6 March 2023).
59. Gabay, G.; Zemel, G.; Moskowitz, H.; Gere, A. Narrative communication messaging in raising public awareness of type 2 diabetes risk—A multi-perspective cartography. *Endocrinol. Diabetes Metab. J.* **2020**, *4*, 1–8.
60. Hastie, T.; Tibshirani, R.; Friedman, J. *The Elements of Statistical Learning*, 1st ed.; Springer Series in Statistics; Springer: New York, NY, USA, 2001; ISBN 9780387848587.
61. Rho, M.J.; Choi, I.Y.; Lee, J. Predictive factors of telemedicine service acceptance and behavioral intention of physicians. *Int. J. Med. Inform.* **2014**, *83*, 559–571. [CrossRef]
62. Gabay, G.; Gere, A.; Moskowitz, H. Uncovering communication messages for health promotion: The case of Arthritis. *Integr. J. Orthop. Traumatol.* **2019**, *2*, 1–13. [CrossRef]
63. Gabay, G.; Gere, A.; Zemel, G.; Sherman, R.; Moskowitz, H.R. Promoting medication-adherence by uncovering patient's mindsets and adjusting clinician-patient communication to mindsets: A Mind Genomics cartography. *J. Clin. Res. Med.* **2019**, *2*, 1–15.
64. Oyalowo, A.; Forde, K.A.; Lamanna, A.; Kochman, M.L. Effect of Patient-Directed Messaging on Colorectal Cancer Screening: A Randomized Clinical Trial. *JAMA Netw. Open* **2022**, *5*, e224529. [CrossRef] [PubMed]
65. Ratanawongsa, N.; Karter, A.J.; Parker, M.M.; Lyles, C.R.; Heisler, M.; Moffet, H.H.; Adler, N.; Warton, E.M.; Schillinger, D. Communication and medication refill adherence: The Diabetes Study of Northern California. *JAMA Intern. Med.* **2013**, *173*, 210–218. [CrossRef] [PubMed]
66. Gabay, G. Exploring perceived control and self-rated health in re-admissions among younger adults: A retrospective study. *Patient Educ. Couns.* **2016**, *99*, 800–806. [CrossRef]
67. Ratanawongsa, N.; Handley, M.A.; Quan, J.; Sarkar, U.; Pfeifer, K.; Soria, C.; Schillinger, D. Quasi-experimental trial of diabetes Self-Management Automated and Real-Time Telephonic Support (SMARTSteps) in a Medicaid managed care plan: Study protocol. *BMC Health Serv. Res.* **2012**, *12*, 22. [CrossRef]
68. Ebbert, J.O.; Ramar, P.; Tulledge-Scheitel, S.M.; Njeru, J.W.; Rosedahl, J.K.; Roellinger, D.; Philpot, L.M. Patient preferences for telehealth services in a large multispecialty practice. *J. Telemed. Telecare* **2021**, *29*, 298–303. [CrossRef] [PubMed]
69. Gabay, G. Patient Self-worth and Communication Barriers to Trust of Israeli Patients in Acute-Care Physicians at Public General Hospitals. *Qual. Health Res.* **2019**, *29*, 1954–1966. [CrossRef] [PubMed]
70. Triantafyllidis, A.; Kondylakis, H.; Votis, K.; Tzovaras, D.; Maglaveras, N.; Rahimi, K. Features, outcomes, and challenges in mobile health interventions for patients living with chronic diseases: A review of systematic reviews. *Int. J. Med. Inform.* **2019**, *132*, 103984. [CrossRef] [PubMed]
71. Saragih, I.D.; Schorr, E.; Porta, C.M.; Batubara, S.O.; Lee, B.-O. Effects of telehealth-assisted interventions for secondary prevention of cardiovascular disease: A systematic review and meta-analysis. *J. Clin. Nurs.* **2022**, *32*, 3613–3629. [CrossRef] [PubMed]

healthcare MDPI

Article

Satisfaction with Teleophthalmology Services: Insights from Remote Areas of Taiwan

Nancy Chen [1], Jen-Hung Wang [2] and Cheng-Jen Chiu [1,3,*]

[1] Department of Ophthalmology, Hualien Tzu Chi Hospital, Buddhist Tzu Chi Medical Foundation, Hualien 970, Taiwan; nancy_chen@tzuchi.com.tw
[2] Department of Medical Research, Hualien Tzu Chi Hospital, Buddhist Tzu Chi Medical Foundation, Hualien 970, Taiwan; paulwang@tzuchi.com.tw
[3] Department of Ophthalmology and Visual Science, Tzu Chi University, Hualien 970, Taiwan
* Correspondence: drcjchiu@outlook.com or drcjchiu@tzuchi.com.tw; Tel.: +886-920-065-865

Abstract: During and after the COVID-19 pandemic, teleophthalmology provided access to eye care for rural populations. This study aimed to assess the efficacy of and satisfaction with an integrated real-time videoconferencing module. This project incorporated ophthalmic instruments and telecommunication devices and provided on-site consultations via videoconferencing. Both patients and healthcare providers completed satisfaction questionnaires. From May 2020 to May 2021, this project provided eye care services to 395 patients (aged 6–90 years). The most frequent eye condition was chronic conjunctivitis (n = 197), followed by senile cataract (n = 163), dry eye (n = 103), and refractive error (n = 95). Among them, 40 (10.1%) patients were referred to secondary or tertiary hospitals for further evaluation or treatment. In total, 181 recruited respondents provided good satisfaction scores in all dimensions, including quality of medical care (4.50 of 5.00), financial aspects of care (4.48), supportive attitude toward the project (4.47), quality of service (4.40), and quality of telecommunication (4.40). Women had a substantially more supportive attitude toward the project, and 25 healthcare providers provided low ratings in areas representing the quality of telecommunication (4.04) and user-friendliness of the instrument (4.00). This teleophthalmology system provided efficient and satisfactory eye care to participants in remote communities. However, better internet access and training in instrument use can reduce obstacles to the future implementation of the project.

Keywords: telemedicine; videoconferencing; teleophthalmology; satisfaction; remote area

1. Introduction

Telemedicine is an emerging paradigm aiming to diminish geographical barriers and disparities in access to medical care resources [1]. During the COVID-19 pandemic, telehealth achieved more acceptance and popularity in various medical fields, as it bridged the gap in patient care, particularly with regard to inconvenient medical visits in rural and urban areas [2,3]. Arguments against the implementation of telemedicine consider that virtual communication is not comparable with in-person physical examinations [1,4]. This perception is even stronger in the field of ophthalmology [5]. Despite these uncertainties, teleophthalmology has been explored as a possible solution for rural and remote areas.

The terrain in eastern Taiwan where indigenous tribes and rural villages are scattered is long, narrow, and mountainous. Considering the large distance between the consulting medical center and associated remote infirmaries, access to specialized medical care, such as eye care, is limited. The nearest township in this study was located 114 km from Hualien Tzu Chi Hospital and the most distant township was Darren, located 224 km away (Figure 1). Among them, residents of Chishang and Guanshan could access urban areas via express train. On the other hand, the ones in other townships would require several different vehicles to reach the urban area for medical attention. For accurate and timely evaluation while setting up the current project, the Public Health Bureau of the Taitung County Government provided ophthalmic instruments and telecommunication devices for local infirmaries. Although most previous studies have focused on the advances in ophthalmic instruments and broadband internet access that have rapidly facilitated the evolution of teleophthalmology [6,7], relatively few studies have addressed the Implementation of teleophthalmology from a patient perspective [8,9], and even fewer studies have surveyed the satisfaction level of healthcare providers practicing telemedicine [10,11]. This study evaluated the patient's and health provider's satisfaction with the application of synchronous videoconference teleophthalmology to determine its effectiveness and identify potential issues for its future implementation.

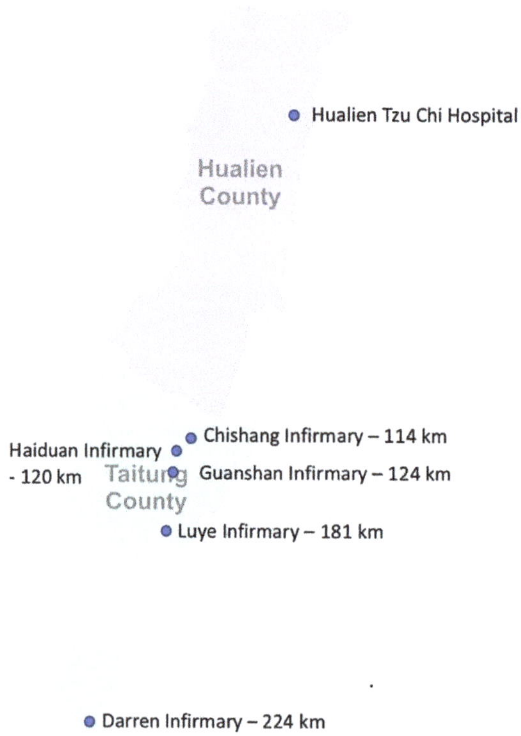

Figure 1. Map of eastern Taiwan showing the involved infirmaries and the distance between these infirmaries and the medical center, Hualien Tzu Chi Hospital.

2. Materials and Methods

2.1. Setting and Participants

Our virtual vision module (VVM) was equipped with ophthalmic instruments, including an auto kerato-refractometer, tonometer, digital ophthalmoscope, digital slit lamp, computers for data storage and transport, and two iPads for videoconferencing. Videoconferencing was performed using software developed by FarEasTone Telecommunications. All telehealth applications, supported by a continuous 80 MHz bandwidth 5G network, were designed to ensure that the remote diagnosis and treatment platform fulfilled the need for privacy protection, medical image transformation, and seamless interactive communications. Images and data were transferred to and stored in our medical center system. The VVM team included 1 general practitioner, 2 to 3 public health nurses from each local infirmary, ophthalmologists, and administrative personnel from the medical center. Ethical approval was obtained from the Institutional Review Board of the Hualien Tzu Chi General

Hospital (IRB109-198-B), which waived the requirement for informed consent because the anonymous questionnaire posed a low or negligible risk to the participants.

The VVM team members of the infirmaries were trained to use the ophthalmic devices and teleophthalmology equipment for 3 months. They collected demographic data, general health information, and eye condition data according to a standardized chart. Patients underwent a comprehensive ophthalmic examination, including visual acuity determination, noncontact tonometry, slit lamp biomicroscopy, and fundoscopy. The ocular examination results, including visual acuity and intraocular pressure, were recorded using a teleophthalmology chart. This chart was photographed and transferred to the videoconferencing platform along with the images acquired by infirmary members using a digital slit lamp and fundoscope. Next, the general practitioner from the infirmary conducted a synchronous video consultation with the ophthalmologist, during which the ophthalmologist input all information collected by the infirmary member into the electronic medical records (EMR). Both images and EMR were subsequently transferred to and stored in the medical center system. After a real-time interview with the patient, the ophthalmologist made a diagnosis and indicated the corresponding treatment, which was administered to the patient at the infirmary. The VVM process is illustrated in detail in Figure 2. The definition of ocular diseases and further details on ocular examinations are available elsewhere [12,13].

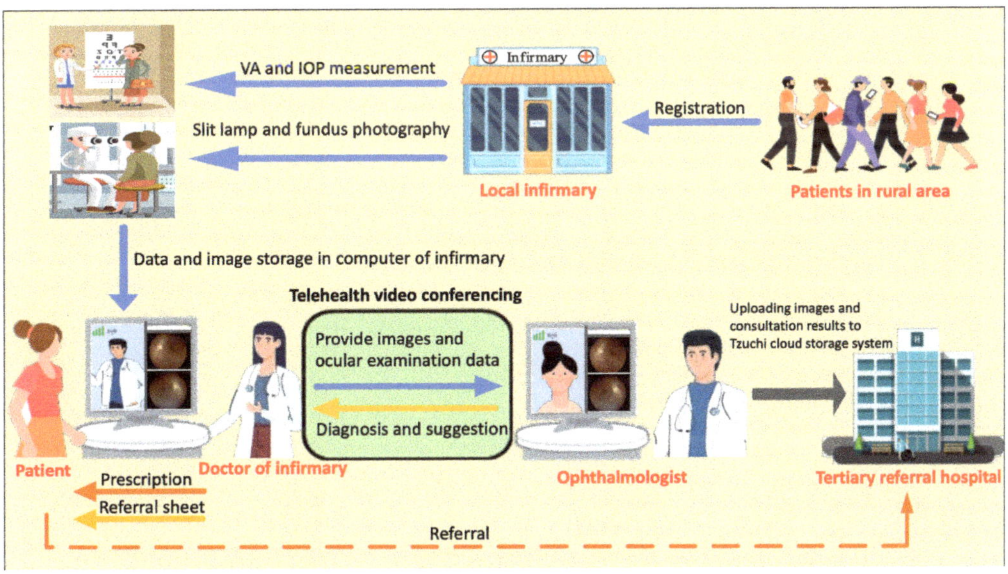

Figure 2. Flowchart showing the virtual vision module process.

When a referral was warranted based on our prior research [14], the public health nurses or infirmary coordinators would arrange appointments at secondary or tertiary hospitals and furnish the necessary referral documents. Patients referred in this manner were eligible to waive their copayment upon presenting the required referral documents.

2.2. Questionnaire Development

The satisfaction survey questionnaires for patients and healthcare providers were developed using a rational methodology [15]. Seven professionals, comprising three physicians and four public health experts, developed the questionnaires based on their expertise in their respective knowledge domains and prior research [9,16,17]. The patient satisfaction survey comprised 15 questions covering 5 key areas: financial aspects of care, quality of medical care, quality of service, supportive attitude toward the project, and quality of telecommunication. Similarly, the healthcare provider satisfaction survey consisted of 13 questions spanning the following 5 domains: user-friendliness of the instrument, quality of medical care, quality of service, supportive attitude toward the project, and quality of telecommunication. Both surveys employed a 5-point Likert scale, with scores ranging from 1 (strongly disagree) to 5 (strongly agree). Patient satisfaction data were collected using convenience sampling through on-site or telephone interviews. This method was conducted based on the accessibility and availability of project participants. Patients with literacy and normal cognitive abilities were approached by a research assistant to ascertain their willingness to participate in a questionnaire.

A Cronbach alpha was used to evaluate the reliability of the responses. The reliability of the responses in the five areas of satisfaction survey questionnaires was 0.88, 0.77, 0.70, 0.87, and 0.75 for patients and 0.90, 0.82, 0.97, 0.80, and 0.77 for healthcare providers, respectively. The scale-level content validity index (S-CVI) was assessed using the viewpoints of a panel of experts comprising seven raters. The S-CVIs of satisfaction survey questionnaires for patients and healthcare providers were 0.92 and 0.95, respectively.

2.3. Statistical Analysis

The participants' baseline characteristics were expressed as frequencies, proportions, or means ± standard deviations, depending on the characteristics of each variable. The independent t-test was used to compare the means of continuous variables, including age and satisfaction score, between different groups. The chi-square test or Fisher's exact test was used to evaluate the association between two categorical variables, including age group, time of visit, referral (yes/no), education level, comorbidities (yes/no), occupation, seniority, and experience of telecommunication. p-values of <0.05 were considered to indicate statistical significance. All statistical analyses were performed using SPSS software version 17.0 (SPSS Inc., Chicago, IL, USA).

3. Results

3.1. Demographic Characteristics of Participants

From 20 May 2020 to 11 May 2021, the VVM project was implemented at five local infirmaries located in five villages in Taitung County, eastern Taiwan (Figure 1). The VVM provided eye care services to 395 patients (mean age, 65.13 ± 15.60 years; range, 6–90 years). Approximately 70% of the patients were aged > 60 years, and the male-to-female ratio was 2:1 (265:130; Table 1).

Table 1. Patient characteristics.

Variables	Male	Female	Total	p-Value
N	130	265	395	
Age (y/o) [a]	65.55 ± 15.90	64.93 ± 15.48	65.13 ± 15.60	0.713
Age group, n (%) [b]				0.714
≤60 y/o	33 (25.4)	80 (30.2)	113 (28.6)	
61–70 y/o	41 (31.5)	72 (27.2)	113 (28.6)	
71–80 y/o	37 (28.5)	77 (29.1)	114 (28.9)	
>80 y/o	19 (14.6)	36 (13.6)	55 (13.9)	
Number of visits, n (%) [b]				0.283
1	111 (85.4)	219 (82.6)	330 (83.5)	
2	17 (13.1)	31 (11.7)	48 (12.2)	
3	1 (0.8)	11 (4.2)	12 (3.0)	
>3	1 (0.8)	4 (1.5)	5 (1.3)	
Referral, n (%) [b]	20 (15.4)	20 (7.5)	40 (10.1)	0.015 *

Data are presented as n (%) or mean ± standard deviation; * p-values of <0.05 were considered to indicate statistical significance; [a]: independent t-test; [b]: chi-square test or Fisher's exact test; y/o: year old.

Examination of the frequency of visits revealed interesting patterns within the patient population (Table 1). Most patients (83.5%; 330) had a single visit, suggesting that a significant proportion of patients sought medical attention for a specific concern. Meanwhile, 12.2% (48) of patients returned for a second visit, indicating a need for ongoing or follow-up care. A smaller proportion of patients (3%; 12) had three visits, indicating a more complex medical situation requiring multiple assessments. Remarkably, an extremely small but notable subset constituting 5 patients (1.3%) had >3 visits, suggesting a consistent and prolonged need for medical attention.

3.2. Frequency of Eye Conditions and Number of Referrals

Based on the International Classification of Diseases 10th Revision (ICD-10 code) reported in the EMR, the most frequent eye condition was chronic conjunctivitis (n = 197), followed by senile cataract (n = 163), dry eye (n = 103), and refractive error (n = 95). Ocular inflammations, such as conjunctivitis, could be readily improved by eyedrops. Senile cataract patients could be followed up according to their visual acuity and slit lamp photos, while patients with refractive errors were referred to an optometrist based on their daily needs, such as presbyopia impeding reading or far vision impairment affecting driving.

One hundred and twenty-two visits were recorded for diabetic retinopathy screening (Figure 3). Among them, those suspected of proliferative retinopathy were referred (n = 11), while others were followed up annually or according to the guideline, along with education about diabetic complication prevention. Forty (10.1%) patients were referred to secondary or tertiary hospitals for further evaluation or treatment. Among the patients referred to our hospital, four underwent surgery for vision-impairing cataracts, while optical coherence tomography (OCT) and fundus angiography (FAG) were performed in four patients with macular degeneration, followed by subsequent treatments. Additionally, three patients with vitreous opacity and two with mild macular puckers were placed under outpatient department follow-up. Two patients underwent irrigation for nasolacrimal duct stenosis, two were prescribed atropine eye drops for myopia, one underwent incision and curettage for a hordeolum, and one was evaluated for an eye contusion. Patients who did not require specialized examinations or treatments were returned to their original infirmary for continued care. Education, suggestions, or medication were provided for those conditions (left side of the entity's bar in Figure 3) that could be effectively managed in the infirmary.

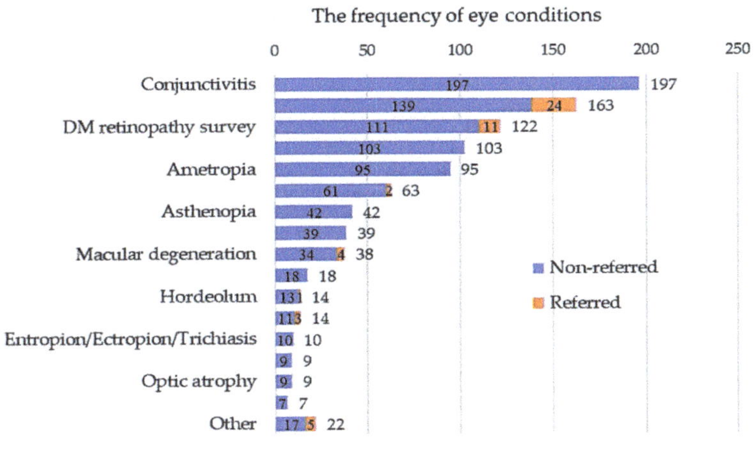

Figure 3. The frequency of eye conditions and the number of referrals.

3.3. Demographic Analysis of Questionnaire Respondents

A research assistant conducted 181 on-site or telephone questionnaire interviews, which provided insights into respondents' demographic characteristics and satisfaction scores, as presented in Table 2. Notably, the age and sex distribution of the respondents closely resembled that of the project participants, with a women-to-men ratio of approximately 2:1 (115 women and 66 men). Additionally, one-third of the female participants were found to be illiterate. The prevailing comorbidities among the respondents included conditions such as hypertension, diabetes, and coronary heart disease.

Table 2. Satisfaction survey of patients.

Variables	Male	Female	Total	*p*-Value
N	66	115	181	
Age group, n (%) [b]				0.719
≤60 y/o	13 (19.7)	31 (27.0)	44 (24.3)	
61–70 y/o	21 (31.8)	31 (27.0)	52 (28.7)	
71–80 y/o	20 (30.3)	32 (27.8)	52 (28.7)	
>80 y/o	12 (18.2)	21 (18.3)	33 (18.2)	
Education, n (%) [b]				<0.001 *
Illiterate	2 (3.0)	36 (31.3)	38 (21.0)	
Primary school	28 (42.4)	44 (38.3)	72 (39.8)	
Junior high school	16 (24.2)	4 (3.5)	20 (11.0)	
Senior high school	13 (19.7)	19 (16.5)	32 (17.7)	
Above college	7 (10.6)	12 (10.4)	19 (10.5)	
Comorbidities, n (%) [b]				
DM (%)	25 (37.9)	28 (24.3)	53 (29.3)	0.054
HTN (%)	30 (45.5)	46 (40.0)	76 (42.0)	0.474
Coronary heart disease (%)	19 (28.8)	22 (19.1)	41 (22.7)	0.135
Satisfaction (maximum score is 5) [a]				
Financial aspects of care (D1)	4.44 ± 0.62	4.5 ± 0.53	4.48 ± 0.56	0.457
Quality of medical care (D2)	4.45 ± 0.46	4.53 ± 0.51	4.50 ± 0.49	0.323
Quality of service (D3)	4.42 ± 0.37	4.38 ± 0.36	4.40 ± 0.37	0.486
Supportive attitude toward the project (D4)	4.31 ± 0.69	4.56 ± 0.56	4.47 ± 0.62	0.009 *
Quality of telecommunication (D5)	4.42 ± 0.56	4.39 ± 0.54	4.40 ± 0.55	0.726

DM, diabetes mellitus; HTN, hypertension; data are presented as n (%) or mean ± standard deviation; * *p*-values of <0.05 were considered to indicate statistical significance; [a]: independent *t*-test ; [b]: chi-square test or Fisher's exact test; y/o: year old.

3.4. Patient Satisfaction

As shown in Table 2 and Figure 4A, the satisfaction survey scores of patients in all five areas were high. The scores were 4.50 of 5 in the quality of medical care (i.e., appropriateness of examination, diagnosis, treatment, and explanation provided by the eye doctor), 4.48 in the financial aspects of care (i.e., time and traffic expense saved), 4.47 in the supportive attitude toward the project (i.e., continued use and willingness to recommend the service), 4.40 in the quality of service (i.e., friendliness and enthusiasm of the healthcare providers and the assistance they provided), and 4.40 in the quality of telecommunication. Women were substantially more supportive of the project (Table 2). We divided the participants into two subgroups to evaluate the study's external validity. Group 1 included participants from Chishang and Guanshan, and group 2 comprised Haiduan, Luye, and Darren participants. The results showed that the satisfaction scores of the two groups were comparable (Table S3).

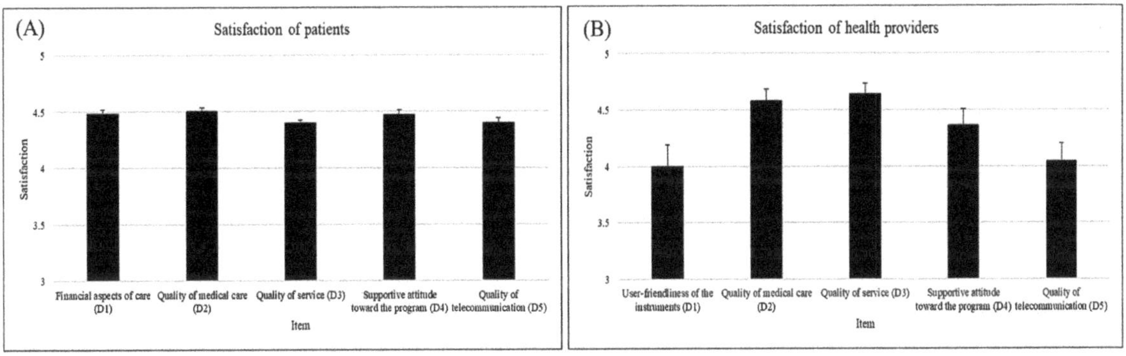

Figure 4. Satisfaction scores of (**A**) patients and (**B**) healthcare providers.

3.5. Satisfaction of Healthcare Providers

The satisfaction survey scores of healthcare providers were good in all five areas (Table 3, Figure 4B). The scores were 4.58 of 5 in the quality of medical care (i.e., diagnosis, treatment, and explanations provided by the eye doctor), 4.46 in the quality of service (i.e., referral arrangements and enthusiasm of the eye doctor), 4.36 in the supportive attitude toward the project, 4.04 in the quality of telecommunication, and 4.00 regarding user-friendliness of the instrument. Nevertheless, the areas representing telecommunication quality (score, 4.04) and user-friendliness of instruments (score, 4.00) were slightly low among healthcare providers. We divided the health providers into two subgroups to evaluate the study's external validity. Group 1 included healthcare providers from Chishang and Guanshan, and group 2 comprised Haiduan, Luye, and Darren healthcare providers. The results showed that the satisfaction scores of the two groups were comparable (Table S4). When comparing the satisfaction scores of patients and healthcare providers, we observed significant differences in two areas: The quality of service was rated lower in the patient group, whereas the quality of telecommunication was rated lower among healthcare providers (Table 4).

Table 3. Satisfaction survey of healthcare providers.

Variables	Male	Female	Total	p-Value
N	2	23	25	
Age group, n (%) [b]				0.597
21–30 y/o	0 (0.0)	2 (8.7)	2 (8.0)	
31–40 y/o	0 (0.0)	11 (47.8)	11 (44.0)	
41–50 y/o	2 (100.0)	9 (39.1)	11 (44.0)	
51–60 y/o	0 (0.0)	1 (4.3)	1 (4.0)	
Occupation, n (%) [b]				0.010 *
Doctor	2 (100.0)	1 (4.3)	3 (12.0)	
Nurse	0 (0.0)	22 (95.7)	22 (88.0)	
Seniority, n (%) [b]				0.680
1–3 years	0 (0.0)	1 (4.3)	1 (4.0)	
4–6 years	0 (0.0)	4 (17.4)	4 (16.0)	
7–10 years	0 (0.0)	8 (34.8)	8 (32.0)	
>10 years	2 (100.0)	10 (43.5)	12 (48.0)	
Experience of telecommunication, n (%) [b]				0.487
1–3 months	0 (0.0)	7 (30.4)	7 (28.0)	
3–6 months	0 (0.0)	7 (30.4)	7 (28.0)	
>6 months	2 (100.0)	9 (39.1)	11 (44.0)	
Satisfaction (maximum score is 5) [a]				
User-friendliness of the instruments (D1)	4.25 ± 1.06	3.98 ± 0.97	4.00 ± 0.96	0.709
Quality of medical care (D2)	5.00 ± 0.00	4.54 ± 0.53	4.58 ± 0.52	0.241
Quality of service (D3)	4.83 ± 0.24	4.62 ± 0.47	4.64 ± 0.46	0.547

Table 3. *Cont.*

Variables	Male	Female	Total	*p*-Value
Supportive attitude toward the project (D4)	4.50 ± 0.71	4.35 ± 0.76	4.36 ± 0.74	0.788
Quality of telecommunication (D5)	3.75 ± 0.35	4.07 ± 0.83	4.04 ± 0.80	0.605

Data are presented as n (%) or mean ± standard deviation; * *p*-values of <0.05 were considered to indicate statistical significance; [a]: independent *t*-test; [b]: chi-square test or Fisher's exact test; y/o: year old.

Table 4. Comparison of satisfaction scores between patients and healthcare providers.

Construct	Patients	Healthcare Providers	*p*-Value
N	181	25	
Quality of medical care [a]	4.50 ± 0.49	4.58 ± 0.52	0.448
Quality of service [a]	4.40 ± 0.37	4.64 ± 0.46	0.004 *
Supportive attitude toward the project [a]	4.47 ± 0.62	4.36 ± 0.74	0.418
Quality of telecommunication [a]	4.40 ± 0.55	4.04 ± 0.80	0.004 *
Financial aspects of care	4.48 ± 0.56	NA	NA
User-friendliness of the instruments	NA	4.00 ± 0.96	NA

Data are presented as mean ± standard deviation. NA, not available; * *p*-values of <0.05 were considered to indicate statistical significance; [a]: independent *t*-test.

4. Discussion

In the context of telemedicine, teleophthalmology, which integrates eye care services into remote healthcare delivery, can be categorized based on its specific applications. These applications encompass various functions, such as disease screening (e.g., fundus assessments for diabetic retinopathy) [18,19], follow-up assessments (e.g., monitoring intraocular pressure in patients with glaucoma and using OCT for age-related macular disease and diabetic macular edema), and triaging of new ocular symptoms [20–22]. Additionally, when ophthalmic consultation is required, it can be provided asynchronously through store-and-forward or synchronously through real-time interactions [23]. In teleophthalmology, integrating emerging technologies is reshaping the landscape of remote eye examinations. In circumstances of ample budget, advanced imaging modalities like OCT, OCT angiography, visual field analyzers, electrophysiologic testing devices, and the advent of non-invasive hybrid ultrasound stimulation of the visual cortex [24] could have significantly enriched the diagnostic armamentarium available to ophthalmologists.

This study implemented a synchronous videoconferencing platform (VVM) that serves multiple functions, including screening, triage, referral, and follow-up, all within a single integrated system. In this study, a general practitioner from the local infirmary accompanied the patients during videoconferences. The general practitioner performed an initial evaluation of the patients, summarized their underlying medical conditions, and clarified the primary concerns related to their ocular issues. Therefore, this module differs from other telemedicine programs as it facilitates communication between recipients (patient and general practitioner) and the provider (ophthalmologist). This integrated approach ensures a comprehensive and efficient delivery of eye care services, thus benefiting patients and healthcare providers.

In comparing face-to-face synchronous videoconferencing teleophthalmology with store-and-forward teleophthalmology (Table 5), several vital considerations arise regarding their advantages and limitations. Face-to-face synchronous videoconferencing allows real-time interaction between the patient and the healthcare provider, facilitating immediate feedback and discussion of findings. This synchronous approach is particularly beneficial for urgent cases requiring prompt assessment and management. However, it may be limited by the need for both parties to be available simultaneously, potentially leading to scheduling challenges. On the other hand, store-and-forward teleophthalmology involves capturing images or data at one location and sending them to another location for later review by a specialist. This asynchronous approach offers flexibility in terms of timing, as experts can review the images at a convenient time. However, store-and-forward teleophthalmology lacks the immediate feedback and interaction provided by synchronous videoconferencing, which may be crucial for specific clinical scenarios.

Table 5. Comparison of two teleophthalmology modalities.

Aspects	Synchronous Video Conference	Store-and-Forward
Technological requirement	Real-time conferencing and examination devices, stable internet connection	Imaging instruments for capturing and transforming examination data
Scalability	Requires simultaneous participation of patient and healthcare providers, less scalable	Does not require simultaneous availability, schedule more flexible, more scalable
Patient engagement	Higher due to interaction with the healthcare providers	Less, no direct interaction during image capture
Diagnostic accuracy	High due to immediate feedback and discussion of findings	Moderate, objective review of images, but lack interaction
Cost-effectiveness	Generally high if operate properly	High, requires less equipment and healthcare staff, lower ongoing cost

During the unprecedented challenges posed by the COVID-19 pandemic, Patel et al. documented various prevalent symptoms observed during teleophthalmology triage visits, encompassing issues such as conjunctivitis, chalazion, scleritis, visual disturbances, and dry eye [20]. Our own experiences within the VVM practice mirrored these findings, where we frequently encountered ICD-10 codes associated with conjunctivitis, senile cataracts, dry eyes, and refractive error. The majority of these conditions demonstrated effective evaluability through teleophthalmology. Our VVM practice notably included 122 visits specifically for diabetic retinopathy screening. A noteworthy study comparing diagnostic accuracy between technology-based eye care services (TECS) and face-to-face (FTF) examinations revealed substantial agreement in the diagnosis of cataracts and diabetic retinopathy [25].

As highlighted in a prior review by Saleem et al. [6], certain subspecialties, including oculoplastics, neuro-ophthalmology, and pediatrics, may be well-suited for telemedicine due to the external nature of many of their examinations. Conversely, addressing anterior segment pathology, such as keratitis and uveitis, through teleophthalmology presents more challenges. Meanwhile, teleophthalmology has demonstrated utility in medicine reconciliation and the assessment of glaucoma medication tolerance. Additionally, the utilization of fundus photography for diabetic retinopathy screening has proven to be both viable and cost-effective in the view of public health [18,26]. A review proposed that the integration of telehealth with in-person care, particularly post-diagnosis, could be valuable in managing chronic conditions [1]. In summary, teleophthalmology in our VVM setting is suitable for managing stable conditions like monitoring glaucoma intraocular pressure, conducting annual fundoscopy screenings for diabetic patients, and addressing mild ocular symptoms such as itchiness, wateriness, dryness, and soreness of the eye. However, acute deteriorations in vision, elevated intraocular pressure, sudden onset diplopia, suspicion of eyelid tumor, eyeball trauma, and intractable eye pain that does not improve after eyedrops should not be managed remotely through teleophthalmology; instead, immediate referral is recommended.

Although higher health literacy and regular internet access have traditionally been associated with patients' interest in using telemedicine in rural areas [2], we found that one-third of the female participants were illiterate. This unexpected finding can be attributed to the dedication and rapport established by the patient-end infirmary staff, who were intimately familiar with the village inhabitants and had earned their trust [23].

Notably, we had more female participants who exhibited a more supportive attitude toward our VVM services. This suggests that the utilization of and satisfaction with our VVM teleophthalmology system were not impeded by factors such as lower educational attainment, gender (female), or older age [27,28]. This highlights that our teleophthalmology system was easily accessible and well-received by the remote population, even by those who may traditionally face barriers to technological advancements and healthcare access.

In addition to the well-established efficacy of telemedicine adaptation owing to increased accessibility of eye care services [29], it is important to recognize that the success of this system depends on the acceptance and robust support from the community [4,23]. Herein, we systematically collected satisfaction data from patients and healthcare providers through a comprehensive questionnaire that delved into various aspects of their telemedicine experience.

Previous research has revealed that high satisfaction levels are closely associated with several factors, including patients' older age, familiarity with the patient-end clinician, interface usability, and appreciation for time and cost savings [9,11,30]. In alignment with these findings, our patients expressed the highest satisfaction levels with the quality of medical care, which assessed the appropriateness of examination, diagnosis, treatment, and explanation provided by the eye doctor. This was closely followed by the financial aspects of care, where patients valued the time and cost savings associated with the teleophthalmology service. Additionally, a supportive attitude toward the project, indicating continued use and willingness to recommend the service, ranked high among satisfaction factors.

Notably, considering that a substantial proportion of our patients were older individuals, on-site videoconferencing consultations, which seamlessly combine examination and treatment in a single session, proved to be a highly convenient and cost-effective approach. This contributed to the high level of satisfaction among our patients, thus underlining the effectiveness of this model in catering to the unique needs of the older population.

In our study, infirmary healthcare providers expressed confidence in the quality of medical care (4.58) and quality of service (4.64). However, they provided slightly low ratings for the quality of telecommunication (4.04) and user-friendliness of instruments (4.0). These findings align with concerns from other studies regarding incomplete assessments using telehealth [10,11] and the need for training and support for using the platform [4,10]. Healthcare providers encountered issues with unstable voice and video quality during real-time videoconferencing. They also faced difficulties transferring patient data from examination instruments to the conferencing device. Some challenges arose in conducting examinations on some patients; for instance, elderly patients might not comply with placing their face on the chin-rest, leading to difficulties in obtaining a clear image of a slit lamp or fundoscopy. Improving internet infrastructure could enhance the quality of telecommunication. Furthermore, on-the-job training and seminars with specialists are essential to mastering the technique comprehensively.

We observed remarkable differences in satisfaction scores between patients and healthcare providers, particularly in the areas of quality of service and quality of telecommunication. From a service quality perspective, infirmary healthcare providers assessed the referral process and the friendliness and enthusiasm of the consulting ophthalmologist. Conversely, patients evaluated the teleophthalmology service as a more complex entity, encompassing aspects such as appointment procedures, referrals, and communication skills of both infirmary healthcare providers and those at the medical center. Therefore, achieving high satisfaction scores in the patients' survey proved to be more challenging.

In this study, healthcare providers, comprising doctors and nurses from local infirmaries, assumed dual responsibilities by serving as service providers for patients and service recipients during interactions with the consulting ophthalmologist. Importantly, these healthcare providers were not employed by the project administration and were not involved in the program's design. This distinctive dual role distinguishes them from participants in conventional satisfaction surveys, where the medical staff generally function solely as care providers. Thus, the scores of such participants hold unique significance [11,17]. Similar to previous studies, the quality of telecommunication was rated high by patients [11,17]. In teleophthalmology, the medical staff bears the responsibility for the preparatory process, ensuring appropriate device setup, whereas patients utilize the equipment once it is ready. The survey findings highlight the importance of enhancing both internet and information technology infrastructures and the development of training programs for the medical staff. These steps are vital to ensure the safe and effective operation of teleophthalmology in the future, aligning with previous research [20,31,32].

Furthermore, although synchronous videoconferencing is a cost-effective approach from the perspective of patients involved in telemedicine [17], pre-consultation preparations place a relatively time-consuming burden on healthcare personnel [20]. Overcoming this challenge necessitates increased manpower support and appropriate reimbursement to streamline and facilitate the process.

To assess the study's external validity, we stratified the five townships into two subgroups based on traffic convenience. Our subgroup analysis also revealed consistent satisfaction scores across all domains for both participants and healthcare providers. This suggests that our VVM model is adaptable across varied populations, ensuring equivalent satisfaction and reinforcing its external validity.

In summary, in our VVM model, teleophthalmology offers significant advantages, including enhanced accessibility to eye care services, improved compliance via infirmaries, and patient-end support to overcome technological barriers. However, notable disadvantages include the high cost of devices, the requirement for substantial training for program setup, and the time-consuming nature of pre-consultation examinations. Common applications of teleophthalmology include vision check-ups, monitoring of intraocular pressure for patients with glaucoma, screening for diabetic retinopathy, and triaging of new-onset eye conditions. Despite these advantages, teleophthalmology has certain limitations, such as the inability to conduct peripheral fundoscopy, provide immediate surgical treatment, and perform comprehensive surveys of patients suspected of glaucoma, age-related macular diseases, or optic neuropathy. In such cases, referrals to secondary or tertiary hospitals become necessary.

There are several limitations in this study. First, our sample size was relatively small; thus, potential bias may exist in patient selection. Nevertheless, the age and sex distribution of respondents closely resembled that of project participants, thus mitigating potential bias. Additionally, the findings of our study may not be universally applicable due to variations in technology and infrastructure. Furthermore, not all referred patients visited the consulting medical centers, resulting in some unknown final diagnoses. In retrospect, we understand that involving an independent panel of international experts could have offered a more objective evaluation. However, due to the project's initiation during the pandemic, these participants were the most viable subjects available without any associated risks. However, they may lack the professional expertise to comprehensively assess the medical system, and their opinions may not align with clinical outcomes. Further research is warranted to overcome these limitations and gain a more comprehensive understanding of the topic.

5. Conclusions

The survey results revealed high satisfaction levels with teleophthalmology services among rural participants and healthcare providers. For the successful future implementation of teleophthalmology, it is crucial to improve telecommunication infrastructure and offer training programs for instrument use. With the ongoing expansion of teleophthalmology during and after the COVID-19 pandemic, VVM videoconferencing has emerged as an efficient alternative for delivering eye care services.

Supplementary Materials: The following supporting information can be downloaded at: https://www.mdpi.com/article/10.3390/healthcare12080818/s1, Table S1: Satisfaction survey questionnaire for patients; Table S2: Satisfaction survey questionnaire for healthcare providers; Table S3: Comparison of satisfaction scores between two groups of patients; Table S4: Comparison of satisfaction scores between two groups of healthcare providers.

Author Contributions: Conceptualization, C.-J.C.; methodology, C.-J.C. and J.-H.W.; software, J.-H.W.; validation, N.C., J.-H.W. and C.-J.C.; investigation, N.C. and C.-J.C.; resources, C.-J.C.; data curation,

N.C., J.-H.W. and C.-J.C.; writing—original draft preparation, N.C.; writing—review and editing, C.-J.C.; visualization, J.-H.W. and N.C; supervision, C.-J.C.; project administration, C.-J.C.; funding acquisition, C.-J.C. All authors have read and agreed to the published version of the manuscript.

Funding: This research was funded by Hualien Tzu Chi General Hospital, grant number TCRD110-53-HHC.

Institutional Review Board Statement: The study was approved by the Institutional Review Board of Hualien Tzu Chi General Hospital (IRB109-198-B, 1 October 2020).

Informed Consent Statement: Patient consent was waived because the anonymous questionnaire posed a low or negligible risk to the participants.

Data Availability Statement: Data are contained within the article and Supplementary Materials.

Conflicts of Interest: The authors declare no conflict of interest. The funders had no role in the design of the study; collection, analyses, or interpretation of data; writing of the manuscript; or decision to publish the results.

References

1. Dorsey, E.R.; Topol, E.J. State of Telehealth. *N. Engl. J. Med* **2016**, *375*, 154–161. [CrossRef] [PubMed]
2. Thomson, M.D.; Mariani, A.C.; Williams, A.R.; Sutton, A.L.; Sheppard, V.B. Factors Associated with Use of and Satisfaction with Telehealth by Adults in Rural Virginia During the COVID-19 Pandemic. *JAMA Netw. Open* **2021**, *4*, e2119530. [CrossRef] [PubMed]
3. Nittari, G.; Savva, D.; Tomassoni, D.; Tayebati, S.K.; Amenta, F. Telemedicine in the COVID-19 Era: A Narrative Review Based on Current Evidence. *Int. J. Environ. Res. Public Health* **2022**, *19*, 5101. [CrossRef] [PubMed]
4. Martin, A.B.; Probst, J.C.; Shah, K.; Chen, Z.; Garr, D. Differences in readiness between rural hospitals and primary care providers for telemedicine adoption and implementation: Findings from a statewide telemedicine survey. *J. Rural Health* **2012**, *28*, 8–15. [CrossRef] [PubMed]
5. Parikh, D.; Armstrong, G.; Liou, V.; Husain, D. Advances in Telemedicine in Ophthalmology. *Semin. Ophthalmol.* **2020**, *35*, 210–215. [CrossRef] [PubMed]
6. Saleem, S.M.; Pasquale, L.R.; Sidoti, P.A.; Tsai, J.C. Virtual Ophthalmology: Telemedicine in a COVID-19 Era. *Am. J. Ophthalmol.* **2020**, *216*, 237–242. [CrossRef] [PubMed]
7. Sommer, A.C.; Blumenthal, E.Z. Telemedicine in ophthalmology in view of the emerging COVID-19 outbreak. *Graefe's Arch. Clin. Exp. Ophthalmol.* **2020**, *258*, 2341–2352. [CrossRef] [PubMed]
8. Golash, V.; Athwal, S.; Khandwala, M. Teleophthalmology and COVID-19: The patient perspective. *Future Healthc. J.* **2021**, *8*, e54–e59. [CrossRef]
9. Host, B.K.; Turner, A.W.; Muir, J. Real-time teleophthalmology video consultation: An analysis of patient satisfaction in rural Western Australia. *Clin. Exp. Optom.* **2018**, *101*, 129–134. [CrossRef]
10. Bouabida, K.; Malas, K.; Talbot, A.; Desrosiers, M.E.; Lavoie, F.; Lebouche, B.; Taghizadeh, N.; Normandin, L.; Vialaron, C.; Fortin, O.; et al. Healthcare Professional Perspectives on the Use of Remote Patient-Monitoring Platforms during the COVID-19 Pandemic: A Cross-Sectional Study. *J. Pers. Med.* **2022**, *12*, 529. [CrossRef]
11. Park, H.Y.; Kwon, Y.M.; Jun, H.R.; Jung, S.E.; Kwon, S.Y. Satisfaction Survey of Patients and Medical Staff for Telephone-Based Telemedicine During Hospital Closing Due to COVID-19 Transmission. *Telemed. e-Health* **2021**, *27*, 724–732. [CrossRef] [PubMed]
12. Chen, N.; Huang, T.L.; Tsai, R.K.; Sheu, M.M. Prevalence and causes of visual impairment in elderly Amis aborigines in Eastern Taiwan (the Amis Eye Study). *Jpn. J. Ophthalmol.* **2012**, *56*, 624–630. [CrossRef] [PubMed]
13. Huang, T.L.; Hsu, S.Y.; Tsai, R.K.; Sheu, M.M. Etiology of ocular diseases in elderly Amis aborigines in Eastern Taiwan (The Amis Eye Study). *Jpn. J. Ophthalmol.* **2010**, *54*, 266–271. [CrossRef] [PubMed]
14. Chen, N.; Hsieh, H.P.; Tsai, R.K.; Sheu, M.M. Eye care services for the populations of remote districts in eastern Taiwan: A practical framework using a Mobile Vision Van Unit. *Rural. Remote Health* **2015**, *15*, 3442. [CrossRef] [PubMed]
15. Oosterveld, P.; Vorst, H.C.M.; Smits, N. Methods for questionnaire design: A taxonomy linking procedures to test goals. *Qual. Life Res.* **2019**, *28*, 2501–2512. [CrossRef] [PubMed]
16. Bakken, S.; Grullon-Figueroa, L.; Izquierdo, R.; Lee, N.J.; Morin, P.; Palmas, W.; Teresi, J.; Weinstock, R.S.; Shea, S.; Starren, J.; et al. Development, validation, and use of English and Spanish versions of the telemedicine satisfaction and usefulness questionnaire. *J. Am. Med. Inform. Assoc.* **2006**, *13*, 660–667. [CrossRef] [PubMed]
17. Nguyen, M.; Waller, M.; Pandya, A.; Portnoy, J. A Review of Patient and Provider Satisfaction with Telemedicine. *Curr Allergy Asthma Rep.* **2020**, *20*, 72. [CrossRef] [PubMed]
18. Daskivich, L.P.; Vasquez, C.; Martinez, C., Jr.; Tseng, C.H.; Mangione, C.M. Implementation and Evaluation of a Large-Scale Teleretinal Diabetic Retinopathy Screening Program in the Los Angeles County Department of Health Services. *JAMA Intern. Med.* **2017**, *177*, 642–649. [CrossRef] [PubMed]

19. Avendano-Veloso, A.; Parada-Hernandez, F.; Gonzalez-Ramos, R.; Dougnac-Osses, C.; Carrasco-Saez, J.L.; Scanlon, P.H. Teleophthalmology: A strategy for timely diagnosis of sight-threatening diabetic retinopathy in primary care, Concepcion, Chile. *Int. J. Ophthalmol.* **2019**, *12*, 1474–1478. [CrossRef] [PubMed]
20. Patel, S.; Hamdan, S.; Donahue, S. Optimising telemedicine in ophthalmology during the COVID-19 pandemic. *J. Telemed. Telecare* **2020**, *28*, 498–501. [CrossRef]
21. Wedekind, L.; Sainani, K.; Pershing, S. Supply and Perceived Demand for Teleophthalmology in Triage and Consultations in California Emergency Departments. *JAMA Ophthalmol.* **2016**, *134*, 537–543. [CrossRef] [PubMed]
22. Gan, K.; Liu, Y.; Stagg, B.; Rathi, S.; Pasquale, L.R.; Damji, K. Telemedicine for Glaucoma: Guidelines and Recommendations. *Telemed. e-Health* **2020**, *26*, 551–555. [CrossRef]
23. Chia, M.A.; Turner, A.W. Benefits of Integrating Telemedicine and Artificial Intelligence into Outreach Eye Care: Stepwise Approach and Future Directions. *Front. Med.* **2022**, *9*, 835804. [CrossRef] [PubMed]
24. Gong, C.; Li, R.; Lu, G.; Ji, J.; Zeng, Y.; Chen, J.; Chang, C.; Zhang, J.; Xia, L.; Nair, D.S.R.; et al. Non-Invasive Hybrid Ultrasound Stimulation of Visual Cortex In Vivo. *Bioengineering* **2023**, *10*, 577. [CrossRef] [PubMed]
25. Maa, A.Y.; Medert, C.M.; Lu, X.; Janjua, R.; Howell, A.V.; Hunt, K.J.; McCord, S.; Giangiacomo, A.; Lynch, M.G. Diagnostic Accuracy of Technology-based Eye Care Services: The Technology-based Eye Care Services Compare Trial Part I. *Ophthalmology* **2020**, *127*, 38–44. [CrossRef] [PubMed]
26. Souza, G.F.; Figueira, R.M.; Alkmim, M.B.; Sousa, L.A.P.; Bonisson, L.; Ribeiro, A.L.P.; Vasconcelos-Santos, D.V. Teleophthalmology Screening for Diabetic Retinopathy in Brazil: Applicability and Economic Assessment. *Telemed. e-Health* **2020**, *26*, 341–346. [CrossRef] [PubMed]
27. Ramirez, A.V.; Ojeaga, M.; Espinoza, V.; Hensler, B.; Honrubia, V. Telemedicine in Minority and Socioeconomically Disadvantaged Communities Amidst COVID-19 Pandemic. *Otolaryngol. Head Neck Surg.* **2021**, *164*, 91–92. [CrossRef] [PubMed]
28. Figueroa, C.A.; Luo, T.; Aguilera, A.; Lyles, C.R. The need for feminist intersectionality in digital health. *Lancet Digit. Health* **2021**, *3*, e526–e533. [CrossRef] [PubMed]
29. Sreelatha, O.K.; Ramesh, S.V. Teleophthalmology: Improving patient outcomes? *Clin. Ophthalmol.* **2016**, *10*, 285–295. [CrossRef] [PubMed]
30. Bartnik, S.E.; Copeland, S.P.; Aicken, A.J.; Turner, A.W. Optometry-facilitated teleophthalmology: An audit of the first year in Western Australia. *Clin. Exp. Optom.* **2018**, *101*, 700–703. [CrossRef] [PubMed]
31. Kumar, G.; Shardha, H.K.; Tariq, W.; Qazi, M.A.; Kumar, K.; Maheshwari, C.; Hussain, A.; Tahir, M.J.; Bai, J.; Asghar, M.S. Assessment of knowledge and attitude of healthcare professionals regarding the use of telemedicine: A cross-sectional study from rural areas of Sindh, Pakistan. *Front. Public Health* **2022**, *10*, 967440. [CrossRef] [PubMed]
32. Bodnar, Z.M.; Schuchard, R.; Myung, D.; Tarver, M.E.; Blumenkranz, M.S.; Afshari, N.A.; Humayun, M.S.; Morse, C.; Nischal, K.; Repka, M.X.; et al. Evaluating New Ophthalmic Digital Devices for Safety and Effectiveness in the Context of Rapid Technological Development. *JAMA Ophthalmol.* **2019**, *137*, 939–944. [CrossRef] [PubMed]

healthcare

MDPI

Review

Utilizing Telemedicine Applications in Celiac Disease and Other Gluten-Free-Diet-Dependent Conditions: Insights from the COVID-19 Pandemic

Motti Haimi [1,2,*] and Aaron Lerner [3,4]

1 Health Systems Management Department, The Max Stern Yezreel Valley College, Yezreel Valley 1930600, Israel
2 Rappaport Faculty of Medicine, Technion-Israel Institute of Technology, Haifa 3109601, Israel
3 Chaim Sheba Medical Center, The Zabludowicz Research Center for Autoimmune Diseases, Ramat Gan 5266202, Israel; aaronlerner1948@gmail.com
4 Research Department, Ariel University, Ariel 407000, Israel
* Correspondence: morx@netvision.net.il

Abstract: Background: Globally, approximately 1.4% of people have celiac disease (CD), induced by gluten sensitivity. If left untreated, it causes small intestinal inflammation and villous atrophy, which can result in failure to thrive, anemia, osteoporosis, malabsorption, and even malignancy. The only treatment option available is a gluten-free diet (GFD). Few studies have looked at the role and perception of telehealth in relation to CD and selective nutrition both before and after the COVID-19 pandemic. Aim: Our goal was to screen and investigate the research conducted both before and after the COVID-19 pandemic concerning the utilization of telehealth applications and solutions in CD and other GFD-dependent circumstances. Methods: We employed a narrative review approach to explore articles that were published in scholarly journals or organizations between the years 2000 and 2024. Only English-language publications were included. PubMed and Google Scholar searches were mainly conducted using the following keywords: telemedicine, telehealth, telecare, eHealth, m-health, COVID-19, SARS-CoV-2, celiac disease, and gluten-free diet (GFD). Manual searches of the references in the acquired literature were also carried out, along with the authors' own personal contributions of their knowledge and proficiency in this field. Results: Only a few studies conducted prior to the COVID-19 outbreak examined the viewpoints and experiences of adult patients with CD with relation to in-person clinic visits, as well as other options such as telehealth. The majority of patients believed that phone consultations were appropriate and beneficial. Video conferencing and telemedicine became more popular during the COVID-19 pandemic, demonstrating the effectiveness of using these technologies for CD on a global basis. In recent years, urine assays for gluten identification have become accessible for use at home. These tests could be helpful for CD monitoring with telemedicine assistance. Conclusions: The extended knowledge gathered from the COVID-19 pandemic is expected to complement pre-COVID-19 data supporting the usefulness of telemedicine even after the emergent pandemic, encouraging its wider adoption in standard clinical practice. The monitoring and follow-up of CD patients and other GFD-dependent conditions can greatly benefit from telemedicine.

Keywords: celiac disease (CD); gluten; gluten-free diet (GFD); telemedicine; eHealth; COVID-19; GFD-dependent; non-celiac gluten sensitivity (NCGS); compliance; diet-adherence

1. Introduction

Celiac disease (CD), an autoimmune condition, affects approximately 1.4% of people worldwide.

It is identified by gluten sensitivity. The target organ is the small intestine, where inflammation injures the mucosa, resulting in a variety of gastrointestinal (GI) and non-GI symptoms [1–4].

Untreated, it induces inflammation in the small intestine, resulting in villous atrophy, which can lead to chronic diarrhea, failure to thrive, malabsorption, anemia, osteoporosis, nutritional deficiencies, and even cancer [5–7]. The sole therapeutic option is to consume a gluten-free diet (GFD) [5–8].

It is generally acknowledged that following a GFD may be difficult; it calls for motivation, knowledge, and altered behavior. The GFD adherence rate might vary from 42% to 91%, depending on the patient category and recruitment strategy. Strict adherence to a gluten-free diet (GFD) is difficult for a variety of reasons, including a lack of awareness, sub-standard labeling, and the high price of gluten-free goods [9,10].

Expert dietitian-led individualized instruction is regarded as the gold standard of care. It takes a lot of money and effort, however. In order to get around these restrictions, other teaching strategies, such as group instruction, have been researched [10–13]. It should be mentioned that GFD has its side effects [14–16] and gluten avoidance can prevent its detrimental effect, not only in celiac patients [16,17]. Improved patient knowledge and comprehensive nutritional education will improve patient compliance [9,15–18].

Across the world, a variety of techniques are employed to help medical professionals monitor and assess patients. These techniques include nutritional and psychological counseling, one-on-one consultations, group meetings, phone clinics, web interfaces, and text messaging, with varying degrees of success documented [19,20].

Educating celiac patients about gluten-free foods, medications, and consumer goods was thought to be a key strategy for improving their adherence to the GFD and reducing the symptoms of the illness [9,14,21].

Transmitting health messages via cellphones has increased recently as a result of the rise in smartphone use worldwide. Utilizing mobile technologies to improve health outcomes is a suitable strategy known as mobile health, or mHealth. This approach is accessible, affordable, and simple to implement. In several studies, this strategy has been employed to encourage behaviors relevant to health [22–31].

Dietary therapy has demonstrated the benefits of smartphone applications for weight loss programs [32–36] and nutrition education for many illnesses, including diabetes [37], kidney ailments [38], and cardiovascular disease [39].

Telephone and smartphone applications have also been reported to be effective for celiac patients [40,41].

Dowd et al. demonstrated that one-month use of the application had a considerably greater favorable effect on GI symptoms in celiac patients than usual therapy [42].

In addition to the gluten content of meals, patients can receive information such as gluten-related labeling and a gluten-free drug list via applications. Previously, a lack of understanding regarding the gluten content of commercial foods and medications was noted as a barrier to GFD compliance [21].

The COVID-19 pandemic has had a considerable detrimental impact on world health and the economy, and it has prompted fresh worries among CD patients [43]. Celiac disease, an immune-mediated ailment, has been related to a higher risk of bacterial pneumonia [44], as well as frequent viral infections including influenza [45] and herpes zoster [46]. These findings have sparked worries about whether celiac patients are more susceptible to contract COVID-19, which can have severe consequences. The pandemic could also potentially harm people who are genetically prone to celiac disease, as viral infections have been found to cause an immune response to dietary antigens [47–49].

Moreover, individuals with CD must deal with pressing issues, including the potential loss of access to medical care and gluten-free food alternatives. Telemedicine has quickly emerged as the main instrument for outpatient assessment as a result of this problem [50].

Only a small number of studies have examined the function and perception of telehealth, in gastroenterology in general, and in CD and nutrition in particular [51–53] before and during the COVID-19 pandemic. These studies typically yielded positive results in favor of telemedicine, with televisits with patients in their homes appearing acceptable for nutritional counseling due to the ease with which patients can submit dietary advice during such in-person consultations [54].

2. Methods

2.1. Search Terms

The following keywords were used to search PubMed and Google Scholar for this narrative review: telemedicine, telehealth, telecare, eHealth, m-health, celiac disease, COVID-19, SARS-CoV-2, gluten-free diet (GFD).

In addition, manual searches of references in the obtained literature were conducted. We also discussed with professionals and experts in the fields of telemedicine and celiac disease. In addition to producing numerous assessments of the relevant literature, we contributed our own expertise and experience in those domains. Table 1 provides a summary of the search terms.

Table 1. Search criteria and sources used for the study.

Type of Review	Narrative Review
Period	2000 to 2024
Keywords used	Telemedicine, telehealth, telecare, eHealth, m-health, celiac disease, COVID-19, SARS-CoV-2, gluten-free diet (GFD).
Sources	• PubMed, Google Scholar. • Manual searches of the obtained literature's references. • Discussion with professionals and experts in the fields of telemedicine and celiac disease. • Bringing our individual experiences and knowledge of that fields' topics.
Language	English only
Types of articles	• Original articles; • Reports of randomized clinical trials; • Observational studies; • Editorials, reviews, and essays by key opinion leaders.

2.2. Selection Criteria

Only English-language publications that were published in scholarly journals or organizations between January 2000 and April 2024 were included.

All types of articles were considered, including original articles, reports of randomized clinical trials, observational studies, and editorials, reviews, or essays by key opinion leaders.

3. Results

3.1. Celiac Disease and Other GFD-Compatible Conditions

As previously mentioned, celiac disease (CD) is an immune-mediated illness that affects people who are genetically susceptible (HLA DQ2 and DQ8 genotypes). It is induced by consuming gluten, which is found in grains including wheat, barley, and rye. About 1.4% of people worldwide are affected with CD, and reports of its prevalence in the US and Europe have been rising over time [55–58]. Furthermore, it seems to be increasing, with a patchy distribution and areas in Saudi Arabia where the sero-prevalence might reach up to 3% [59,60].

The only proven method for treating CD patients' symptoms, returning their immune systems to normal, as well as the normalization of serological markers and healing their intestinal mucosa, is a life-long gluten-free diet (GFD) [9,14,61–64].

The histologic and serological criteria of classic CD are not met in some borderline instances that have received a lot of attention lately, but it appears that gluten may contribute to the symptoms. A gluten-free diet appears to help this diverse group, known as "non-celiac gluten sensitivity" (NCGS), at least symptomatically. Their histopathologic analysis also reveals milder villus architectural alterations. These symptoms are typically milder than those of classic CD [65–69]. Survey study data indicate that the prevalence rates of NCGS range from 0.49% to 14.9%, exceeding nearly all estimates of CD or WA (wheat allergy) prevalence rates [70].

A subset of this group, known as lymphocytic doudenosis, is identified by elevated intraepithelial lymphocytes (IELs) in the small intestine biopsy, without any other histopathologic characteristics of the CD and negative serology [71].

In addition to gluten proteins, other parts of wheat have been suggested by researchers to trigger symptoms in NCGS patients and activate the innate immune system [72,73].

Furthermore, a few trials have demonstrated relief in individuals with non-specific enteropathies, dyspepsia, or IBS-like symptoms after a GFD, indicating that a GFD may have uses beyond treating people with classic CD [74–76]. Notably, GFD was recently reported to benefit patients with non-celiac autoimmune conditions [17].

It is generally acknowledged that the consumption of grains such as wheat, rye, and barley by individuals in whom CD has been conclusively ruled out can be linked to extraintestinal symptoms such as fatigue, as well as typical IBS-like symptoms such as bloating, abdominal pain, and irregular bowel habits. Consequently, diagnoses of NCGS have been performed for individuals who do not have wheat allergy or CD but who experience gastrointestinal symptoms similar to IBS after eating gluten-containing foods and who see improvements in these symptoms after following a GFD [77].

According to estimates, the prevalence of NCGS ranges from 0.6% to 13.0%. Wheat allergy, and gluten ataxia, are other illnesses that have benefited from GFD. However, a lot of people would rather limit or completely avoid consuming gluten. Up to 50% of some groups, including athletes, report varying degrees of adherence to a GFD [78,79].

Atopic illnesses and nongrain food allergies in children have been found to be more common in patients with NCGS and IBS symptoms [80].

The outcomes of the first trial using a GFD for fibromyalgia were published in a recent study by Slim and colleagues [81]. In this study, over the course of 24 weeks, 75 adult patients with fibromyalgia were randomized to either a GFD or a hypocaloric diet (HCD). Similar positive effects in lowering the symptoms of gluten sensitivity and other secondary outcomes were linked to both dietary treatments.

The effects of a GFD in patients with endometriosis and persistent pelvic discomfort have been assessed in two studies. Following the application of a GFD for six or twelve months, both trials reported an improvement in pain scores [82,83].

3.2. Telehealth Application for Celiac Patients

Very few studies in the literature have assessed the function and perception of telehealth, specifically televisits in gastroenterology and even fewer in celiac disease, both before and after the COVID-19 pandemic.

None of these studies explore the perspective of patients' trust in telemedicine and televisits, despite the fact that similar studies conducted in other disciplines have generally shown positive results in terms of satisfaction and cost-effectiveness [51–54].

Across the world, a variety of techniques are employed to allow medical professionals to monitor and assess patients, such as individual consultations, group meetings, phone clinics, and web-based tools [20,21].

According to Kurien et al. [84], efforts must be made to develop a financially sensible method of providing a CD follow-up treatment that is well-received by patients and medical professionals.

Thirty-four persons with CD participated in qualitative interviews [75] to discuss their preferences for the kind of intervention that would be designed to increase dietary adherence. In addition to being easy, flexible, and convenient, the participants thought that telephone clinics were just as helpful as in-person clinics when it came to GF dietary adherence. This study showed that a six-month intervention using a telephone clinic increases GF dietary adherence. The participants' understanding of nutrition increased, especially with regard to their awareness of what gluten-free items they could eat. The study also showed that individuals who did not strictly follow a GFD needed to be regularly followed up with because the improvements showed maximum benefit after six months [85].

Muhammad et al. conducted another study to learn more about the perspectives and experiences of adult CD patients regarding in-person clinic visits and other options such as telehealth. Based on simplicity and convenience, most patients thought that telephone consultations were acceptable and useful [86].

Nikniaz et al. [41] created a Persian-language application for CD patients and evaluated the impact of a three-month educational intervention given via smartphone application on gastrointestinal symptom rating scale (GSRS) score in patients with CD in comparison with routine care.

The findings showed that, in comparison to standard clinic teaching, utilizing a smartphone application to educate patients with CD significantly improved their symptoms of indigestion. The CD-GSRS mean score ($p = 0.001$) and the indigestion sub score ($p < 0.001$) in the intervention group were both significantly lower than the baseline.

3.3. The Effect of the COVID-19 Pandemic

The COVID-19 pandemic has led to an increase in the use of video conferencing and telemedicine in place of in-person consultations, which has proven the efficacy of employing these technologies for CD on a global scale [87].

Telemedicine was adopted for CD patients during the countrywide lockdown during the COVID-19 pandemic in Italy [54]. Phone calls were conducted between March 2020 and May 2020 for follow-up appointments that were previously planned but never completed at the tertiary referral center (Centre for Prevention and Diagnosis of Celiac Disease in Milan, Italy). In addition to phone calls, televisits were suggested for any patient exhibiting symptoms (such as diarrhea, abdominal pain, or weight loss) or for those exhibiting changed blood test results. Patients were also given the option of televisits for nutritional counseling on GFD and CD. Depending on the preferences of each patient, video calling services from Microsoft Teams or Google (Hangouts or Meet) were employed. According to this study, telemedicine was a viable option, and CD patients had a positive attitude towards it. Most patients trusted the combined gastroenterological and nutritional televisits. Gluten detection tests were shown to be useful in helping patients and caregivers verify GFD compliance from a distance.

Researchers have worked to determine whether CD patients are more likely to experience severe COVID-19 outcomes during the pandemic. Undoubtedly, the pandemic has altered how CD is managed; for example, lockdowns have necessitated the use of new technologies to provide medical care during this time [88].

It was first thought that those who have autoimmune diseases including type 1 diabetes and CD would be more susceptible to catching COVID-19. Furthermore, there was a concern that these people would experience more serious COVID-19-infection-related outcomes [89].

A study conducted in Italy in March 2020 found that patients with celiac disease who are older or have other chronic illnesses perceive a larger risk of contracting COVID-19 infection [52]. Nevertheless, elderly adults may benefit from an increased awareness of celiac disease [90].

CD has been associated with an increased risk of respiratory infection outcomes, such as pneumococcal pneumonia and influenza, as well as a greater mortality rate from respiratory causes [44,91,92].

Hospitalization and death rates for people with CD were comparable to those in the general population, according to studies carried out before COVID-19 vaccinations were made available. In addition, CD patients did not have higher COVID-19-related morbidity or mortality, according to early American research [93–95].

In conclusion, there is currently universal agreement that individuals with celiac disease do not have an increased chance of developing symptomatic COVID-19, despite initial worries that this patient population might be more affected by the virus than the general population [89].

In relation to obtaining gluten-free food and adhering to a GFD, early in 2020, as COVID-19 spread over the world, many households bought a lot of long-lasting products, which had a big impact on access to particular products. Furthermore, there was restricted entry to restaurants due to strict lockdowns in numerous nations. Due to their dietary limitations, those with CD were particularly burdened by this, and compared to the general population, people with CD reported higher degrees of food insecurity [96].

The purposeful consumption of gluten-containing items increased as a result of a decrease in the availability of gluten-free meals, according to a study conducted on American families [97]. More recently diagnosed CD patients had more trouble following a GFD, according to a Turkish study [98].

People in Chile stated that maintaining a GFD was challenging because of rising prices for gluten-free goods, job losses, and food shortages [99].

Two significant ways that environmental factors can impact a GFD were brought to light by the COVID-19 pandemic. Some reported sticking to a GFD more closely since they were unable to eat during the severe lockdown [100]. On the other hand, other CD patients reported more difficulty paying for gluten-free food and more obstacles to sticking to a GFD [99].

In a study conducted by Siniscalchi et al. [52], the researchers sought to understand how persons with CD from Veneto and Campania, Italy, for whom food supplies are a daily concern, saw the COVID-19 pandemic during the lockdown. Significant percentages of respondents to a quality-of-life questionnaire related to CD stated that they felt generally intimidated and depressed as a result of their condition. Concerns about their celiac illness, which increases the risk of infection and serious CD consequences, were more prevalent among older responders. However, the main finding was that individuals with CD did not believe they were at a heightened risk of contracting the SARS-CoV-2 virus. Another noteworthy conclusion is that the majority of CD patients were content with remote consultations and were not concerned about the lack of gluten-free food in stores or pharmacies. According to the findings, CD healthcare may eventually adopt remote consulting as normal practice.

During the first phase of the COVID-19 pandemic, a cross-sectional questionnaire-based study involving 37 Dutch pediatric patients with CD and their parents was conducted to learn more about the experiences of children with CD and their families regarding their GFD, symptoms, and CD management. The majority said that eating more meals at home made it simpler to stick to the diet during the pandemic and reported strong compliance with the GFD. Some found that online purchasing offered a wider selection of GF items, which could increase the GFD's cost. In terms of overall eating patterns, 21.6% reported a healthier pattern, compared to 37.8% and 10.8% who, respectively, had fewer fruits and vegetables and more unhealthy snacks than usual over the pandemic [101].

In certain cases, the pandemic also affected the diagnosis of CD. The British Society for Gastroenterology released a non-biopsy-based protocol for CD diagnosis in 2020 in an attempt to reduce exposure to COVID-19. Villus atrophy on endoscopy appears to be substantially correlated with laboratory data, particularly increased IgA tissue transglutaminase levels 10 times the upper limit of normal or above. Those guidelines state that a positive endomysial antibody and a highly elevated IgA tissue transglutaminase (tTG; $\geq$10 times the upper limit of normal) in individuals under 55 years of age can be regarded as a confirmed diagnosis of CD [102].

3.4. Future Use in a Non-Pandemic Scenario

Even after the emergency pandemic, the experience gained from the COVID-19 pandemic is likely to support pre-COVID-19 evidence regarding the efficacy and good performance of telemedicine and encourage its wider adoption in routine clinical practice.

During the pandemic, telehealth made it possible for those with celiac disease to obtain dietary counseling, which is essential in adopting GFD. In places with limited healthcare resources, telehealth will probably make dietitians more accessible. During the pandemic, telehealth had additionally made high-quality gastrointestinal treatment more accessible. Given its widespread use, telemedicine is expected to become more prevalent in medicine as long as technological advancements keep pace. Using telemedicine, a larger patient group may be able to receive specialist care [103].

Early in the COVID-19 pandemic, a lack of access to endoscopy resulted in modifications to the diagnostic standards for celiac disease, which are probably going to be followed in non-pandemic times as well. Outside of this context, a non-biopsy method to the diagnosis of adult CD is not commonly used; however, this may be beginning to change. A very elevated tTG IgA in adults (10 times the upper normal limit) had a 95% positive predictive value, according to a multicenter investigation [104,105].

Technology for self-monitoring health may have become more popular as a result of the COVID-19 pandemic. Urine assays that can be performed at home to identify gluten have been available in recent years. The presence of gluten immunogenic peptides (GIPs) in the urine and stool may make it possible to monitor compliance and identify individuals who were not following a GFD. These tests might be useful for telemedicine-assisted CD monitoring [54,106,107].

Individuals who have CD must deal with pressing issues such as the potential loss of access to healthcare and gluten-free dietary alternatives. Due to this latter problem, telemedicine has quickly emerged as the main instrument for outpatient assessment. For this patient group, telemedicine is a popular technology that provides a means of giving people who live outside of cities access to subspecialists in CD. Telemedicine holds great potential in the monitoring and follow-up of these patients, especially considering the relative lack of specialist knowledge in the field in general, and qualified dietitians in particular [50].

4. Discussion

Genetically vulnerable people worldwide are affected with celiac disease (CD), a life-long, gluten-sensitive autoimmune illness of the small intestine. In people with CD, symptoms may be extraintestinal, gastrointestinal, or absent. Diarrhea, steatorrhea, and weight loss from malabsorption are among the gastrointestinal symptoms that are considered classical. Anemia, osteoporosis, dermatitis herpetiformis, neurological issues, and hypoplasia of the tooth enamel are extraintestinal or atypical symptoms that over 50% of CD patients experience. Genetic and immunological bases contribute to the diverse clinical picture of CD; factors influencing the disease's clinical expression include the age at onset, degree of mucosal injury, dietary habits, and gender [108,109].

While the amount of people worldwide who suffer from celiac disease is only 1.4%, there are locations where this percentage is much higher. The area of birth, a family history of celiac disease, female sex, and the amount of gluten taken in early life are significant risk factors for the development of this autoimmune illness. Roughly twice as many women as men are impacted. The increased incidence of celiac disease and the number of cases of gluten sensitivity in the general population are worrying [2–4,108,110].

A lifetime GFD is the only established way to alleviate the symptoms of CD patients, restore their immune systems to normal, and heal their intestinal mucosa [61,62].

Telemedicine is widely acknowledged as a useful tool with enormous potential. Individual consultations, group meetings, phone clinics, and web-based tools are among the strategies used globally by medical professionals to monitor and assess patients [19,20].

However, its use in daily clinical practice may still be limited because most patient communication takes place via emails and texts, which patients frequently find unsatisfactory because of the offline interaction and response latency [111,112].

Remote monitoring may be crucial given that the only treatment available to individuals with CD (except from those with refractory celiac disease) is rigorous adherence to a GFD. However, it has taken a global epidemic to spur the widespread adoption of telemedicine, even though it has long shown promise in the treatment of CD [54].

Health care professionals can now communicate with patients over long distances using synchronous and asynchronous modalities, primarily live videoconferencing that enables interactive consultation and prompt interventions, thanks to sophisticated communication technologies, most commonly computers and mobile phones. However, patients who are unfamiliar with digital technologies may hinder the spread of telemedicine [113].

Furthermore, the necessity for improved diagnostic standards, the scarcity of specialists, and the high cost of gluten-free food make the management of this patient group problematic. In many European nations, the condition progresses for an average of eight years before a diagnosis is made, during which time the patient's body deteriorates due to a variety of factors and cannot be healed. Thus, suggestions to use cellphones to monitor the amount of gluten in food products and to contact specialists give many patients—especially those who live in small towns far from specialist centers and those with low socioeconomic status—great hope for a better quality of life [21,50,114–116].

Research has shown that CD patients have a favorable attitude toward telemedicine and that it was a feasible option. A vital requirement for feeling confident in suggesting this strategy and seeing it through to effective implementation is the good trust rate in televisits among CD patients [51–54,85,86].

In-person visits were kept for people who were either incapable of using technology or did not have access to the internet or other electronic devices. As an alternative, the patient's caregiver could provide support for the subset of patients who are ultimately ineligible for remote help [113].

Nevertheless, the experience gained from the COVID-19 pandemic is likely to support pre-COVID-19 evidence regarding the efficacy and good performance of telemedicine and encourage its wider integration into routine clinical practice in general, and in CD patients in particular [52,54,87,88].

Furthermore, in certain situations, self-administered and point-of-care assays (such urinary GIP, or gluten immunogenic peptides) that monitor GFD may be a valuable resource for patients with CD.

They have been shown to be an invaluable tool for celiac patients to monitor their GFD, enhancing adherence and ensuring that no unintentional gluten ingestion occurs. Even during distant televisits, these point-of-care tests can be used as simple, affordable, accurate, and reliable instruments to confirm potential gluten contamination [106,117,118].

Since a GFD appears to help also in group of conditions, known as "non-celiac gluten sensitivity" (NCGS), these people can also benefit from the telehealth solutions described here [65–77].

Regardless of the patients' financial situation, the telehealth systems discussed here offer a great basis for creating and enduringly implementing an efficient system into the care of patients with gluten sensitivity and celiac disease around the globe. Furthermore, the task of specialists in the treatment of this patient group will be made easier by such a system [40,86,114,119].

5. Conclusions

Across the world, a variety of techniques are employed to allow medical professionals to monitor and assess patients with CD.

During the COVID-19 pandemic, people with CD experienced urgent concerns to address, such as the loss of access to healthcare and gluten-free food options. Telemedicine has therefore swiftly become the primary tool for outpatient assessment.

The extended knowledge gathered from the COVID-19 pandemic is expected to complement pre-COVID-19 data supporting the usefulness of telemedicine even after the emergent pandemic, encouraging its wider adoption in standard clinical practice.

The monitoring and follow-up of these patients can greatly benefit from telemedicine, especially in light of the relative dearth of specialized knowledge in this area.

6. Limitations

Although this narrative review was thorough, as with all narrative evaluations, selection bias cannot be completely eliminated.

Since we mainly included publications that discussed favorable telemedicine experiences in CD, this could potentially have led to confirmation bias.

Author Contributions: Conceptualization, M.H. and A.L.; methodology, M.H.; validation, M.H. and A.L.; formal analysis, M.H. and A.L.; investigation, M.H. and A.L.; resources, M.H. and A.L.; data curation, M.H. and A.L.; writing—original draft preparation, M.H.; writing—review and editing, M.H. and A.L.; visualization, M.H. and A.L.; supervision, A.L.; project administration, M.H.; funding acquisition, M.H. All authors have read and agreed to the published version of the manuscript.

Funding: This research received no external funding.

Institutional Review Board Statement: Not applicable.

Informed Consent Statement: Not applicable.

Data Availability Statement: All data are available on request.

Conflicts of Interest: The authors declare no conflicts of interest.

References

1. Lerner, A.; Matthias, T.; Wusterhausen, P. Autoimmunity in celiac disease: Extra-intestinal manifestations. *Autoimmun. Rev.* **2019**, *18*, 241–246. [CrossRef] [PubMed]
2. Makovicky, P.; Makovicky, P.; Caja, F.; Rimarova, K.; Samasca, G.; Vannucci, L. Celiac disease and gluten-free diet: Past, present, and future. *Gastroenterol. Hepatol. Bed Bench* **2020**, *13*, 1–7. [PubMed]
3. Singh, P.; Arora, A.; Strand, T.A.; Leffler, D.A.; Catassi, C.; Green, P.H.; Kelly, C.P.; Ahuja, V.; Makharia, G.K. Global Prevalence of Celiac Disease: Systematic Review and Meta-analysis. *Clin. Gastroenterol. Hepatol.* **2018**, *16*, 823–836. [CrossRef] [PubMed]
4. Reilly, N.R.; Fasano, A.; Green, P.H.R. Presentation of celiac disease. *Gastrointest. Endosc. Clin. N. Am.* **2012**, *22*, 613–621. [CrossRef] [PubMed]
5. Mahadev, S.; Laszkowska, M.; Sundström, J.; Björkholm, M.; Lebwohl, B.; Green, P.H.R.; Ludvigsson, J.F. Prevalence of celiac disease in patients with iron deficiency Anemia—A systematic review with meta-analysis. *Gastroenterology* **2018**, *155*, 374–382. [CrossRef]
6. Meyer, D.; Stavropolous, S.; Diamond, B.; Shane, E.; Green, P.H. Osteoporosis in a North American adult population with celiac disease. *Am. J. Gastroenterol.* **2001**, *96*, 112–119. [CrossRef] [PubMed]
7. Emilsson, L.; Semrad, C.; Lebwohl, B.; Green, P.H.R.; Ludvigsson, J.F. Risk of small bowel adenocarcinoma, adenomas, and carcinoids in a nationwide cohort of individuals with celiac disease. *Gastroenterology* **2020**, *159*, 1686–1694.e2. [CrossRef] [PubMed]
8. Rubio-Tapia, A.; Hill, I.D.; Kelly, C.P.; Calderwood, A.H.; Murray, J.A. ACG clinical guidelines: Diagnosis and management of celiac disease. *Am. J. Gastroenterol.* **2013**, *108*, 656–676. [CrossRef]
9. Samasca, G.; Lerner, A.; Girbovan, A.; Sur, G.; Lupan, I.; Makovicky, P.; Matthias, T.; Freeman, H.J. Challenges in gluten-free diet in coeliac disease: Prague consensus. *Eur. J. Clin. Investig.* **2017**, *47*, 394–397. [CrossRef]
10. Muhammad, H.; Reeves, S.; Jeanes, Y.M. Identifying and improving adherence to the gluten-free diet in people with coeliac disease. *Proc. Nutr. Soc.* **2019**, *78*, 418–425. [CrossRef]
11. Hall, N.J.; Rubin, G.; Charnock, A. Systematic review: Adherence to a gluten-free diet in adult patients with coeliac disease. *Aliment. Pharmacol. Ther.* **2009**, *30*, 315–330. [CrossRef] [PubMed]
12. Akbari Namvar, Z.; Mahdavi, R.; Shirmohammadi, M.; Nikniaz, Z. The effect of group-based education on knowledge and adherence to a gluten-free diet in patients with celiac disease: Randomized controlled clinical trial. *Int. J. Behav. Med.* **2021**, *28*, 583–590. [CrossRef] [PubMed]
13. Sainsbury, K.; Mullan, B.; Sharpe, L. A randomized controlled trial of an online intervention to improve gluten-free diet adherence in celiac disease. *Off. J. Am. Coll. Gastroenterol. ACG* **2013**, *108*, 811–817. [CrossRef] [PubMed]
14. Lerner, A.; Matthias, T. Gluten-free Diet—Tough Alley in Torrid Time. *Internat J. Celiac Dis.* **2017**, *5*, 50–55. [CrossRef]
15. Lerner, A.; O'Bryan, T.; Matthias, T. Navigating the Gluten-Free Boom: The Dark Side of Gluten Free Diet. *Front. Pediatr.* **2019**, *7*, 414. [CrossRef] [PubMed]

16. Lerner, A.; Shoenfeld, Y.; Matthias, T. Adverse effects of gluten ingestion and advantages of gluten withdrawal in nonceliac autoimmune disease. *Nutr. Rev.* **2017**, *75*, 1046–1058. [CrossRef]
17. Lerner, A.; Freire de Carvalho, J.; Kotrova, A.; Shoenfeld, Y. Gluten-free diet can ameliorate the symptoms of non-celiac autoimmune diseases. *Nutr. Rev.* **2022**, *80*, 525–543. [CrossRef] [PubMed]
18. Bascunan, K.A.; Vespa, M.C.; Araya, M. Celiac disease: Understanding the gluten-free diet. *Eur. J. Nutr.* **2017**, *56*, 449–459. [CrossRef]
19. Sainsbury, K.; Mullan, B.; Sharpe, L. Predicting intention and behaviour following participation in a theory-based intervention to improve gluten free diet adherence in coeliac disease. *Psychol. Health* **2015**, *30*, 1063–1074. [CrossRef]
20. Kallos, S.; Jeanes, Y. Cross-Sectional survey of the dietetic provision for adults with coeliac disease in the UK. *J. Hum. Nutr. Diet.* **2020**, *33*, 6–15.
21. Rajpoot, P.; Sharma, A.; Harikrishnan, S.; Baruah, B.J.; Ahuja, V.; Makharia, G.K. Adherence to gluten-free diet and barriers to adherence in patients with celiac disease. *Indian. J. Gastroenterol.* **2015**, *34*, 380–386. [CrossRef] [PubMed]
22. LeBeau, K.; Huey, L.G.; Hart, M. Assessing the quality of mobile apps used by occupational therapists: Evaluation using the user version of the mobile application rating scale. *JMIR mHealth uHealth* **2019**, *7*, e13019. [CrossRef] [PubMed]
23. Kumar, S.; Nilsen, W.J.; Abernethy, A.; Atienza, A.; Patrick, K.; Pavel, M.; Riley, W.T.; Shar, A.; Spring, B.; Spruijt-Metz, D.; et al. Mobile health technology evaluation: The mHealth evidence workshop. *Am. J. Prev. Med.* **2013**, *45*, 228–236. [CrossRef] [PubMed]
24. Díaz-Hellín, P.; Fontecha, J.; Hervás, R.; Bravo, J. NFC as a childhood obesity treatment tool. *J. Med. Syst.* **2015**, *39*, 96. [CrossRef] [PubMed]
25. El-Gayar, O.; Timsina, P.; Nawar, N.; Eid, W. Mobile applications for diabetes self-management: Status and potential. *J. Diabetes Sci. Technol.* **2013**, *7*, 247–262. [CrossRef]
26. Semper, H.; Povey, R.; Clark-Carter, D. A systematic review of the effectiveness of smartphone applications that encourage dietary self-regulatory strategies for weight loss in overweight and obese adults. *Obes. Rev.* **2016**, *17*, 895–906. [CrossRef] [PubMed]
27. Cook, K.A.; Modena, B.D.; Simon, R.A. Improvement in asthma control using a minimally burdensome and proactive smartphone application. *J. Allergy Clin. Immunol. Pract.* **2016**, *4*, 730–737.e1. [CrossRef] [PubMed]
28. Licskai, C.J.; Sands, T.W.; Ferrone, M. Development and pilot testing of a mobile health solution for asthma self-management: Asthma action plan smartphone application pilot study. *Can. Respir. J.* **2013**, *20*, 301–306. [CrossRef]
29. Zeltzer, D.; Einav, L.; Rashba, J.; Waisman, Y.; Haimi, M.; Balicer, R.D. Adoption and utilization of device-assisted telemedicine. *J. Health Econ.* **2023**, *90*, 102780. [CrossRef] [PubMed]
30. Haimi, M.; Goren, U.; Grossman, Z. Barriers and challenges to telemedicine usage among the elderly population in Israel in light of the COVID-19 era: A qualitative study. *Digit. Health* **2024**, *10*. [CrossRef]
31. Haimi, M.; Sergienko, R. Adoption and Use of Telemedicine and Digital Health Services Among Older Adults in Light of the COVID-19 Pandemic: Repeated Cross-Sectional Analysis. *JMIR Aging* **2024**, *7*, e52317. [CrossRef] [PubMed]
32. Carter, M.C.; Burley, V.J.; Nykjaer, C.; Cade, J.E. Adherence to a smartphone application for weight loss compared to website and paper diary: Pilot randomized controlled trial. *J. Med. Internet Res.* **2013**, *15*, e32. [CrossRef]
33. Gilliland, J.; Sadler, R.; Clark, A.; O'Connor, C.; Milczarek, M.; Doherty, S. Using a smartphone application to promote healthy dietary behaviours and local food consumption. *BioMed Res. Int.* **2015**, 841368. [CrossRef]
34. Laing, B.Y.; Mangione, C.M.; Tseng, C.H.; Leng, M.; Vaisberg, E.; Mahida, M.; Bholat, M.; Glazier, E.; Morisky, D.E.; Bell, D.S. Effectiveness of a smartphone application for weight loss compared with usual care in overweight primary care patients: A randomized, controlled trial. *Ann. Intern. Med.* **2014**, *161* (Suppl. 10), S5–S12. [CrossRef]
35. Stephens, J.D.; Yager, A.M.; Allen, J. Smartphone technology and text messaging for weight loss in young adults: A randomized controlled trial. *J. Cardiovasc. Nurs.* **2017**, *32*, 39–46. [CrossRef] [PubMed]
36. Allen, J.K.; Stephens, J.; Dennison Himmelfarb, C.R.; Stewart, K.J.; Hauck, S. Randomized controlled pilot study testing use of smartphone technology for obesity treatment. *J. Obes.* **2013**, 151597. [CrossRef]
37. Holmen, H.; Torbjørnsen, A.; Wahl, A.K.; Jenum, A.K.; Småstuen, M.C.; Arsand, E.; Ribu, L. A mobile health intervention for self-management and lifestyle change for persons with type 2 diabetes, part 2: One-year results from the Norwegian randomized controlled trial RENEWING HEALTH. *JMIR mHealth uHealth* **2014**, *2*, e3882. [CrossRef]
38. Chang, A.R.; Bailey-Davis, L.; Hetherington, V.; Ziegler, A.; Yule, C.; Kwiecen, S.; Graboski, E.; Melough, M.M.; Collins, C.; Anderson, C. Remote dietary counseling using smartphone applications in patients with stages 1-3a chronic kidney disease: A mixed methods feasibility study. *J. Ren. Nutr.* **2020**, *30*, 53–60. [CrossRef] [PubMed]
39. Eyles, H.; McLean, R.; Neal, B.; Jiang, Y.; Doughty, R.N.; McLean, R.; Ni Mhurchu, C. A salt-reduction smartphone app supports lower-salt food purchases for people with cardiovascular disease: Findings from the SaltSwitch randomised controlled trial. *Eur. J. Prev. Cardiol.* **2017**, *24*, 1435–1444. [CrossRef]
40. Muhammad, H.; Reeves, S.; Ishaq, S.; Mayberry, J.F.; Jeanes, Y.M. Telephone clinic improves gluten free dietary adherence in adults with coeliac disease: Sustained at 6 months. *Frontline Gastroenterol.* **2021**, *12*, 586–592. [CrossRef]
41. Nikniaz, Z.; Namvar, Z.A.; Shirmohammadi, M.; Maserat, E. Smartphone Application for Celiac Patients: Assessing Its Effect on Gastrointestinal Symptoms in a Randomized Controlled Clinical Trial. *Int. J. Telemed. Appl.* **2022**, *2022*, 8027532. [CrossRef] [PubMed]

42. Dowd, A.J.; Warbeck, C.B.; Tang, K.T.; Fung, T.; Culos-Reed, S.N. MyHealthyGut: Findings from a pilot randomized controlled trial on adherence to a gluten-free diet and quality of life among adults with celiac disease or gluten intolerance. *Digit. Health* **2020**, *6*, 205520762090362. [CrossRef] [PubMed]
43. Lebwohl, B.; Sanders, D.; Green, P.H.R. Celiac disease. *Lancet* **2018**, *391*, 70–81. [CrossRef] [PubMed]
44. Simons, M.; Scott-Sheldon, L.A.J.; Risech-Neyman, Y. Celiac disease and increased risk of pneumococcal infection: A systematic review and meta-analysis. *Am. J. Med.* **2018**, *131*, 83–89. [CrossRef] [PubMed]
45. Kårhus, L.L.; Gunnes, N.; Størdal, K. Influenza and risk of later celiac disease: A cohort study of 2.6 million people. *Scand. J. Gastroenterol.* **2018**, *53*, 15–23. [CrossRef] [PubMed]
46. Ludvigsson, J.F.; Choung, R.S.; Marietta, E.V. Increased risk of herpes zoster in patients with coeliac disease—Nationwide cohort study. *Scand. J. Public Health* **2018**, *46*, 859–866. [CrossRef]
47. Bouziat, R.; Biering, S.B.; Kouame, E. Murine norovirus infection induces TH1 inflammatory responses to dietary antigens. *Cell Host Microbe* **2018**, *24*, 677–688. [CrossRef] [PubMed]
48. Samasca, G.; Lerner, A. Celiac disease in COVID-19 pandemic. *J. Transl. Autoimmun.* **2021**, *4*, 100120. [CrossRef]
49. Lerner, A. Are My Patients with Celiac Disease at Higher Risk of COVID-19 Virus? *Int. J. Celiac Dis.* **2020**, *8*, 35–38.
50. Ines Pinto-Sanchez, M.; Lebwohl, B. Delivery of care remotely through telemedicine in celiac disease: Thinking beyond COVID-19: Commentary on: "COVID-19 pandemic perception in adults with celiac disease: An impulse to implement the use of telemedicine" by Siniscalchi M et al. Dig Liv Dis 2020;52:1071-5. *Dig. Liver Dis.* **2020**, *52*, 1069–1070. [CrossRef] [PubMed] [PubMed Central]
51. Vriezinga, S.; Borghorst, A.; van den Akker-van Marle, E.; Benninga, M.; George, E.; Hendriks, D.; Hopman, E.; de Meij, T.; van der Meulen-de Jong, A.; Putter, H.; et al. E-Healthcare for celiac disease a multicenter randomized controlled trial. *J. Pediatr.* **2018**, *195*, 154–160.e7. [CrossRef] [PubMed]
52. Siniscalchi, M.; Zingone, F.; Savarino, E.V.; D'Odorico, A.; Ciacci, C. COVID-19 pandemic perception in adults with celiac disease: An impulse to implement the use of telemedicine. *Dig. Liver Dis.* **2020**, *52*, 1071–1075. [CrossRef] [PubMed]
53. Rollo, M.E.; Hutchesson, M.J.; Burrows, T.L.; Krukowski, R.A.; Harvey, J.R.; Hoggle, L.B.; Collins, C.E. Video consultations and virtual nutrition care for weight management. *J. Acad. Nutr. Diet.* **2015**, *115*, 1213–1225. [CrossRef] [PubMed]
54. Costantino, A.; Roncoroni, L.; Noviello, D.; Nandi, N.; Lombardo, V.; Scricciolo, A.; Scaramella, L.; Vecchi, M.; Elli, L. Nutritional and Gastroenterological Monitoring of Patients With Celiac Disease During COVID-19 Pandemic: The Emerging Role of Telemedicine and Point-of-Care Gluten Detection Tests. *Front. Nutr.* **2021**, *8*, 622514. [CrossRef]
55. Di Sabatino, A.; Corazza, G.R. Coeliac disease. *Lancet* **2009**, *373*, 1480–1493. [CrossRef] [PubMed]
56. Catassi, C. The world map of celiac disease. *Acta Gastroenterol. Latinoam.* **2005**, *35*, 37–55. [PubMed]
57. Rubio-Tapia, A.; Kyle, R.A.; Kaplan, E.L.; Johnson, D.R.; Page, W.; Erdtmann, F.; Brantner, T.L.; Kim, W.R.; Phelps, T.K.; Lahr, B.D.; et al. Increased prevalence and mortality in undiagnosed celiac disease. *Gastroenterology* **2009**, *137*, 88–93. [CrossRef] [PubMed]
58. Lohi, S.; Mustalahti, K.; Kaukinen, K.; Laurila, K.; Collin, P.; Rissanen, H.; Lohi, O.; Bravi, E.; Gasparin, M.; Reunanen, A.; et al. Increasing prevalence of coeliac disease over time. *Aliment. Pharmacol. Ther.* **2007**, *26*, 1217–1225. [CrossRef]
59. King, J.A.; Jeong, J.; Underwood, F.E.; Quan, J.; Panaccione, N.; Windsor, J.W.; Coward, S.; DeBruyn, J.; Ronksley, P.E.; Shaheen, A.A.; et al. Incidence of Celiac Disease Is Increasing Over Time: A Systematic Review and Meta-analysis. *Am. J. Gastroenterol.* **2020**, *115*, 507–525. [CrossRef]
60. Ashtari, S.; Najafimehr, H.; Pourhoseingholi, M.A.; Rostami, K.; Asadzadeh-Aghdaei, H.; Rostami-Nejad, M.; Tavirani, M.R.; Olfatifar, M.; Makharia, G.K.; Zali, M.R. Prevalence of celiac disease in low and high-risk population in Asia-Pacific region: A systematic review and meta-analysis. *Sci. Rep.* **2021**, *11*, 2383. [CrossRef]
61. Green, P.H.; Cellier, C. Celiac disease. *N. Engl. J. Med.* **2007**, *357*, 1731–1743. [CrossRef] [PubMed]
62. Rubio-Tapia, A.; Murray, J.A. Classification and management of refractory coeliac disease. *Gut* **2010**, *59*, 547–557. [CrossRef] [PubMed] [PubMed Central]
63. Mazzola, A.M.; Zammarchi, I.; Valerii, M.C.; Spisni, E.; Saracino, I.M.; Lanzarotto, F.; Ricci, C. Gluten-Free Diet and Other Celiac Disease Therapies: Current Understanding and Emerging Strategies. *Nutrients* **2024**, *16*, 1006. [CrossRef] [PubMed]
64. Niewinski, M.M. Advances in Celiac Disease and Gluten-Free Diet. *J. Am. Diet. Assoc.* **2008**, *108*, 661–672. [CrossRef] [PubMed]
65. Hurley, J.J.; Lee, B.; Turner, J.K.; Beale, A.; Jenkins, H.R.; Swift, G.L. Incidence and presentation of reported coeliac disease in Cardiff and the Vale of Glamorgan: The next 10 years. *Eur. J. Gastroenterol. Hepatol.* **2012**, *24*, 482–486. [CrossRef] [PubMed]
66. Volta, U.; Villanacci, V. Celiac disease: Diagnostic criteria in progress. *Cell Mol. Immunol.* **2011**, *8*, 96–102. [CrossRef] [PubMed]
67. Aziz, I.; Sanders, D.S. Emerging concepts: From coeliac disease to non-coeliac gluten sensitivity. *Proc. Nutr. Soc.* **2012**, *71*, 576–580. [CrossRef] [PubMed]
68. Troncone, R.; Jabri, B. Coeliac disease and gluten sensitivity. *J. Intern. Med.* **2011**, *269*, 582–590. [CrossRef]
69. Mansueto, P.; Seidita, A.; D'Alcamo, A.; Carroccio, A. Non-celiac gluten sensitivity: Literature review. *J. Am. Coll. Nutr.* **2014**, *33*, 39–54. [CrossRef]
70. Cárdenas-Torres, F.I.; Cabrera-Chávez, F.; Figueroa-Salcido, O.G.; Ontiveros, N. Non-Celiac Gluten Sensitivity: An Update. *Medicina* **2021**, *57*, 526. [CrossRef] [PubMed] [PubMed Central]
71. Walker, M.M.; Murray, J.A.; Ronkainen, J.; Aro, P.; Storskrubb, T.; D'Amato, M.; Lahr, B.; Talley, N.J.; Agreus, L. Detection of celiac disease and lymphocytic enteropathy by parallel serology and histopathology in a population-based study. *Gastroenterology* **2010**, *139*, 112–119. [CrossRef] [PubMed]

72. Talaie, R. Does gluten free diet have more implications than treatment of celiac disease? *Gastroenterol. Hepatol. Bed Bench.* **2015**, *8*, 160–166. [PubMed] [PubMed Central]
73. Fasano, A.; Sapone, A.; Zevallos, V.; Schuppan, D. Nonceliac gluten sensitivity. *Gastroenterology* **2015**, *148*, 1195–1204. [CrossRef] [PubMed]
74. Newnham, E.D. Does gluten cause gastrointestinal symptoms in subjects without coeliac disease? *J. Gastroenterol. Hepatol.* **2011**, *26*, S132–S134. [CrossRef] [PubMed]
75. Esteve, M.; Carrasco, A.; Fernandēz-Bañares, F. Is a gluten-free diet necessary in Marsh I intestinal lesions in patients with HLADQ2, DQ8 genotype and without gastrointestinal symptoms? *Curr. Opin. Clin. Nutr. Metab. Care.* **2012**, *15*, 505–510. [CrossRef] [PubMed]
76. Rostami Nejad, M.; Dabiri, R.; Ehsani-Ardakani, M.J.; Nazemalhosseini Mojarad, E.; Derakhshan, F.; Telkabadi, M.; Rostami, K. Gluten associated dyspepsia; serology and histological characteristics. *Gastroenterol. Hepatol. Bed Bench.* **2012**, *5*, 197–201. [PubMed]
77. Niland, B.; Cash, B.D. Health Benefits and Adverse Effects of a Gluten-Free Diet in Non-Celiac Disease Patients. *Gastroenterol. Hepatol.* **2018**, *14*, 82–91. [PubMed] [PubMed Central]
78. Lis, D.M.; Stellingwerff, T.; Shing, C.M.; Ahuja, K.D.; Fell, J.W. Exploring the popularity, experiences, and beliefs surrounding gluten-free diets in nonceliac athletes. *Int. J. Sport. Nutr. Exerc. Metab.* **2015**, *25*, 37–45. [CrossRef] [PubMed]
79. Aziz, I.; Dwivedi, K.; Sanders, D.S. From coeliac disease to noncoeliac gluten sensitivity; should everyone be gluten free? *Curr. Opin. Gastroenterol.* **2016**, *32*, 120–127. [CrossRef]
80. Bucci, C.; Zingone, F.; Russo, I.; Morra, I.; Tortora, R.; Pogna, N.; Scalia, G.; Iovino, P.; Ciacci, C. Gliadin does not induce mucosal inflammation or basophil activation in patients with nonceliac gluten sensitivity. *Clin. Gastroenterol. Hepatol.* **2013**, *11*, 1294–1299.e1. [CrossRef]
81. Slim, M.; Calandre, E.P.; Garcia-Leiva, J.M.; Rico-Villademoros, F.; Molina-Barea, R.; Rodriguez-Lopez, C.M.; Morillas-Arques, P. The effects of a gluten-free diet versus a hypocaloric diet among patients with fibromyalgia experiencing gluten sensitivity-like symptoms: A pilot, open-label randomized clinical trial. *J. Clin. Gastroenterol.* **2017**, *51*, 500–507. [CrossRef] [PubMed]
82. Marziali, M.; Venza, M.; Lazzaro, S.; Lazzaro, A.; Micossi, C.; Stolfi, V.M. Gluten-free diet: A new strategy for management of painful endometriosis related symptoms? *Minerva Chir.* **2012**, *67*, 499–504. [PubMed]
83. Marziali, M.; Capozzolo, T. Role of gluten-free diet in the management of chronic pelvic pain of deep infiltrating endometriosis. *J. Minim. Invasive Gynecol.* **2015**, *22*, S51–S52. [CrossRef]
84. Kurien, M.; Trott, N.; Sanders, D.S. Long-Term care for patients with coeliac disease in the UK: A review of the literature and future directions. *J. Hum. Nutr. Diet.* **2016**, *29*, 617–623. [CrossRef]
85. Muhammad, H.; Reeves, S.; Jeanes, Y. Qualitative Interviews to Explore patient Preference for Health Care Led Interventions to Promote Gluten Free Dietary Adherence. Coeliac, U.K. 2019. Available online: https://pure.roehampton.ac.uk/portal/en/publications/qualitative-interviews-to-explore-patient-preference-for-health-c (accessed on 4 May 2024).
86. Muhammad, H.; Reeves, S.; Ishaq, S.; Jeanes, Y. Experiences of Outpatient Clinics and Opinions of Telehealth by Caucasian and South Asian Patients with Celiac Disease. *J. Patient Exp.* **2021**, *8*. [CrossRef]
87. Alrubaiy, L. Gastroenterology services in the time of COVID-19 pandemic. *Frontline Gastroenterol.* **2020**, *11*, 257–258. [CrossRef]
88. Cohen, B.S.; Lebwohl, B. COVID-19 and celiac disease: A review. *Ther. Adv. Gastroenterol.* **2023**, *16*. [CrossRef] [PubMed]
89. Zhen, J.; Stefanolo, J.P.; Temprano, M.P.; Seiler, C.L.; Caminero, A.; de-Madaria, E.; Huguet, M.M.; Santiago, V.; Niveloni, S.I.; Smecuol, E.G.; et al. Risk perception and knowledge of COVID-19 in patients with celiac disease. *World J. Gastroenterol.* **2021**, *27*, 1213–1225. [CrossRef]
90. Lerner, A.; Matthias, T. Increased knowledge and awareness of celiac disease will benefit the elderly. *Intern. J. Celiac Dis.* **2015**, *3*, 112–114. [CrossRef]
91. Mårild, K.; Fredlund, H.; Ludvigsson, J.F. Increased risk of hospital admission for influenza in patients with celiac disease: A nationwide cohort study in Sweden. *Am. J. Gastroenterol.* **2010**, *105*, 2465–2473. [CrossRef]
92. Lebwohl, B.; Green, P.H.R.; Söderling, J.; Roelstraete, B.; Ludvigsson, J.F. Association between celiac disease and mortality risk in a Swedish population. *JAMA* **2020**, *323*, 1277–1285. [CrossRef] [PubMed]
93. Mansoor, E.; Alikhan, M.M.; Perez, J.A.; Schlick, K.; Abou Saleh, M.; Rubio-Tapia, A. Clinical characteristics, hospitalisation and mortality rates of COVID-19 among patients with coeliac disease in the USA: A multicentre network study. *Gut* **2022**, *71*, 1691–1692. [CrossRef] [PubMed]
94. Lebwohl, B.; Larsson, E.; Söderling, J.; Roelstraete, B.; Murray, J.A.; Green, P.H.R.; Ludvigsson, J.F. Risk of severe COVID-19 in patients with celiac disease: A population-based cohort study. *Clin. Epidemiol.* **2021**, *13*, 121–130. [CrossRef] [PubMed]
95. Hadi, Y.B.; Sohail, A.H.; Lakhani, D.A.; Naqvi, S.F.; Kupec, J.T.; Pervez, A. Outcomes of SARS-CoV-2 infection in patients with celiac disease: A multicenter research network study. *Ann. Gastroenterol.* **2022**, *35*, 164–168. [PubMed]
96. Guillaume, J.D.; Jagai, J.S.; Makelarski, J.A.; Abramsohn, E.M.; Lindau, S.T.; Verma, R.; Ciaccio, C.E. COVID-19-related food insecurity among households with dietary restrictions: A national survey. *J. Allergy Clin. Immunol. Pract.* **2021**, *9*, 3323–3330.e3. [CrossRef] [PubMed]
97. Du, N.; Mehrotra, I.; Weisbrod, V.; Regis, S.; Silvester, J.A. Survey-based study on food insecurity during COVID-19 for households with children on a prescribed gluten-free diet. *Am. J. Gastroenterol.* **2022**, *117*, 931–934. [CrossRef] [PubMed]

98. Gokden, Y.; Hot, S.; Adas, M.; Ogutmen Koc, D.; Atak, S.; Hot, A.B. Celiac disease and COVID-19 pandemic: Should we worry? *Acta Gastroenterol. Belg.* **2020**, *83*, 517–525. [PubMed]
99. Bascuñán, K.A.; Rodríguez, J.M.; Osben, C.; Fernández, A.; Sepúlveda, C.; Araya, M. Pandemic effects and gluten-free diet: An adherence and mental health problem. *Nutrients* **2021**, *13*, 1822. [CrossRef]
100. Falcomer, A.L.; Farage, P.; Pratesi, C.B.; Pratesi, R.; Gandolfi, L.; Nakano, E.Y.; Raposo, A.; Zandonadi, R.P. Health-related quality of life and experiences of brazilian celiac individuals over the course of the SARS-CoV-2 pandemic. *Nutrients* **2021**, *13*, 1582. [CrossRef]
101. Kreutz, J.M.; Heynen, L.; Arayess, L.; Vreugdenhil, A.C.E. Celiac Disease and the Gluten Free Diet during the COVID-19 Pandemic: Experiences of Children and Parents. *Medicina* **2023**, *59*, 425. [CrossRef]
102. British Society of Gastroenterology. BSG Interim Guidance 2022: COVID-19 Specific Non-Biopsy Protocol for Those with Suspected Coeliac Disease. Available online: https://www.bsg.org.uk/covid-19-advice/covid-19-specific-non-biopsy-protocol-guidance-for-those-with-suspected-coeliac-disease/ (accessed on 4 May 2024).
103. Elli, L.; Barisani, D.; Vaira, V.; Bardella, M.T.; Topa, M.; Vecchi, M.; Doneda, L.; Scricciolo, A.; Lombardo, V.; Roncoroni, L. How to manage celiac disease and gluten-free diet during the COVID-19 era: Proposals from a tertiary referral center in a high-incidence scenario. *BMC Gastroenterol.* **2020**, *20*, 387. [CrossRef] [PubMed]
104. Penny, H.A.; Raju, S.A.; Lau, M.S.; Marks, L.J.S.; Baggus, E.M.R.; Bai, J.C.; Bassotti, G.; Bontkes, H.J.; Carroccio, A.; Danciu, M.; et al. Accuracy of a no-biopsy approach for the diagnosis of coeliac disease across different adult cohorts. *Gut* **2021**, *70*, 876–883. [CrossRef] [PubMed]
105. Rubio-Tapia, A.; Hill, I.D.; Semrad, C.; Kelly, C.P.; Greer, K.B.; Limketkai, B.N.; Lebwohl, B. American college of gastroenterology guidelines update: Diagnosis and management of celiac disease. *Am. J. Gastroenterol.* **2023**, *118*, 59–76. [CrossRef] [PubMed]
106. Moreno, M.L.; Cebolla, Á.; Muñoz-Suano, A.; Carrillo-Carrion, C.; Comino, I.; Pizarro, Á.; León, F.; Rodríguez-Herrera, A.; Sousa, C. Detection of gluten immunogenic peptides in the urine of patients with coeliac disease reveals transgressions in the gluten-free diet and incomplete mucosal healing. *Gut* **2017**, *66*, 250–257. [CrossRef] [PubMed]
107. Ciacci, C.; Gagliardi, M.; Siniscalchi, M.; Ruotolo, M.; Santonicola, A.; Hajji, N.; Zingone, F. Gluten immunogenic peptides (GIP) point-of-care urine test in coeliac disease follow-up before and during the COVID-19 lockdown in Italy. *Clin. Exp. Gastroenterol.* **2021**, *14*, 451–456. [CrossRef] [PubMed]
108. Gujral, N.; Freeman, H.J.; Thomson, A.B. Celiac disease: Prevalence, diagnosis, pathogenesis and treatment. *World J. Gastroenterol.* **2012**, *18*, 6036–6059. [CrossRef] [PubMed] [PubMed Central]
109. Bai, D.; Brar, P.; Holleran, S.; Ramakrishnan, R.; Green, P.H. Effect of gender on the manifestations of celiac disease: Evidence for greater malabsorption in men. *Scand. J. Gastroenterol.* **2005**, *40*, 183–187. [CrossRef] [PubMed]
110. Catassi, C.; Yachha, S.K. The global village of celiac disease. In *Frontiers in Celiac Disease*; Fasano, A., Troncone, R., Branski, D., Eds.; Karger: Basel, Switzerland, 2008; pp. 23–31.
111. Daschle, T.; Dorsey, E.R. The return of the house call. *Ann. Intern. Med.* **2015**, *162*, 587–588. [CrossRef] [PubMed]
112. Welch, B.M.; Harvey, J.; O'Connell, N.S.; McElligott, J.T. Patient preferences for direct-to-consumer telemedicine services: A nationwide survey. *BMC Health Serv. Res.* **2017**, *17*, 784. [CrossRef]
113. Wilson, L.S.; Maeder, A.J. Recent directions in telemedicine: Review of trends in research and practice. *Healthc. Inform. Res.* **2015**, *21*, 213–222. [CrossRef]
114. Hanci, O.; Jeanes, Y.M. Are gluten-free food staples accessible to all patients with coeliac disease? *Frontline Gastroenterol.* **2019**, *10*, 222–228. [CrossRef] [PubMed] [PubMed Central]
115. Alavinejad, P.; Hajiani, E.; Masjedizadeh, R.; Hashemi, S.J.; Faramarzi, M.; Sebghatollahi, V.; Shayesteh, A.A.; Kadkhodae, A.; Jasemi Zergani, F.; Asghari, S.; et al. Epidemiologic and demographic survey of celiac disease in khuzestan province. *Middle East. J. Dig. Dis.* **2014**, *6*, 98–103. [PubMed] [PubMed Central]
116. Mustalahti, K.; Catassi, C.; Reunanen, A.; Fabiani, E.; Heier, M.; McMillan, S.; Murray, L.; Metzger, M.-H.; Gasparin, M.; Bravi, E.; et al. Prevalence of celiac disease in Europe: Results of a centralized, international mass screening project. *Ann. Med.* **2010**, *42*, 587–595. [CrossRef] [PubMed]
117. Elli, L.; Bascuñán, K.; di Lernia, L.; Bardella, M.T.; Doneda, L.; Soldati, L.; Orlando, S.; Ferretti, F.; Lombardo, V.; Barigelletti, G.; et al. Safety of occasional ingestion of gluten in patients with celiac disease: A real-life study. *BMC Med.* **2020**, *18*, 42. [CrossRef] [PubMed]
118. Soler, M.; Estevez, M.C.; Moreno, M.L.; Cebolla, A.; Lechuga, L.M. Label-free SPR detection of gluten peptides in urine for non-invasive celiac disease follow-up. *Biosens. Bioelectron.* **2016**, *79*, 158–164. [CrossRef] [PubMed]
119. Wieser, H.; Ruiz-Carnicer, Á.; Segura, V.; Comino, I.; Sousa, C. Challenges of Monitoring the Gluten-Free Diet Adherence in the Management and Follow-Up of Patients with Celiac Disease. *Nutrients* **2021**, *13*, 2274. [CrossRef] [PubMed] [PubMed Central]

healthcare

MDPI

Article

Investigating Physicians' Adoption of Telemedicine in Romania Using Technology Acceptance Model (TAM)

Abigaela Bîlbîie [1], Andreea-Ionela Puiu [2,*], Viorel Mihăilă [3] and Marin Burcea [3]

1 Faculty of Theoretical and Applied Economics, The Academy of Economic Studies, 010552 Bucharest, Romania; bilbiieabigaela@gmail.com
2 Department of Applied Economics and Quantitative Analysis, Faculty of Business and Administration, University of Bucharest, 030018 Bucharest, Romania
3 Department of Public Administration, Faculty of Business and Administration, University of Bucharest, 030018 Bucharest, Romania; viorel.mihaila@faa.unibuc.ro (V.M.); marin.burcea@faa.unibuc.ro (M.B.)
* Correspondence: ionela-andreea.puiu@faa.unibuc.ro

Abstract: This study investigates Romanian physicians' acceptance of telemedicine using the Technology Acceptance Model. We analyzed 1093 responses to an online survey distributed nationwide to physicians via email by the National Authority of Quality Management in Health, employing the partial least squares algorithm to estimate the relationship between the behavioral intention to adopt telemedicine and its potential determinants. Our findings reveal that the model accounts for 84.6% of the variance in behavioral intention to use telemedicine. Among the two constructs of the TAM model, perceived usefulness is a stronger predictor of behavioral intention than perceived ease of use. Additionally, subjective norms positively and significantly influence physicians' intention to use telemedicine and their perception of its usefulness. Furthermore, perceived incentives and accessibility to medical records also positively impact the behavioral intention to use telemedicine.

Keywords: telemedicine acceptance; physicians telemedicine acceptance; technology acceptance model; perceived usefulness; perceived ease of use

1. Introduction

The emergence of COVID-19 brought public health back into focus, and there was a collective global effort to tackle this issue as effectively as possible [1]. A major driving force behind this worldwide endeavor was the widely recognized fact that public health is a vital and basic human right, as well as a significant factor that influences economic growth [2]. Healthy individuals exhibit higher productivity and enhanced physical and mental robustness, enabling them to work more efficiently and positively contributing to overall economic performance [3]. In addition to the emphasis on public health, the COVID-19 pandemic has compelled governments and international organizations to seriously consider the impact of this crisis on science, technology, and innovation [4]. As a result, healthcare stakeholders have had to acknowledge the importance of the digital transformation of the healthcare system [5] not only to address patients' needs [6], but also "to improve healthcare industry's efficiency, productivity and overall value" [7].

In a wide sense, digital transformation in healthcare encompasses all digital technologies and Internet-related adjustments that aim to improve health management procedures, including the development of new therapies and best practices [8]. The digitalization of the healthcare system focuses on the development of two main aspects of public health, namely patients' experience and healthcare infrastructure [9]. The post-pandemic healthcare industry is confronted with the new "consumer of health care" who desires more integrated, effortless, and holistic healthcare services [10], along with an improved healthcare experience characterized by customization, comfort, and speed [8]. Regarding the impact of digitalization in healthcare infrastructure, Gjellebæk et al. [9] suggest that it could enhance employee productivity and the efficiency and effectiveness of health units and decrease their operational expenses.

In the sphere of digital health, telemedicine is a component that makes "use of information and communication technologies to improve patient outcomes by increasing access to care and medical information" [11]. More precisely, telemedicine involves the provision of healthcare services from a distance. During the COVID-19 pandemic, telemedicine was the only option for minimizing the spread of the disease by remotely monitoring and treating patients, including those infected with COVID-19 as well as those with other chronic conditions. From a medical standpoint, telemedicine has enabled doctors to remotely monitor patients, facilitating the early detection of COVID-19 and timely treatment of infected individuals. It has also ensured the uninterrupted care of vulnerable patients with other medical conditions [12].

This study aims to investigate the level of telemedicine adoption among physicians in Romania and identify the factors or drivers that influence their acceptance of this technology.

For this study, we adapted the third version of the Technology Acceptance Model (TAM3) to apply to telemedicine services. We also introduce additional constructs, namely clinical factors, and regulatory factors, to gain a better understanding of how physicians perceive telemedicine. Using partial least squares path modeling, conducted in WarpPLS, version 8.0, the study not only examines the statistical relevance of the predictive factors proposed by an adapted version of TAM3 but also identifies the most appropriate determinants that can be used to enhance the intention of physicians to adopt telemedicine services.

The rest of the paper is organized as follows: Section 2 of this scientific article aims to provide a comprehensive understanding of the existing research landscape, identify gaps, and establish the theoretical foundation for the current study, encompassing both the theoretical framework and hypotheses development. Moving into Section 3, detailed information is presented regarding the acquisition of data, the chosen metrics and instruments, as well as the research design and statistical techniques applied, while Section 4 presents the results. Section 5 critically interprets and contextualizes the findings in relation to the theoretical framework and the prior literature.

2. Literature Review

2.1. Telemedicine in the Healthcare Sector

During this challenging period, health specialists had to recognize the significance of telemedicine in healthcare, not only during pandemics or epidemics but also in the routine delivery of healthcare services. Furthermore, the public health crisis precipitated by the pandemic has generated heightened interest from patients and an increased demand for healthcare delivery through virtual means. To illustrate this impact more comprehensively, we can look at pertinent statistics from the United States where, over the period spanning 2019 to 2022, there was a remarkable 63-fold increase in the number of virtual medical consultations [7,13].

The primary factors that have led to the increased attention towards telemedicine among healthcare providers include its capacity to enhance access to healthcare [14], increase convenience [15], reduce treatment costs [16], and decrease hospital admissions [17] or readmissions, especially in the Accident and Emergency department, where a patient visit could be much more expensive [18,19]. Telemedicine can enhance hospital efficiency by automating routine tasks using AI, which allows medical personnel to allocate more time to other aspects of their work [20]. A 2019 study suggests that the National Health Service (NHS) could reduce staff costs by GBP 12.5 billion annually through automation, while the social care industry could save GBP 5.9 billion [21].

Furthermore, telemedicine has the potential to improve patient–physician interactions and reduce misunderstandings, which account for around 80% of severe medical injuries [7]. The healthcare sector generates vast amounts of data annually, including clinical records, medical imagery, genomic information, and health behavior data from patients, organizations, and monitoring devices [22]. Therefore, using big data in healthcare can reduce medication or medical mistakes, improve comprehension of patient trends, provide accurate staffing predictions, examinate real-time alerts, and develop preventive care strategies [7].

The medical fields where telemedicine is used the most include radiology [23], psychiatry, mental health [24], and cardiology, while the lowest usage of telemedicine is recorded in allergology/immunology, gastroenterology, and obstetrics/gynecology [25]. Also, emergency physicians, pathologists, and radiologists are among the healthcare professionals who use telemedicine the most to communicate with other healthcare providers [25].

In Romania, before 2020, telemedicine was not a priority for the Romanian government or public health system, and existing pilot projects were underdeveloped. However, the pandemic prompted authorities to establish a legal framework to promote telemedicine [26,27]. Based on a 2021 study, Romania has the highest proportion of telemedicine enthusiasts among E.U. countries (69%), yet only 28% believe that telemedicine functions effectively in the country [28].

Regarding physicians' acceptance of telemedicine services, previous research has indicated that medical professionals from developing countries are less inclined to adopt telemedicine [29]. In a particular county in Romania, a cross-sectional study conducted in 2020 revealed that 61% of surveyed physicians found telemedicine consultations more time-consuming than in-person visits, and 64% were concerned about the reliability of telemedicine diagnostics [30].

2.2. Technology Acceptance Model

The Technology Acceptance Model (TAM) was initially proposed by Davis [31] in 1989 as part of his doctoral research, drawing upon the foundations of the Theory of Reasoned Action [32]. The basic technology acceptance model framework assumes that people's behavioral intention to use information technology (IT) is influenced by two personal beliefs, namely perceived usefulness (PU) and perceived ease of use (PEOU), along with the attitude towards technology adoption. Perceived usefulness and perceived ease of use also play a role in how other external factors affect the intention to use IT [33]. According to [31], perceived usefulness refers to how much an individual believes that using IT will improve their job performance, while perceived ease of use is the extent to which an individual believes that using IT will be effortless or without much effort.

Venkatesh and Davis [34] expanded the TAM into TAM2, identifying and conceptualizing determinants affecting perceived usefulness such as subjective norm, image, job relevance, output quality, result demonstrability, and perceived ease of use, with experience and voluntariness as moderators. Further, Venkatesh [35] formulated a model that explores the determinants influencing perceived ease of use, based on the anchoring and adjustment framing of human decision-making processes. In this model, computer self-efficacy, computer anxiety, computer playfulness, and perceived external control were explored as anchors, while perceived enjoyment and objective usability were framed as adjustments. TAM3 represents the integrated model of TAM2 and the model of determinants of perceived ease of use.

The extensive popularity of the TAM model and its extensions relies on its ability to explain and predict human behavior in the acceptance of technology across various disciplines, contexts, and geographical locations. This is achieved through the concise structure of perceived usefulness and perceived ease of use, as well as the determinants that directly impact these constructs.

2.3. Hypotheses Development

The TAM and its extensions have been widely used to explain people's behaviors in an Information System and technology acceptance [36]. For example, TAM3 has been successfully applied to explain a variety of behavioral intentions, such as the acceptance of technology in the construction industry [37], digital banking channel acceptance [38], the social network impact on learning [39], the behavioral intention to use a smart village [40], m-commerce adoption [41], and many more. TAM3 is also used to investigate different areas of the healthcare industry, such as understanding key factors influencing the adoption of hospital electronic health records [42], identifying factors that predict the likelihood to adopt tele-neurorehabilitation [43], determining factors influencing nurses' acceptance of a hospital information system [44], or the factors influencing the acceptance of teleorthodontic technology [45]. Over time, the TAM framework has been extensively used to analyze the perceptions and adoption of health information technology by healthcare providers [46,47], especially in health services such as telemedicine, electronic health records, and mobile health applications [48].

In this research, we adapt to telemedicine services the third iteration of the technology acceptance model (TAM3) introduced by Venkatesh and Bala [33]. We specifically choose this model due to its inclusive methodology in examining the factors that influence perceived ease of use, and that is because when individuals perceive a technology as being user-friendly, it enhances their confidence and competence in adopting and using the technology effectively [49].

In addition to TAM3, our study includes two constructs derived from clinical factors identified in previous studies [50–52], namely accessibility to medical records and accessibility to patients.

Based on Venkatesh and Bala's [33] findings, the original TAM3 predicts behavioral intention over various periods and models with 40% to 53% accuracy, with perceived usefulness and perceived ease of use as significant predictors of behavioral intention—this finding is also supported by various other researchers [53–55]. Among these two predictors, perceived usefulness has a stronger predictive power than perceived ease of use [33,56,57]. Additionally, perceived ease of use not only influences behavioral intention but also plays a role in determining perceived usefulness. This is because a system that requires less effort to use can enhance people's belief in its usefulness [34]. Based on these considerations, it is also assumed that the following research hypotheses hold true in this study case too:

H1. *Perceived usefulness has a positive influence on the behavioral intention to use telemedicine.*

H2. *Perceived ease of use has a positive influence on the behavioral intention to use telemedicine.*

H3. *Perceived ease of use has a positive influence on perceived usefulness.*

In addition to examining perceived usefulness and perceived ease of use as main predictors of the behavioral intention to use telemedicine, our study also incorporates the construct of perceived incentives. This construct, classified as a regulatory factor, refers to the "extent to which an individual believes that the provision of telemedicine services would be rewarded with financial support or compensation for medical expenses" [58] and can directly influence the behavioral intention towards telemedicine, either positively or negatively. A lack of clear regulations or incentives often hinders telemedicine adoption [33,51,59], while high incentives increase healthcare professionals' willingness to embrace a new technology [58]. Thus, to better understand the role of perceived incentives among Romanian physicians, we set the following hypothesis:

H4. *Perceived incentives positively influence the behavioral intention to use telemedicine.*

Perceived usefulness can be influenced by different determinants, including subjective norms [34], and clinical factors like accessibility of medical records and accessibility of patients [51]. Subjective norms represent the extent to which individuals perform a certain behavior to obtain approval from a referent group and are expected to positively influence perceived usefulness and behavioral intention [33]. Previous studies show that the accessibility of medical records and patients enhances physician satisfaction, speeds up care delivery, reduces healthcare service time, and lowers costs [50,52]. Rho et al. [51] found that the accessibility of patients affects both perceived usefulness and the behavioral intention to use telemedicine. In this study, we want to examine whether the accessibility of medical records can directly influence the behavioral intention to use telemedicine services. We therefore set the following hypotheses:

H5. *Subjective norms have a positive influence on perceived usefulness.*

H6. *Accessibility of medical records has a positive influence on perceived usefulness.*

H7. *Accessibility of patients has a positive influence on perceived usefulness.*

H8. *Subjective norms have a positive influence on behavioral intention.*

H9. *Accessibility of medical records has a positive influence on behavioral intention.*

H10. *Accessibility of patients has a positive influence on behavioral intention.*

The factors contributing to perceived ease of use, as proposed by Venkatesh [35], based on the anchoring framing of human decision-making, include computer self-efficacy, computer anxiety, and perceptions of external control. These factors are based on the idea that individuals' perceptions of how easy technology is to use are anchored to their past computer experiences. Computer self-efficacy refers to one's belief in their ability to effectively use a system, such as telemedicine [33]. Conversely, computer anxiety involves fear of the unknown, frustration, embarrassment, failure, or disappointment, which can lead to avoidance of using the technology [60]. Perceptions of external control relate to the belief that organizational and technical resources will provide adequate support for using the system [33,61]. Taking this into account, we set the research hypotheses outlined below:

H11. *Computer self-efficacy has a positive influence on perceived ease of use.*

H12. *Perceived external control has a positive influence on perceived ease of use.*

H13. *Computer anxiety has a negative influence on perceived ease of use.*

Understanding these determinants and their influence on Romanian physicians' adoption of telemedicine can help policymakers pinpoint areas for improvement, boosting telemedicine use and productivity. Moreover, integrating TAM3 with other factors can offer a more detailed explanation of physicians' acceptance and use of telemedicine services [51]. The conceptual model is presented in Figure 1.

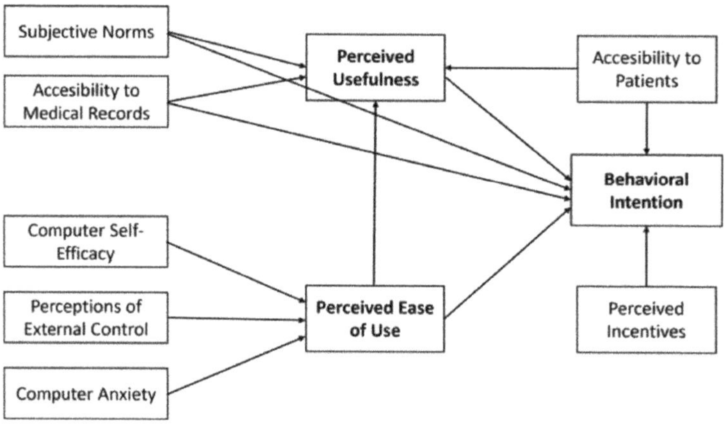

Figure 1. The research model.

3. Materials and Methods

3.1. Data

Data were gathered from 8th February to 26th February 2023, through a self-reported survey created on Google Forms. The survey was distributed to physicians nationwide via email by the National Authority of Quality Management in Health (ANMCS). The privacy and anonymity of the participants were ensured during the data collection process, and no ethical issues were identified, following established practices in socioeconomic research. Out of 5200 distinct emails sent to different physicians throughout Romania by the ANMCS, 1093 completed the questionnaire. Participants did not receive reminders to complete the questionnaire. The survey response rate was 21.02%. All variables' questions were measured using a 7-point Likert scale because it supplies a better accuracy estimate of participants' evaluation, compared to a 5-point Likert scale, and is more suitable for electronically distributed and unsupervised usability questionnaires [62,63].

3.2. Measurement

This study aims to investigate the determinants that influence the acceptance of telemedicine among physicians in Romania and the impact of these determinants on their intention to use this service. By comprehending these aspects, we can gain a clearer understanding of the feasibility of implementing telemedicine in Romania and its potential to enhance efficiency and productivity in public healthcare systems.

In this research, we adapted the TAM3 framework to suit the context of telemedicine services and adjusted the variables employed. Among the factors measuring TAM3 dimensions, we excluded one moderator, namely experience. We proceeded this way because, in the TAM3 model [33], 'experience' is mentioned as a moderator but is not listed as a variable. Instead, the model includes a variable called 'use'. Our study uses a similar question under the variable 'Telemed', asking if respondents have provided telemedicine services in the past year. However, this variable does not show statistical significance in our results. Additionally, we excluded image construct, which influences perceived usefulness, as well as computer playfulness, a variable that affects perceived ease of use. We also excluded the constructs of perceived enjoyment and objective usability, comprising related adjustment. Although we collected data on variables such as voluntariness, job relevance, output quality, and result demonstrability, we decided not to include them in the analysis due to identified endogeneity issues with behavioral intention. The questionnaire employed in this study incorporates items drawn from the work of Rho et al. [51] for assessing behavioral intention to use, perceived usefulness, perceived ease of use, perceived incentives, accessibility of medical records, and accessibility of patients. Additionally, items proposed by Venkatesh and Bala [33] are employed to measure computer self-efficacy, perceptions of external control, computer anxiety, and subjective norms. The questionnaire is available for reference in Appendix C.

3.3. Method

To assess the extent to which the predictors of the TAM, along with clinical and regulatory factors, account for variability in the outcome, we employed the partial least squares (PLS) algorithm [64]. The PLS algorithm consists of two main components: the inner model, which examines the connections between the latent variables within the PLS model, and the outer model, which explores the relationship between the latent variables and the observed variables in the PLS model. To conduct the analysis, we used WarpPLS, version 8.0.

4. Results

Our study encompasses 300 hospitals, predominantly located in urban areas, out of a total of 704 hospitals nationwide. Our sample consists of 1093 respondents (759 women and 334 men) with an average age of 46 years old. The largest age group within our sample, accounting for 33.4% of respondents, falls within the 40 to 49-year-old range. A total of 89.7% of the respondents have their provenience in urban areas. According to the national data provided by the National Institute of Statistics (INSSE) in their 2022 report [65], Romania has 71,293 physicians, with 92.3% practicing in urban areas and 7.7% in rural areas. Among these physicians, 70.8% are female. Subsequently, these comparisons validate the representativeness of our sample at the national level.

Also, 56.9% of them are primary care physicians, which can explain why around 69% of them have an income above RON 10,000 (EUR ~2000). As per the updated law 153/2017 in 2023, the base salary for a primary care physician is approximately RON 15,567 (EUR ~3100) [66]. A detailed description of our sample is available in Table 1.

Table 1. Descriptive statistics.

	Participants in Current Study N = 1093 (%)
Sex	
Male	334 (30.6%)
Female	759 (69.4%)
Age	
18–29 years old	14 (1.3%)
30–39 years old	311 (28.5%)
40–49 years old	365 (33.4%)
50–59 years old	274 (25.1%)
60–69 years old	119 (10.9%)
70–79 years old	10 (0.9%)
Over 80 years old	None
Provenience	
Rural	113 (10.3%)
Urban	980 (89.7%)
Education	
Medical school	161 (14.7%)
Medical Residency	343 (31.4%)
Ph.D. in medicine	285 (26.1%)
Post-university studies	282 (25.8%)

Table 1. *Cont.*

	Participants in Current Study N = 1093 (%)
Income	
Under RON 4000 (EUR 806)	2 (0.2%)
RON 4000–6000 (EUR 807–1208 euro)	48 (4.4%)
RON 6001–8000 (EUR 1209–1610)	100 (9.1%)
RON 8001–10,000 (EUR 1611–2013)	172 (15.7%)
RON 10,001–12,000 (EUR 2014–2416)	234 (21.4%)
RON 12,001–14,000 (EUR 2417–2819)	161 (14.7%)
RON 14,001–16,000 (EUR 2820–3221)	149 (13.6%)
Above RON 16,000 (EUR 3221)	212 (19.4%)
Refuse to answer	15 (1.4%)
Specialization	
Resident physician	21 (1.9%)
Specialist physician	315 (28.8%)
Primary care physician	622 (56.9%)
Doctor in medical sciences	135 (12.4%)

4.1. The Measurement (Outer) Model

Table 2 presents the measurement reliability of each construct used in the study. The composite reliability values range between 0.866 and 0.971, exceeding the recommended threshold of 0.70 [67]. Moreover, the Cronbach's alpha values for most variables are higher than 0.80 indicating a high level of internal consistency, except for the perceived incentives variable which has a Cronbach's alpha of 0.768 However, this value is still above the threshold of 0.70 [68], which is considered acceptable in many research situations [67]. Additionally, Table 2 indicates that all variables have an average variance extracted (AVE) greater than 0.50 [69], indicating strong convergent validity. The composite reliability, Cronbach's alpha values, and AVE results suggest that the variables employed in our study possess both reliable and high-quality measurement questions.

Table 2. The reliability of measurement.

Variable	Composite Reliability	Cronbach's Alpha	Average Variance Extracted (AVE)
Behavioral Intention	0.967	0.954	0.879
Perceived Usefulness	0.946	0.923	0.814
Perceived Ease of Use	0.918	0.864	0.788
Computer Self-Efficacy	0.900	0.851	0.694
Perceptions of External Control	0.954	0.927	0.873
Accessibility of Medical Records	0.955	0.929	0.875
Accessibility of Patients	0.971	0.955	0.917
Perceived Incentives	0.866	0.768	0.683
Computer Anxiety	0.951	0.922	0.865
Subjective Norms	0.920	0.883	0.741

Table 3 demonstrates that the measurement exhibits discriminant validity, as indicated by the higher values on the diagonal compared to the corresponding off-diagonal values. While only a few off-diagonal correlations slightly exceed the recommended threshold of 0.8 [70], it is important to note that discriminant validity, as assessed by the cross-loadings, is influenced by various factors. These factors include the correlations between constructs, the measurement process, and the characteristics of the sample. Each of these factors has distinct implications for determining which values should be considered high and potentially problematic [71].

Table 3. Square roots of AVE.

	BI	PU	PEOU	CSE	PEC	AMR	AP	PI	CANX	SN
BI	0.937	0.802	0.745	0.614	0.729	0.802	0.819	0.600	−0.229	0.780
PU	0.802	0.902	0.739	0.547	0.721	0.750	0.716	0.481	−0.158	0.729
PEOU	0.745	0.739	0.888	0.703	0.814	0.695	0.720	0.517	−0.283	0.629
CSE	0.614	0.547	0.703	0.833	0.637	0.555	0.601	0.469	−0.188	0.548
PEC	0.729	0.721	0.814	0.637	0.934	0.724	0.702	0.480	−0.286	0.617
AMR	0.802	0.750	0.695	0.555	0.724	0.935	0.726	0.489	−0.204	0.676
AP	0.819	0.716	0.720	0.601	0.702	0.726	0.958	0.533	−0.255	0.660
PI	0.600	0.481	0.517	0.469	0.480	0.489	0.533	0.827	−0.177	0.484
CANX	−0.229	−0.158	−0.283	−0.188	−0.286	−0.204	−0.225	−0.177	0.930	−0.108
SN	0.780	0.729	0.629	0.548	0.617	0.676	0.660	0.484	−0.108	0.861

The loadings of all reflective items fall within the range of 0.753 to 0.968, surpassing the minimum threshold of 0.7 [72–74], which indicates that the constructs capture the variance of the considered items. Additionally, the off-diagonal values for each set of measurement items are lower than the corresponding diagonal values, indicating good discriminant validity among the indicators. The combined loadings and cross-loadings of the indicator items for the latent construct are available in Appendix B.

4.2. *The Inner Model*

Appendix A presents the estimated coefficients of the model, while Appendix B shows the effect sizes for direct, indirect, and total effects. The analysis indicates that the model explains 84.6% of the behavioral intention to use telemedicine, as well as 71.5% of the variance in perceived usefulness and 72.7% of the variance in perceived ease of use. The overall model has a Tenenhaus Goodness of Fit (GoF) value of 0.82, exceeding the recommended threshold of 0.36 In the absence of other studies using a model similar to ours for comparison, we can also highlight the good performance of the TAM3 model developed by Venkatesh and Bala [33], which served as the foundation for our model, along with the model of Rho et al. [51], from which we incorporated two variables: accessibility of medical records and accessibility of patients. This can serve as further evidence that our model effectively captures the underlying patterns and relationships present in the data. Also, the model demonstrates an absence of endogeneity, signifying that the variables are not subjected to biased and inefficient estimates in statistical analyses. We checked for multicollinearity, and the average block VIF (AVIF), an index that tends to increase if new latent variables are added to the model and they overlap in meaning with existing latent variables, is 1.998, which is below the recommended threshold of 3.3 [75–77]. Therefore, full collinearity was not identified.

4.2.1. Predictors of Behavioral Intention

Perceived usefulness ($\beta = 0.179$, $p < 0.001$) and perceived ease of use ($\beta = 0.098$, $p < 0.001$) demonstrate a significant positive association with the intention to use telemedicine, supporting H1 and H2. In terms of predictive power, perceived usefulness exhibits a higher effect size (0.146) compared to perceived ease of use (0.073), indicating that perceived usefulness has a stronger impact on the behavioral intention to use telemedicine than perceived ease of use. Additionally, perceived ease of use positively and significantly influences perceived usefulness ($\beta = 0.283$, $p < 0.001$), providing support for H3.

Perceived incentives, our regulatory factor in the study, positively influence behavioral intention ($\beta = 0.120$, $p < 0.001$), supporting H4. Additionally, subjective norms ($\beta = 0.303$, $p < 0.001$) and accessibility of patients ($\beta = 0.278$, $p < 0.001$) demonstrate a positive predictive effect on the behavioral intention to use telemedicine. Hence, H8 and H9 are supported.

As we expected, the accessibility of medical records ($\beta = 0.254$, $p < 0.001$) also emerged as a variable that positively influences the behavioral intention to adopt telemedicine services, supporting the H10 hypothesis.

Out of all the variables that influence the behavioral intention to use telemedicine services, subjective norms have the greatest effect size (0.243) followed by accessibility of patients (0.228) and accessibility of medical records (0.204).

4.2.2. Predictors of Perceived Usefulness

Subjective norms ($\beta = 0.287$, $p < 0.001$), accessibility of medical records ($\beta = 0.255$, $p < 0.001$), as well as accessibility of patients ($\beta = 0.142$, $p < 0.001$), significantly predict perceived usefulness, exerting a positive influence on this construct. Thus, H5, H6, and H7 are supported. Of all these variables, subjective norms and perceived ease of use (both with an effect size of 0.211) demonstrate a stronger predictive ability for perceived usefulness compared to accessibility of medical records (effect size = 0.191) or accessibility of patients (effect size = 0.103).

4.2.3. Predictors of Perceived Ease of Use

Computer self-efficacy ($\beta = 0.280$, $p < 0.001$) and perceptions of external control ($\beta = 0.613$, $p < 0.001$) are positively and significantly associated with perceived ease of use, while computer anxiety ($\beta = -0.078$, $p = 0.005$) is negatively and significantly correlated with perceived ease of use ($\beta = -0.078$, $p = 0.005$). Therefore, we can confirm support for H11, H12, and H13. Among the three predictors of perceived ease of use, perceptions of external control exhibit the highest effect size (0.505), indicating that it has a stronger predictive power compared to the other two predictors.

Regarding age ($\beta = 0.007$, $p = 0.406$), previous use of telemedicine ($\beta = 0.033$, $p = 0.135$), and gender ($\beta = -0.005$, $p = 0.430$), their influences on behavioral intention are positive and negative, respectively. However, none of these variables yield statistically significant effects on the intention to use telemedicine.

5. Discussion

We explored the factors influencing Romanian physicians' intention to use telemedicine, using the third version of the Technology Acceptance Model (TAM) as our theoretical framework, with clinical and regulatory factors as additional variables. Our model explains 84.6% of the behavioral intention to use telemedicine, higher than the 53% identified in the work of Venkatesh and Bala [33]. Similarly, perceived usefulness (70.7% vs. 67%) and perceived ease of use (72.7% vs. 52%) were also higher than in the work of Venkatesh and Bala [33].

Our findings show that perceived usefulness and perceived ease of use, key variables in the Technology Acceptance Model (TAM), significantly and positively impact physicians' intention to use telemedicine, with perceived usefulness being the stronger predictor. This result is supported by previous studies [33,51,78]. Additionally, a study carried out by Kohnke [79], focusing on telehealth use by patients, reached a similar conclusion. They found that both perceived usefulness and perceived ease of use were important factors in predicting the intention to use telehealth services. Between the two, the ease-of-use factor plays a more significant role in determining the intention to use telemedicine. Physicians, particularly those with prior experience in using medical technologies, hold a stronger belief in the usefulness of various e-health technologies, perceiving their advantages to outweigh any potential challenges or drawbacks [80].

Furthermore, our findings indicate that subjective norms play a positive and significant role in shaping physicians' intention to use telemedicine, but also in the perceived usefulness of this technology. According to Venkatesh and Bala [33], subjective norms played a key role in predicting perceived usefulness and their impact on behavioral intention was influenced by factors such as experience and voluntariness. As individuals gained more experience, particularly in a voluntary setting, the influence of subjective norms became less significant. A study conducted in Senegal [81] also identified subjective norms as significant factors influencing physicians' intentions to incorporate telemedicine into their professional practices. Specifically, their behavioral intention to adopt telemedicine is greatly influenced by the thoughts and actions of their reference group, such as family, friends, colleagues, and other significant ones [82].

However, in another study on Iranian medical students, subjective norms were not statistically significant in influencing students' intention to use mobile health applications [83]. Also, in the study of Cohen et al. [84] on a South African population concerning electronic prescribing, subjective norms (or social influence) had a low impact on the usage of this technology. Those inconsistent findings can be interpreted considering Lee and Wan's [85] perspective, which proposes that the varying results concerning the impact of subjective norms on technology adoption may be influenced by the individuals' cultural context. Specifically, the distinction between individualistic and collectivist cultures may play a role in shaping the influence of subjective norms on technology adoption.

Individuals in individualistic societies pay less attention to the opinions of those around them, while those in collectivist societies value the opinions of their reference groups. By using a country comparison tool, we can observe that both Romania and Senegal (where subjective norms significantly influenced the behavioral intention to use technology) have scores of 30 and 25, respectively, on the Individualism dimension. This suggests that both countries are collectivist societies that rely on social networks for their identity. Conversely, South Africa (where subjective norms did not significantly impact intention to use) records a score of 65 on Individualism, indicating that South African individuals may have lower interpersonal connections with individuals outside their core "family" group [86,87]. Thus, it is essential to consider the various social and cultural contexts when interpreting the impact of subjective norms on the intention to use telemedicine.

The accessibility of medical records significantly influences Romanian physicians' inclination to adopt telemedicine and its perceived usefulness. This is primarily because Romania lacks a well-designed database capable of providing comprehensive medical data about patients. The Romanian healthcare system is marked by a lack of integration between different health sectors and a lack of progress in ensuring uninterrupted and interconnected healthcare services [88], leading to a higher risk of medical errors [89].

In 2014, the Romanian National Health Insurance House launched the project "The Patient's Electronic Health Record" to consolidate all patient's medical records, including consultations, referrals, analyses, prescriptions, observation sheets, and medical history, into a single platform [90]. However, the implementation of the electronic file was rushed and poorly prepared, presenting serious issues regarding protection of personal data of a medical nature contained in the Electronic Health Record, as the Ombudsman signaled to the Constitutional Court of Romania [91]. Consequently, shortly after its launch, the "Patient's Electronic Health Record" encountered significant functionality issues for three and a half years, mostly due to data security vulnerabilities [92].

An updated version of The Patient's Electronic Health Record was introduced in November 2021, but awareness among doctors and patients was low. Currently, 27,219 doctors from over 12,261 medical units (approximately 40% of Romania's doctors) have submitted data [93], and only 0.07% of patients have accessed the medical information stored in these records. Most submissions within the Electronic Health Record come from family doctors, while very few hospitals share this information with the National Health Insurance House. The reason behind this issue is the lack of connectivity between the software systems used by medical units and those employed by the National Health Insurance House [94].

The accessibility of patients, the other clinical factor observed in our research, also exerts a significant positive effect on both behavioral intention and the perceived usefulness of using telemedicine. According to a European Commission's report from 2022, Romania faces considerable healthcare accessibility challenges due to staff shortages, underdeveloped primary care, and high unmet needs (4.4%, one of the highest in EU). Additionally, the country experiences lower rates of consultations in primary and ambulatory care compared to the EU average. Despite producing many medical graduates, the healthcare system faces significant staff shortages and distribution imbalances due to workforce emigration, with 12% of doctors and 11% of nurses trained in Romania working elsewhere in the EU [95]. Romania has significantly limited healthcare access in rural areas, and this issue is further exacerbated by differences in demographic coverage (e.g., the Roma population and homeless people have very low access to healthcare) [88]. Therefore, healthcare professionals, particularly physicians who are deeply engaged in public health, experienced the greatest difficulties in delivering healthcare services to these vulnerable populations. As a result, telemedicine emerges as a potential solution that could enhance healthcare accessibility for patients who face obstacles in attending in-person medical consultations.

In this study, we also observed three determinants that previous studies have indicated could influence perceived ease of use [33,35]: perceptions of external control, computer self-efficacy, and computer anxiety. Our study reinforces that these factors significantly influence the extent to which a technology is perceived as being easy to use.

Perceptions of external control positively influence perceived ease of use and exert the highest influence on perceived ease of use, followed by computer self-efficacy. Perceptions of external control positively influence perceived ease of use and exert the highest influence on perceived ease of use, followed by computer self-efficacy. Healthcare technologies, encompassing various systems from health data management to diagnosis and care delivery, possess unique complexities compared to other technological domains. Understanding the technological landscape and user (i.e., physicians, medical staff, etc.) dynamics, along with their perspectives and concerns about these technologies, is essential for proposing context-specific solutions tailored to healthcare systems. Moreover, the integration of new health technology in healthcare requires adequate guidance to minimize complexity in its usage.

Comparing our results with previous findings, we observed that in the study conducted by Rho et al. [51] on South Korean physicians, computer self-efficacy was the dominant predictor of telemedicine acceptance. However, both constructs, as proposed by Venkatesh [35], represent different dimensions of control, which refers to "the individual's perception of the availability of knowledge, resources, and opportunities required to perform the specific behavior". While control has traditionally been seen as a unidimensional concept in research, Ajzen [96] revolutionized its conceptualization by introducing a bidimensional approach: internal control (i.e., knowledge/self-efficacy) and external control (i.e., environment). In the context of technology usage, internal control is represented by computer self-efficacy, whereas external control corresponds to perceptions of external control [35]. As the same study suggests, considering the broad conceptualization of perceived ease of use, we might also expect that people will incorporate both internal and external dimensions of control into their perceptions of external control.

Computer anxiety has a notable detrimental impact on technology usage, which is consistent with earlier research conducted by [33,35,97]. This implies that individuals with higher levels of technology anxiety are less likely to have the intention to use any form of technology.

Conversely, it appears that perceived incentives significantly and positively impact the adoption of telemedicine, consistent with the studies conducted in [51,80]. In addition, research conducted on Nigerian physicians by Adenuga et al. [98] revealed that financial incentives were influential in their propensity to use telemedicine services. Similarly, healthcare professionals from Morocco, as studied by Mohammed et al. [58], expressed that "appropriate support from governmental bodies, financial support for institutions that adopt this technology, and reimbursement for procedures conducted through the digital platform" had the potential to increase telemedicine usage. The significant role of incentives in healthcare was also highlighted by Glaser [99], who found low technology adoption in institutions with insufficient or nonexistent incentives. Additionally, Chaix-Couturier et al. [100] discovered that the inclusion of financial incentives led to an increase in night calls.

The minimal or non-significant effects of the control variables "age" and "gender" can be attributed to the fact that physicians, regardless of age and gender, receive professional training and ongoing education that often includes exposure to new technologies and practices, enhancing their confidence and willingness to adopt new technologies [61,101]. Thus, their acceptance of telemedicine might be more influenced by professional, institutional, or practical considerations than by their demographic characteristics, as this study's findings have already suggested above.

6. Limitations and Future Directions

There is no doubt that this study has provided valuable insights regarding telemedicine acceptance by physicians in Romania, since the research on telemedicine acceptance in Romania is almost nonexistent, and therefore our results cannot be judged against local theoretical backgrounds or previous findings. However, we must consider the limitations and future directions of this study, which will be briefly discussed below.

First, most of the study participants (~89.7%) were from urban areas. This is because the study was based on the database of the National Authority of Quality Management in Health, which primarily includes physicians from urban medical units. However, having a study sample predominantly composed of physicians from urban areas can impact the generalizability of the study's findings, since they may not accurately represent the attitudes, behaviors, and challenges faced by physicians from rural areas. Moreover, the healthcare delivery and patient demographics can vary significantly between urban and rural areas. This is particularly relevant given that rural areas often have a higher proportion of older patients compared to urban areas [102]. These older patients may find technology too complicated to understand [103], which can influence the adoption of telemedicine among both patients and physicians. Taking these aspects into account, future research might consider a deliberate sampling from diverse geographic locations, ensuring a more representative reflection of physicians across urban and rural settings.

Second, telemedicine is currently underdeveloped in Romania [26] and this may be a limitation of this study in the way that physicians may have limited exposure to telemedicine practices in the public health system, impacting their perceptions and attitudes and making it challenging to draw comprehensive conclusions about telemedicine acceptance. In addition to the previously mentioned National Electronic Health Record, which has significant shortcomings, the Ministry of Health initiated a bid in 2023 [104] to procure comprehensive telemedicine solutions, intended to outfit 131 Emergency Reception Units. However, this initiative represents a relatively small step forward and is insufficient to establish an integrated telemedicine system in Romania. Furthermore, the insufficient overall technological assistance and resources for various digital healthcare solutions implemented in Romania (i.e., the Electronic Health Record) thus far may foster uncertainty, resistance, or skepticism among physicians regarding the adoption of telemedicine. Consequently, these characteristics pose limitations on the generalizability of findings to other countries or contexts. Future research in regions with diverse telemedicine implementations can provide a more comprehensive understanding of the factors influencing telemedicine acceptance among physicians.

Third, the model employed in this study did not measure constructs associated with trust, data protection concerns, and cybersecurity within the telemedicine context. Evaluating physicians' levels of trust in telemedicine has the potential to yield a more comprehensive understanding of the psychological and attitudinal factors that either contribute to or impede its adoption. Furthermore, trust and security considerations are often interconnected with policy and implementation decisions in telemedicine, providing a more nuanced comprehension of the factors influencing physicians' acceptance of telemedicine and facilitating the development of strategies to address potential barriers. Therefore, to enhance the study's robustness and applicability, future research should consider integrating measurements for trust in telemedicine and variables related to personal data and cybersecurity.

7. Conclusions

This research is timely, with a consistent practical footprint. The Romanian legislation on telemedicine services has been steadily updated from 2020 onward, with EMERGENCY ORDINANCE no. 196 of 18 November 2020 for the amendment and completion of Law no. 95/2006 regarding health reform, followed by the DECISION no. 1133 of 14 September 2022 regarding the approval of the Methodological Norms for the implementation of the provisions of the Government Emergency Ordinance no. 196/2020 for the amendment and completion of Law no. 95/2006 on health reform. Moreover, within Romania's recovery and resilience plan, funded by the EU till 2026, the Romanian government will fund the implementation of e-health and telemedicine systems within the digital transformation pillar. Some other initiatives have also been supported by the EU in the previous years, such as the project POSCCE 49472—"Increasing the quality of the medical act in rural areas by implementing a Telemedicine Information System"—financed by The European Regional Development Fund under the Increase of Economic Competitiveness, Sectorial Operational Program 2007–2013.

While the policy perspectives have started to be better articulated, as always, in real life, things are a bit more complicated. For the researched area of medical professionals working in urban areas in hospital settings, the adoption of telemedicine services as a routine act is still in its infancy. Uncovering the intricacies of medical professionals' decision-making processes when contemplating telemedicine services will help the authorities speed up the process.

Telemedicine is a promising field that offers numerous opportunities for innovation and investment, having the potential to enhance the quality of healthcare services through technological advancements in the coming years. However, the successful implementation of telemedicine relies on the willingness of both physicians and patients to embrace this digital healthcare feature, as well as on the government and healthcare institutions. This study serves as an initial step in gaining a deeper comprehension of the factors that encourage or impede Romanian physicians from adopting telemedicine services. Our study not only aims to uncover the perceptions, motivations, and barriers specific to Romanian physicians but also seeks to compare our findings with those from similar or more developed countries. By doing so, we aim to gain a broader understanding of the factors that truly influence the acceptance of telemedicine among physicians.

Author Contributions: Conceptualization, A.B., V.M. and M.B.; methodology, V.M.; software, A.-I.P.; formal analysis, A.-I.P.; data curation, M.B.; writing—original draft preparation, A.B.; writing—review and editing, A.-I.P. and V.M. All authors have read and agreed to the published version of the manuscript.

Funding: This research received no external funding.

Institutional Review Board Statement: This study was approved by the Ethics Committee of Autoritatea Națională de Management al Calității în Sănătate (ANMCS) (30 January 2023).

Informed Consent Statement: Informed consent was obtained from all subjects involved in the study. Written informed consent for publication has been waived due to the privacy and anonymity of the data collection process, and the participants cannot be identified.

Data Availability Statement: The data presented in this study are available on request from the corresponding author.

Acknowledgments: We would like to thank Elena Druică for her support in managing this research.

Conflicts of Interest: The authors declare no conflicts of interest.

Appendix A

Table A1. Path Coefficients of the Structural Model.

Estimated Coef.	Direct Effects			Indirect Effects		Total Effects		
Model	**BI**	**PU**	**PEOU**	**BI**	**PU**	**BI**	**PU**	**PEOU**
BI	-	-		-	-	-	-	-
PU	0.179 *** ($p < 0.001$)	-		-	-	0.179 *** ($p < 0.001$)	-	-
PEOU	0.047 ($p = 0.059$)	0.283 *** ($p < 0.001$)		0.051 ** ($p = 0.009$)	-	0.098 *** ($p < 0.001$)	0.283 *** ($p < 0.001$)	-
CSE	-	-	0.280 *** ($p < 0.001$)	0.013 ($p = 0.268$)	0.079 *** ($p < 0.001$)	0.027 ($p = 0.100$)	0.079 *** ($p < 0.001$)	0.280 *** ($p < 0.001$)
PEC	-	-	0.613 *** ($p < 0.001$)	0.029 ($p = 0.088$)	0.173 *** ($p < 0.001$)	0.060 ** ($p = 0.002$)	0.173 *** ($p < 0.001$)	0.613 *** ($p < 0.001$)
AMR	0.209 *** ($p < 0.001$)	0.255 *** ($p < 0.001$)		0.046 * ($p = 0.016$)		0.254 *** ($p < 0.001$)	0.255 *** ($p < 0.001$)	
AP	0.252 *** ($p < 0.001$)	0.142 *** ($p < 0.001$)		0.025 ($p = 0.117$)		0.278 *** ($p < 0.001$)	0.142 *** ($p < 0.001$)	
PI	0.120 *** ($p < 0.001$)	-				0.120 *** ($p < 0.001$)		
CANX	-	-	−0.078 ** ($p = 0.005$)	−0.004 ($p = 0.432$)	−0.022 ($p = 0.151$)	−0.008 ($p = 0.361$)	−0.022 ($p = 0.151$)	−0.078 ** ($p = 0.005$)
SN	0.252 *** ($p < 0.001$)	0.287 *** ($p < 0.001$)		0.051 ** ($p = 0.008$)		0.303 *** ($p < 0.001$)	0.287 *** ($p < 0.001$)	
Age	0.007 ($p = 0.406$)	-				0.007 ($p = 0.406$)		
Gender	−0.005 ($p = 0.430$)	-				−0.005 ($p = 0.430$)		
Telemed	0.033 ($p = 0.135$)					0.033 ($p = 0.135$)		
R2/ Adjusted R2	84.6%/ 84.4%	71.5%/ 71.4%	72.7%/ 72.6%					
Tenehaus GoF	0.821 (large)							

*** *p*-value < 0.001; ** *p*-value < 0.01; * *p*-value < 0.05.

Appendix B

Table A1. Effect Sizes for Direct, Indirect, and Total Effects.

Estimated Coef.	Direct Effects			Indirect Effects		Total Effects		
Model	**BI**	**PU**	**PEOU**	**BI**	**PU**	**BI**	**PU**	**PEOU**
BI	-	-	-	-	-	-	-	-
PU	0.146	-	-	-	-	0.146	-	-
PEOU	0.035	0.211	-	0.038	-	0.073	0.211	-
CSE	-	-	0.198	0.008	0.043	0.017	0.043	0.198
PEC	-	-	0.505	0.021	0.125	0.044	0.125	0.505
AMR	0.168	0.191	-	0.037	-	0.204	0.191	-
AP	0.207	0.103	-	0.021	-	0.228	0.103	-
PI	0.073	-	-	-	-	0.073	-	-
CANX	-	-	0.024	0.001	0.003	0.002	0.003	0.024
SN	0.202	0.211	-	0.041	-	0.243	0.211	-
Age	0.000	-	-	-	-	0.000	-	-
Gender	0.000	-	-	-	-	0.000	-	-
Telemed	0.009	-	-	-	-	0.009	-	-

Appendix C

Table A2. The Questionnaire.

Construct	Items	
Behavioral Intention	BI1. I have a positive intention to adopt the telemedicine service. BI2. I will care for my patients through telemedicine service. BI3. I will gain accurate patient information and treatment histories. BI4. I will provide telemedicine services and share the information through this service.	
Perceived Usefulness	PU1. It will positively affect the treatment plan. PU2. It is possible to provide a more comprehensive care service. PU3. It is efficient for diagnosing patients and scheduling. PU4. I can precisely monitor the patient's condition.	[51]
Perceived Ease of Use	PEOU1. It is easy to use the device for telemedicine service. PEOU2. It is easy to learn how to use the new device for telemedicine. PEOU3. It is easy to perform my job by using the telemedicine service.	
Computer Self−Efficacy	I could complete the job using a software package. CSE1. if there was no one around to tell me what to do as I go. CSE2. if I had just the built−in help facility for assistance. CSE3. if someone showed me how to do it first. CSE4. if I had used similar packages before this one to do the same job	[33]
Perceptions of External Control	PEC1. I have control over using the system. PEC2. I have the resources necessary to use the system. PEC3. Given the resources. opportunities. and knowledge it takes to use the system. it would be easy for me to use the system. PEC4. The system is not compatible with other systems I use.	
Accessibility to Medical Records	AMR1. I can gather correct information about the patient. AMR2. I can easily record a patient's health condition. AMR3. Because of the precise record of the patients. it enables me to provide proper healthcare service to my patients.	
Accessibility to Patients	AP1. I am able to care for patients living at further distances. AP2. I am able to be in contact with patients who seldom come to the clinic. AP3. I am able to be in contact with patients who cannot be easily delivered to the clinic.	[51]
Perceived Incentives	PI1. This service needs proper government policy and support. PI2. It needs monetary incentives. PI3. It would be meaningful. if financial support were given.	
Computer Anxiety	CANX1. Computers do not scare me at all. CANX2. Working with a computer makes me nervous. CANX3. Computers make me feel uncomfortable. CANX4. Computers make me feel uneasy.	[33]
Subjective Norms	SN1.People who influence my behavior think that I should use the system. SN2. People who are important to me think that I should use the system. SN3. The senior management of this business has been helpful in the use of the system. SN4. In general. the organization has supported the use of the system.	

Appendix D

Table A3. The Combined Loadings and Cross-Loadings of the Indicator Items.

	BI	PU	PEOU	CSE	PEC	AMR	AP	PI	CANX	SN
BI_1	0.950	0.008	0.042	0.017	0.011	−0.169	−0.037	0.020	−0.007	0.019
BI_2	0.955	−0.064	0.026	0.000	0.067	−0.196	0.072	−0.022	0.005	0.030
BI_3	0.892	0.043	−0.110	0.040	−0.089	0.469	−0.150	0.039	−0.010	−0.056
BI_4	0.952	0.016	0.035	−0.055	0.005	−0.074	0.106	−0.035	0.010	0.004
PU_1	0.044	0.927	0.129	−0.009	−0.086	−0.049	−0.009	−0.005	0.006	0.003
PU_2	0.085	0.931	−0.022	0.010	−0.091	−0.024	−0.056	−0.022	−0.010	−0.023
PU_3	−0.130	0.881	0.024	−0.019	−0.012	0.065	−0.060	0.081	−0.002	0.045
PU_4	−0.006	0.868	−0.138	0.018	0.203	0.012	0.131	−0.053	0.006	−0.024
$PEOU_1$	−0.084	−0.190	0.931	0.008	0.079	0.048	0.009	0.002	−0.012	−0.008
$PEOU_2$	−0.130	−0.244	0.914	0.037	0.041	−0.006	0.067	0.089	−0.031	−0.044
$PEOU_3$	0.242	0.491	0.814	−0.050	−0.136	−0.047	−0.086	−0.102	0.048	0.060
CSE_1	0.034	−0.174	0.427	0.753	0.330	−0.140	0.037	−0.133	−0.045	0.063
CSE_2	−0.029	0.007	0.134	0.888	0.027	−0.083	0.061	−0.046	−0.016	0.020
CSE_3	0.047	0.027	−0.204	0.869	−0.172	0.112	0.002	0.058	0.037	−0.078
CSE_4	−0.051	0.124	−0.324	0.815	−0.151	0.100	−0.102	0.111	0.020	0.003
PEC_1	0.012	0.094	0.067	0.045	0.926	0.010	−0.027	−0.010	−0.006	−0.004
PEC_2	−0.005	−0.053	−0.149	−0.059	0.937	0.007	0.024	−0.023	0.035	0.012
PEC_3	−0.006	−0.040	0.083	0.014	0.940	0.004	0.003	0.033	−0.029	−0.009
AMR_1	−0.010	0.012	−0.044	0.041	−0.037	0.934	−0.075	−0.005	0.030	−0.036
AMR_2	−0.073	−0.134	0.072	−0.012	0.075	0.938	0.067	−0.010	−0.036	0.036
AMR_3	0.084	0.123	−0.028	−0.028	−0.039	0.935	0.007	0.016	0.006	0.000
AP_1	0.014	0.127	−0.055	0.005	−0.011	0.003	0.942	−0.019	0.020	0.006
AP_2	−0.035	−0.064	0.026	−0.006	0.000	0.031	0.968	0.005	−0.015	0.021
AP_3	0.022	−0.060	0.028	0.002	0.010	−0.034	0.962	0.013	−0.005	−0.026
PI_1	−0.105	−0.243	0.227	0.057	−0.017	0.015	0.086	0.804	−0.067	−0.047
PI_2	−0.379	0.096	−0.207	−0.004	0.060	0.025	0.043	0.838	0.037	0.062
PI_3	0.480	0.137	−0.011	−0.050	−0.044	−0.039	−0.126	0.837	0.027	−0.017
$CANX_2$	0.037	−0.020	−0.050	−0.029	−0.017	0.006	0.012	0.000	0.905	0.037
$CANX_3$	−0.029	0.005	0.041	0.011	−0.005	0.000	0.012	0.025	0.939	−0.024
$CANX_4$	−0.007	0.014	0.007	0.016	0.021	−0.005	−0.023	−0.025	0.947	−0.012
SN_1	−0.665	0.028	−0.198	0.003	0.217	0.091	0.061	0.000	0.014	0.812
SN_2	−0.478	0.042	−0.072	−0.054	0.128	0.129	0.040	−0.005	0.010	0.879
SN_3	0.445	−0.015	0.099	0.022	−0.153	−0.115	−0.008	0.018	0.000	0.879
SN_4	0.653	−0.053	0.158	0.029	−0.176	−0.100	−0.089	−0.013	−0.023	0.871

References

1. Wang, J.; Xu, Y. Digitalization, Income Inequality, and Public Health: Evidence from Developing Countries. *Technol. Soc.* **2023**, *73*, 102210. [CrossRef]
2. Guzel, A.E.; Arslan, U.; Acaravci, A. The Impact of Economic, Social, and Political Globalization and Democracy on Life Expectancy in Low-Income Countries: Are Sustainable Development Goals Contradictory? *Environ. Dev. Sustain.* **2021**, *23*, 13508–13525. [CrossRef]
3. Huang, S.; Zhou, T.; Xu, C.; Zheng, J. Does Public Health Influence Economic Performance? Investigating the Role of Governance and Greener Energies for the Case of China. *Front. Public Health* **2022**, *10*, 864736. [CrossRef]
4. Paunov, C.; Planes-Satorra, S. *What Future for Science, Technology and Innovation after COVID-19?* OECD Science, Technology and Industry Policy Papers; OECD: Paris, France, 2021; Volume 107.

5. Smith, A.C.; Thomas, E.; Snoswell, C.L.; Haydon, H.; Mehrotra, A.; Clemensen, J.; Caffery, L.J. Telehealth for Global Emergencies: Implications for Coronavirus Disease 2019 (COVID-19). *J. Telemed. Telecare* **2020**, *26*, 309–313. [CrossRef]
6. Golinelli, D.; Boetto, E.; Carullo, G.; Nuzzolese, A.G.; Landini, M.P.; Fantini, M.P. Adoption of Digital Technologies in Health Care During the COVID-19 Pandemic: Systematic Review of Early Scientific Literature. *J. Med. Internet Res.* **2020**, *22*, e22280. [CrossRef]
7. How Digital Transformation in Healthcare Improves Efficiency and Patient Care. 2021. Available online: https://sidebench.com/digital-transformation-healthcare-improves-efficiency-patient-care/ (accessed on 12 June 2024).
8. Stoumpos, A.I.; Kitsios, F.; Talias, M.A. Digital Transformation in Healthcare: Technology Acceptance and Its Applications. *Int. J. Environ. Res. Public Health* **2023**, *20*, 3407. [CrossRef]
9. Gjellebæk, C.; Svensson, A.; Bjørkquist, C.; Fladeby, N.; Grundén, K. Management Challenges for Future Digitalization of Healthcare Services. *Futures* **2020**, *124*, 102636. [CrossRef]
10. CVSHealth. 2022 Health Care Insights Study. Available online: https://www.cvshealth.com/content/dam/enterprise/cvs-enterprise/pdfs/cvs-health-care-insights-study-2022-report-executive-summary.pdf (accessed on 12 June 2024).
11. Hyder, M.A.; Razzak, J. Telemedicine in the United States: An Introduction for Students and Residents. *J. Med. Internet Res.* **2020**, *22*, e20839. [CrossRef]
12. Omboni, S.; Padwal, R.S.; Alessa, T.; Benczúr, B.; Green, B.B.; Hubbard, I.; Kario, K.; Khan, N.A.; Konradi, A.; Logan, A.G.; et al. The Worldwide Impact of Telemedicine during COVID-19: Current Evidence and Recommendations for the Future. *Connect. Health* **2022**, *1*, 7. [CrossRef]
13. Li, J. Telemedicine and Telehealth in 2023 and beyond: From Leveling Out to Leveling Up. 2022. Available online: https://www.forbes.com/sites/forbestechcouncil/2022/12/27/telemedicine-and-telehealth-in-2023-and-beyond-from-leveling-out-to-leveling-up/ (accessed on 12 June 2024).
14. Barbosa, W.; Zhou, K.; Waddell, E.; Myers, T.; Dorsey, E.R. Improving Access to Care: Telemedicine Across Medical Domains. *Annu. Rev. Public Health* **2021**, *42*, 463–481. [CrossRef]
15. Haleem, A.; Javaid, M.; Singh, R.P.; Suman, R. Telemedicine for Healthcare: Capabilities, Features, Barriers, and Applications. *Sens. Int.* **2021**, *2*, 100117. [CrossRef]
16. Atmojo, J.T.; Sudaryanto, W.T.; Widiyanto, A.; Ernawati; Arradini, D. Telemedicine, Cost Effectiveness, and Patients Satisfaction: A Systematic Review. *J. Health Policy Manag.* **2020**, *5*, 103–107. [CrossRef]
17. Lasslo, J.A.; Anthony, K.E.; Reif, C.E.; Bell, N.H. Overcoming Health Disparities. In *Health Professionals' Education in the Age of Clinical Information Systems, Mobile Computing and Social Networks*; Elsevier: London, UK, 2017; pp. 35–62. ISBN 978-0-12-805362-1.
18. Williams, R.M. The Costs of Visits to Emergency Departments. *N. Engl. J. Med.* **1996**, *334*, 642–646. [CrossRef]
19. Tapia, A.D.; Howard, J.T.; Bebo, N.L.; Pfaff, J.A.; Chin, E.J.; Trueblood, W.A.; April, M.D.; Long, B.J.; Long, A.N.; Fernandez, W.G.; et al. A Retrospective Review of Emergency Department Visits That May Be Appropriate for Management in Non-Emergency Settings. *Mil. Med.* **2022**, *187*, e1153–e1159. [CrossRef]
20. Hazarika, I. Artificial Intelligence: Opportunities and Implications for the Health Workforce. *Int. Health* **2020**, *12*, 241–245. [CrossRef]
21. Ramanauskas, B. Better and Cheaper Public Services 2018. Available online: https://d3n8a8pro7vhmx.cloudfront.net/taxpayersalliance/pages/9468/attachments/original/1529499259/Automation_Paper_1.pdf?1529499259 (accessed on 10 June 2024).
22. Batko, K.; Ślęzak, A. The Use of Big Data Analytics in Healthcare. *J. Big Data* **2022**, *9*, 3. [CrossRef]
23. Koff, D.A.; Doyle, T.E. Imaging Informatics. In *Encyclopedia of Biomedical Engineering*; Elsevier: Amsterdam, The Netherlands, 2019; pp. 551–560, ISBN 978-0-12-805144-3.
24. Hasselberg, M.J. The Digital Revolution in Behavioral Health. *J. Am. Psychiatr. Nurses Assoc.* **2020**, *26*, 102–111. [CrossRef] [PubMed]
25. Robeznieks, A. Which Medical Specialties Use Telemedicine the Most? 2019. Available online: https://www.ama-assn.org/practice-management/digital/which-medical-specialties-use-telemedicine-most (accessed on 30 May 2024).
26. Scîntee, S.G.; Vlădescu, C. Implementation of Telemedicine in Romania. European Observatory of Health Systems and Policies. 30 September 2022. Available online: https://eurohealthobservatory.who.int/monitors/health-systems-monitor/updates/hspm/romania-2016/implementation-of-telemedicine-in-romania (accessed on 12 June 2024).
27. Market Data Forecast Telemedicine Market. Market Data Forecast. 2023. Available online: https://www.marketdataforecast.com/market-reports/telemedicine-market (accessed on 4 May 2024).
28. Observatoire Cetelem. Contactless Solutions Are Taking Hold Of Our Lives: Telemedicine 2021. Available online: https://observatoirecetelem.com/en/lobservatoire-cetelem-de-la-consommation/contactless-solutions-are-taking-hold-of-our-lives/telemedicine (accessed on 12 June 2024).
29. Bagchi, A.D. Telemedicine Delivery for Urban Seniors with Low Computer Literacy: A Pilot Study. *Online J. Nurs. Inform.* **2018**, *22*, 1–7.
30. Florea, M.; Lazea, C.; Gaga, R.; Sur, G.; Lotrean, L.; Puia, A.; Stanescu, A.M.A.; Lupsor-Platon, M.; Florea, H.; Sur, M.L. Lights and Shadows of the Perception of the Use of Telemedicine by Romanian Family Doctors During the COVID-19 Pandemic. *IJGM* **2021**, *14*, 1575–1587. [CrossRef]
31. Davis, F.D. Perceived Usefulness, Perceived Ease of Use, and User Acceptance of Information Technology. *MIS Q.* **1989**, *13*, 319. [CrossRef]

32. Help University, Malaysia; Lai, P. The Literature Review of Technology Adoption Models and Theories for the Novelty Technology. *JISTEM* **2017**, *14*, 21–38. [CrossRef]
33. Venkatesh, V.; Bala, H. Technology Acceptance Model 3 and a Research Agenda on Interventions. *Decis. Sci.* **2008**, *39*, 273–315. [CrossRef]
34. Venkatesh, V.; Davis, F.D. A Theoretical Extension of the Technology Acceptance Model: Four Longitudinal Field Studies. *Manag. Sci.* **2000**, *46*, 186–204. [CrossRef]
35. Venkatesh, V. Determinants of Perceived Ease of Use: Integrating Control, Intrinsic Motivation, and Emotion into the Technology Acceptance Model. *Inf. Syst. Res.* **2000**, *11*, 342–365. [CrossRef]
36. Chen, S.-C.; Li, S.-H.; Li, C.-Y. Recent related research in technology acceptance model: A literature review. *AJBMR* **2012**, *1*, 124–127. [CrossRef]
37. Elshafey, A.; Saar, C.C.; Aminudin, E.B.; Gheisari, M.; Usmani, A. Technology Acceptance Model for Augmented Reality and Building Information Modeling Integration in the Construction Industry. *ITcon* **2020**, *25*, 161–172. [CrossRef]
38. Musyaffi, A.M.; Mulyani, S.; Suraida, I.; Sukmadilaga, C. Lack of readiness of digital banking channel acceptance: Study on TAM 3 and technology readiness. *Acad. Strateg. Manag. J.* **2021**, *20*, 1–18.
39. Barabadi, S.A.; Shams, A.; Wise, N. Social Network Sites Impact on Learning: Extending the TAM3 Model to Assess Academic Performance in Higher Education. *JAST* **2022**, *24*, 1073–1086.
40. Mayasari, R.; Febriantoko, J.; Putra, R.R.; Hadiwijaya, H.; Kurniawan, D. Analysis of Behavioral Intention Towards the Use of Smart Village Ogan Ilir (SVOI) Using Technology Acceptance Model (TAM) 3 Method. In Proceedings of the International Conference of Economics, Business, and Entrepreneur (ICEBE 2022), Palembang, Indonesia, 26 October 2022; Nairobi, Yuliansyah, Jimad, H., Perdana, R., Putrawan, G.E., Septiawan, T.Y., Eds.; Advances in Economics, Business and Management Research. Atlantis Press SARL: Paris, France, 2023; Volume 241, pp. 545–553, ISBN 978-2-38476-063-3.
41. Salimon, M.G.; Kareem, O.; Mokhtar, S.S.M.; Aliyu, O.A.; Bamgbade, J.A.; Adeleke, A.Q. Malaysian SMEs M-Commerce Adoption: TAM 3, UTAUT 2 and TOE Approach. *JSTPM* **2023**, *14*, 98–126. [CrossRef]
42. Ebnehoseini, Z.; Tara, M.; Tabesh, H.; Dindar, F.; Hasibian, S. Understanding Key Factors Affecting on Hospital Electronic Health Record (EHR) Adoption. *J. Fam. Med. Prim. Care* **2020**, *9*, 4348. [CrossRef]
43. Klaic, M.; Galea, M.P. Using the Technology Acceptance Model to Identify Factors That Predict Likelihood to Adopt Tele-Neurorehabilitation. *Front. Neurol.* **2020**, *11*, 580832. [CrossRef] [PubMed]
44. Barzegari, S.; Arpaci, I.; Marznaki, Z.H. Determining Factors Affecting Nurses' Acceptance of a Hospital Information System Using a Modified Technology Acceptance Model 3. In *International Conference on Information Systems and Intelligent Applications*; Al-Emran, M., Al-Sharafi, M.A., Shaalan, K., Eds.; Lecture Notes in Networks and Systems; Springer International Publishing: Cham, Switzerland, 2023; Volume 550, pp. 449–456. ISBN 978-3-031-16864-2.
45. Yazdanpanahi, F.; Shahi, M.; Vossoughi, M. Investigating the Effective Factors on the Acceptance of Teleorthodontic Technology Based on the Technology Acceptance Model 3 (TAM3). *J. Dent.* **2024**, *25*. [CrossRef]
46. Holden, R.J.; Karsh, B.-T. The Technology Acceptance Model: Its Past and Its Future in Health Care. *J. Biomed. Inform.* **2010**, *43*, 159–172. [CrossRef] [PubMed]
47. AlQudah, A.A.; Al-Emran, M.; Shaalan, K. Technology Acceptance in Healthcare: A Systematic Review. *Appl. Sci.* **2021**, *11*, 10537. [CrossRef]
48. Rahimi, B.; Nadri, H.; Lotfnezhad Afshar, H.; Timpka, T. A Systematic Review of the Technology Acceptance Model in Health Informatics. *Appl. Clin. Inf.* **2018**, *9*, 604–634. [CrossRef] [PubMed]
49. He, Y.; Chen, Q.; Kitkuakul, S. Regulatory Focus and Technology Acceptance: Perceived Ease of Use and Usefulness as Efficacy. *Cogent Bus. Manag.* **2018**, *5*, 1459006. [CrossRef]
50. Martínez, A.; Everss, E.; Rojo-Álvarez, J.L.; Figal, D.P.; García-Alberola, A. A Systematic Review of the Literature on Home Monitoring for Patients with Heart Failure. *J. Telemed. Telecare* **2006**, *12*, 234–241. [CrossRef]
51. Rho, M.J.; Choi, I.Y.; Lee, J. Predictive Factors of Telemedicine Service Acceptance and Behavioral Intention of Physicians. *Int. J. Med. Inform.* **2014**, *83*, 559–571. [CrossRef] [PubMed]
52. Whitten, P.; Doolittle, G.; Mackert, M. Providers' Acceptance of Telehospice. *J. Palliat. Med.* **2005**, *8*, 730–735. [CrossRef]
53. Gagnon, M.P.; Orruño, E.; Asua, J.; Abdeljelil, A.B.; Emparanza, J. Using a Modified Technology Acceptance Model to Evaluate Healthcare Professionals' Adoption of a New Telemonitoring System. *Telemed. E-Health* **2012**, *18*, 54–59. [CrossRef]
54. Kowitlawakul, Y. The Technology Acceptance Model: Predicting Nurses' Intention to Use Telemedicine Technology (eICU). *CIN Comput. Inform. Nurs.* **2011**, *29*, 411–418. [CrossRef] [PubMed]
55. Molfenter, T.; Roget, N.; Chaple, M.; Behlman, S.; Cody, O.; Hartzler, B.; Johnson, E.; Nichols, M.; Stilen, P.; Becker, S. Use of Telehealth in Substance Use Disorder Services During and After COVID-19: Online Survey Study. *JMIR Ment. Health* **2021**, *8*, e25835. [CrossRef] [PubMed]
56. Croteau, A.-M.; Vieru, D. Telemedicine Adoption by Different Groups of Physicians. In Proceedings of the 35th Annual Hawaii International Conference on System Sciences, Big Island, HI, USA, 10 January 2002; pp. 1985–1993.
57. Cilliers, L.; Flowerday, S. User Acceptance of Telemedicine by Health Care Workers A Case of the Eastern Cape Province, South Africa. *Electron. J. Inf. Syst. Dev. Ctries.* **2014**, *65*, 1–10. [CrossRef]
58. Mohammed, R.; Elmajid, E.A.; Amine, H.; Khadija, C. Acceptance Factors of Telemedicine Technology during COVID-19 Pandemic among Health Professionals: A Qualitative Study. *Healthc. Technol. Lett.* **2023**, *10*, 23–33. [CrossRef]

59. Olver, I.N.; Selva-Nayagam, S. Evaluation of a Telemedicine Link Between Darwin and Adelaide to Facilitate Cancer Management. *Telemed. J.* **2000**, *6*, 213–218. [CrossRef] [PubMed]
60. Achim, N.; Kassim, A.A. Computer Usage: The Impact of Computer Anxiety and Computer Self-Efficacy. *Procedia Soc. Behav. Sci.* **2015**, *172*, 701–708. [CrossRef]
61. Venkatesh, V.; Morris, M.G.; Davis, G.B.; Davis, F.D. User Acceptance of Information Technology: Toward a Unified View. *MIS Q.* **2003**, *27*, 425. [CrossRef]
62. Korkut Altuna, O.; Arslan, F.M. Impact of the Number of Scale Points on Data Characteristics and Respondents' Evaluations: An Experimental Design Approach Using 5-Point and 7-Point Likert-Type Scales. *İstanbul Üniversitesi Siyasal Bilgiler Fakültesi Derg.* **2016**. [CrossRef]
63. Finstad, K. Response Interpolation and Scale Sensitivity: Evidence Against 5-Point Scales. *J. Usability Stud.* **2010**, *5*, 104–110.
64. Jöreskog, K.G.; Wold, H.O.A. (Eds.) *Systems under Indirect Observation: Causality, Structure, Prediction*; Contributions to economic analysis; North-Holland: Amsterdam, The Netherlands; Sole distributors for the U.S.A. and Canada: New York, NY, USA; Elsevier Science Publishers: New York, NY, USA, 1982; ISBN 978-0-444-86301-0.
65. Ioniță, A.; Rădoi, M.F.; Gusicov, D.M.; Anca, M. Activitatea Rețelei Sanitare Și de Ocrotire a Sănătății 2023. Available online: https://insse.ro/cms/ro/content/activitatea-re%C8%9Belei-sanitare-%C8%99i-de-ocrotire-s%C4%83n%C4%83t%C4%83%C8%9Bii-%C3%AEn-anul-2023 (accessed on 12 June 2024).
66. lege5.ro. ANEXA Nr II | Lege 153/2017. 2023. Available online: https://lege5.ro/Gratuit/ge3dkmzyga3a/anexa-nr-ii-lege-153-2017?dp=giydanzzga3dmny (accessed on 13 June 2024).
67. Shrestha, N. Factor Analysis as a Tool for Survey Analysis. *AJAMS* **2021**, *9*, 4–11. [CrossRef]
68. Cortina, J.M. What Is Coefficient Alpha? An Examination of Theory and Applications. *J. Appl. Psychol.* **1993**, *78*, 98–104. [CrossRef]
69. Fornell, C.; Larcker, D.F. Evaluating Structural Equation Models with Unobservable Variables and Measurement Error. *J. Mark. Res.* **1981**, *18*, 39–50. [CrossRef]
70. Kennedy, P. *A Guide to Econometrics*, 6th ed.; Blackwell Pub: Malden, MA, USA, 2008; ISBN 978-1-4051-8258-4.
71. Rönkkö, M.; Cho, E. An Updated Guideline for Assessing Discriminant Validity. *Organ. Res. Methods* **2022**, *25*, 6–14. [CrossRef]
72. Henseler, J.; Ringle, C.M.; Sinkovics, R.R. The Use of Partial Least Squares Path Modeling in International Marketing. In *Advances in International Marketing*; Sinkovics, R.R., Ghauri, P.N., Eds.; Emerald Group Publishing Limited: Bingley, UK, 2009; Volume 20, pp. 277–319. ISBN 978-1-84855-468-9.
73. Hair, J.F. (Ed.) *Multivariate Data Analysis*, 7th ed.; Prentice Hall: Upper Saddle River, NJ, USA, 2010; ISBN 978-0-13-813263-7.
74. Hair, J.F.; Hult, G.T.M.; Ringle, C.M.; Sarstedt, M.; Danks, N.P.; Ray, S. *Partial Least Squares Structural Equation Modeling (PLS-SEM) Using R: A Workbook*; Classroom Companion: Business; Springer International Publishing: Cham, Switzerland, 2021, ISBN 978-3-030-80518-0.
75. Kock, N.; Lynn, G. Lateral Collinearity and Misleading Results in Variance-Based SEM: An Illustration and Recommendations. *JAIS* **2012**, *13*, 546–580. [CrossRef]
76. Kock, N. WarpPLS User Manual: Version 8.0. Laredo. 2023. Available online: https://scriptwarp.com/warppls/UserManual_v_8_0.pdf (accessed on 24 April 2023).
77. Kock, N. Common Structural Variation Reduction in PLS-SEM: Replacement Analytic Composites and the One Fourth Rule. *Data Anal. Perspect. J.* **2021**, *2*, 1–6.
78. Zin, K.S.L.T.; Kim, S.; Kim, H.-S.; Feyissa, I.F. A Study on Technology Acceptance of Digital Healthcare among Older Korean Adults Using Extended Tam (Extended Technology Acceptance Model). *Adm. Sci.* **2023**, *13*, 42. [CrossRef]
79. Kohnke, A.; Cole, M.L.; Bush, R. Incorporating UTAUT Predictors for Understanding Home Care Patients' and Clinician's Acceptance of Healthcare Telemedicine Equipment. *J. Technol. Manag. Innov.* **2014**, *9*, 29–41. [CrossRef]
80. Ruiz Morilla, M.D.; Sans, M.; Casasa, A.; Giménez, N. Implementing Technology in Healthcare: Insights from Physicians. *BMC Med. Inf. Decis. Mak.* **2017**, *17*, 92. [CrossRef] [PubMed]
81. Ly, B.A.; Kristjansson, E.; Labonté, R.; Bourgeault, I.L. Determinants of the Intention of Senegal's Physicians to Use Telemedicine in Their Professional Activities. *Telemed. E-Health* **2018**, *24*, 897–898. [CrossRef] [PubMed]
82. Conner, M.; Armitage, C.J. Extending the Theory of Planned Behavior: A Review and Avenues for Further Research. *J. Appl. Soc. Pyschol.* **1998**, *28*, 1429–1464. [CrossRef]
83. Garavand, A.; Samadbeik, M.; Nadri, H.; Rahimi, B.; Asadi, H. Effective Factors in Adoption of Mobile Health Applications between Medical Sciences Students Using the UTAUT Model. *Methods Inf. Med.* **2019**, *58*, 131–139. [CrossRef] [PubMed]
84. Cohen, J.; Bancilhon, J.-M.; Jones, M. South African Physicians' Acceptance of e-Prescribing Technology: An Empirical Test of a Modified UTAUT Model. *SACJ* **2013**, *50*, 43–54. [CrossRef]
85. Lee, C.; Wan, G. Including Subjective Norm and Technology Trust in the Technology Acceptance Model: A Case of e-Ticketing in China. *SIGMIS Database* **2010**, *41*, 40–51. [CrossRef]
86. Hofstede Insights. Country Comparison Tool 2023. Available online: https://www.hofstede-insights.com/country-comparison-tool (accessed on 30 May 2024).
87. Hofstede, G.; Hofstede, G.J.; Minkov, M. *Cultures and Organizations: Software of the Mind: Intercultural Cooperation and Its Importance for Survival*; Revised and expanded third edition; McGraw-Hill: New York, NY, USA, 2010; ISBN 978-0-07-177015-6.
88. *European Observatory on Health Systems and Policies State of Health in the EU: Romania*; The European Commission: Brussels, Belgium, 2017.

89. Alhur, A. An Exploration of Nurses' Perceptions of the Usefulness and Easiness of Using EMRs. *J. Public Health Sci.* **2023**, *2*, 20–31. [CrossRef]
90. CNAS Ce Este Dosarul Electronic de Sănatate? 2023. Available online: http://www.des-cnas.ro/pub/ (accessed on 12 June 2024).
91. Constitutional Court of Romania. Decizia Nr.498 Din 17 Iulie 2018 Referitoare La Excepția de Neconstituționalitate a Dispozițiilor Art.30 Alin.(2) Și (3), Precum Și a Sintagmei "sistemul Dosarului Electronic de Sănătate al Pacientului" Din Cuprinsul Art.280 Alin.(2) Din Legea Nr.95/2006. 2018. Available online: https://legislatie.just.ro/Public/DetaliiDocumentAfis/203149 (accessed on 13 June 2024).
92. Șomănescu, C. Dosarul Electronic de Sănătate, Un Şir Lung de Rateuri la Doi Ani Şi Jumătate de Când e Obligatoriu. Economica.net. 2019. Available online: https://www.economica.net/dosar-electronic-de-sanatate-al-pacietului-probleme-si-beneficii_168361.html (accessed on 12 June 2024).
93. CNAS COMUNICAT. Dosarul Electronic de Sănătate a Redevenit Funcțional. CNAS. 2021. Available online: https://cnas.ro/2021/12/22/comunicat-dosarul-electronic-de-sanatate-a-redevenit-functional/ (accessed on 12 June 2024).
94. Borcea, Ș. Dosarul Electronic al Pacientului, Un Instrument Util, Dar Ignorat de Spitale. Ce Spun Autoritățile. adevarul.ro. 26 November 2022. Available online: https://adevarul.ro/stiri-interne/societate/dosarul-electronic-al-pacientului-un-instrument-2223162.html (accessed on 12 June 2024).
95. European Commission. *Commission Staff Working Document: 2023 Country Report—Romania*; European Commission: Brussels, Belgium, 2023.
96. Ajzen, I. From Intentions to Actions: A Theory of Planned Behavior. In *Action Control*; Kuhl, J., Beckmann, J., Eds.; Springer: Berlin/Heidelberg, Germany, 1985; pp. 11–39. ISBN 978-3-642-69748-7.
97. Nov, O.; Ye, C. Resistance to Change and the Adoption of Digital Libraries: An Integrative Model. *J. Am. Soc. Inf. Sci.* **2009**, *60*, 1702–1708. [CrossRef]
98. Adenuga, K.I.; Iahad, N.A.; Miskon, S. Towards Reinforcing Telemedicine Adoption amongst Clinicians in Nigeria. *Int. J. Med. Inform.* **2017**, *104*, 84–96. [CrossRef] [PubMed]
99. Glaser, J. Financial Incentives for Healthcare IT Adoption. *Healthc. Financ. Manag.* **2007**, *61*, 118–120.
100. Chaix-Couturier, C.; Durand-Zaleski, I.; Jolly, D.; Durieux, P. Effects of Financial Incentives on Medical Practice: Results from a Systematic Review of the Literature and Methodological Issues. *Int. J. Qual. Health Care* **2000**, *12*, 133–142. [CrossRef] [PubMed]
101. Gagnon, M.-P.; Desmartis, M.; Labrecque, M.; Car, J.; Pagliari, C.; Pluye, P.; Frémont, P.; Gagnon, J.; Tremblay, N.; Légaré, F. Systematic Review of Factors Influencing the Adoption of Information and Communication Technologies by Healthcare Professionals. *J. Med. Syst.* **2012**, *36*, 241–277. [CrossRef]
102. Iftimoaei, C. Aspecte Sociodemografice Privind Calitatea Vieții În Mediul Rural. In *Provocări Rurale Contemporane. Studii de Agro-economie și Antropologie Rurală*; Presa Universitară Clujeană: Cluj-Napoca, Romania, 2021; pp. 39–55. ISBN 978-606-37-1280-7.
103. Lee, H.Y.; Kanthawala, S.; Choi, E.Y.; Kim, Y.S. Rural and Non-Rural Digital Divide Persists in Older Adults: Internet Access, Usage, and Attitudes toward Technology. *Gerontechnology* **2021**, *20*, 1–9. [CrossRef]
104. MINISTERUL SĂNĂTĂȚII. 131 de Spitale Dotate Cu Sistem de Telemedicină Pentru Serviciul de Urgență. 2023. Available online: https://www.ms.ro/ro/centrul-de-presa/131-de-spitale-dotate-cu-sistem-de-telemedicin%C4%83-pentru-serviciul-de-urgen%C8%9B%C4%83/ (accessed on 19 May 2024).

healthcare

MDPI

Article

Telehealth Outreach Program for Child Traumatic Stress: Strategies for Long-Term Sustainability

Emily Johnson [1,*], Ryan Kruis [2], Rosaura Orengo-Aguayo [3], Rebecca Verdin [2], Kathryn King [4], Dee Ford [5] and Regan Stewart [6]

[1] College of Nursing, Medical University of South Carolina, Charleston, SC 29425, USA
[2] Center for Telehealth, Medical University of South Carolina, Charleston, SC 29425, USA
[3] Department of Psychiatry and Behavioral Sciences, National Crime Victims Research and Treatment Center, Medical University of South Carolina, Charleston, SC 29425, USA
[4] Department of Pediatrics, Center for Telehealth, Medical University of South Carolina, Charleston, SC 29425, USA
[5] Department of Pulmonary and Critical Care Medicine, Center for Telehealth, Medical University of South Carolina, Charleston, SC 29425, USA
[6] Department of Psychiatry and Behavioral Sciences, Mental Health Disparities and Diversity Division, Medical University of South Carolina, Charleston, SC 29425, USA
* Correspondence: johnsoem@musc.edu

Abstract: Background: There are high documented rates of exposure to traumatic events and mental health disorders among youths yet existing disparities in access to care for racial and ethnic minority youths and youths in rural communities. Trauma-Focused Cognitive Behavioral Therapy (TF-CBT) is an evidence-based behavioral health therapy for children. The delivery of TF-CBT via telehealth can decrease access to care barriers. An interdisciplinary clinical team developed a training program to guide clinicians to effectively provide TF-CBT via telehealth. The goal of this study was to describe variation in implementation processes of the telehealth TF-CBT program and identify barriers and facilitators to program implementation post-training, which were utilized to develop implementation strategies for intervention sustainability. Methods: Using a mixed-methods approach, data were collected on telehealth implementation processes and facilitators and barriers to the delivery of telehealth TF-CBT. This study was guided by an adapted implementation science framework, namely the Exploration, Preparation, Implementation, Sustainment model. Interviews and surveys were completed with clinical site leaders who had participated in the telehealth TF-CBT training. Results: Throughout clinical sites, there was varied adoption and penetration of the telehealth TF-CBT program. Facilitators to implementation included leadership and site staff buy in, community needs, and training resources, while barriers included funding, available logistical resources, and child and family involvement. Conclusions: The feedback gained from this project assisted in the development of implementation strategies for increased adoption and sustainment of TF-CBT delivered via telehealth. Strategies include ongoing interactive assistance and resource support, enhanced training for stakeholders, and program adaptations, with the goal to increase access to quality mental health care for underserved populations.

Keywords: trauma care; disparities; implementation evaluation; implementation strategy; telehealth

1. Introduction

Childhood trauma is prevalent and can have significant lifelong effects on children and their families and communities. It is estimated that 34 million children, nearly half of all children in the United States, have experienced at least one trauma in their lives, and at least 16 million have experienced more than one type of traumatic event [1,2]. Research on the relationship between adverse childhood experiences and adult health outcomes shows strong connections between stress and trauma in childhood and serious long-term behavioral and physical health outcomes, including post-traumatic stress disorder (PTSD), depression, anxiety disorders, substance use, and physical health problems [3–5].

Children living in rural communities are particularly vulnerable to trauma effects because of geographic isolation, poverty, and lack of access to mental health services [6]. Despite high rates of trauma exposure and subsequent mental health outcomes, many children in need of mental health care still do not receive it or do not receive evidence-based care [7–9]. Even greater disparities in access to care are seen across geographies (rural locations) and among racial and ethnic minority youths and those whose primary language is not English [10–12].

For many years, telehealth (also tele-mental health, telemedicine, and telepsychology) has offered an innovative way to address gaps in care access. Telehealth can reduce barriers to care for populations that need mental health treatment but may not typically receive it due to a lack of available providers or the costs associated with traveling to appointments [7]. In addition to distance and time barriers, children and families also report that they utilize telehealth to decrease mental health care stigma by connecting with providers via child-friendly locations such as schools and primary care centers [13]. Current research provides support that mental health services delivered via telehealth are effective in addressing numerous mental health disorders in children and adolescents, including PTSD [13–16].

Trauma-Focused Cognitive Behavioral Therapy (TF-CBT) is an evidence-based, manualized treatment protocol designed to treat post-traumatic stress and co-occurring symptoms such as depression and anxiety in trauma-exposed children aged 3–18 [17]. Over 23 randomized controlled trials across the U.S. and worldwide have documented TF-CBT's effectiveness in treating post-traumatic stress symptoms in children and adolescents [17,18]. TF-CBT has also been shown to be feasible and effective when delivered via telehealth to trauma-exposed youths, including racial/ethnic minority youths and youths in rural locations, via published case studies and open pilot feasibility trials [19–22].

Prior studies have illustrated that while tele-mental health programs are beneficial to patient outcomes [23] and improving access to care [24], implementation can be complex and challenging [24]. Implementation science methods can identify barriers and facilitators to tele-mental health program adoption [25] and thus guide strategies to improve the widespread implementation of these programs. This is one of the first studies to utilize implementation science methods to comprehensively and systematically identify barriers and facilitators to a telehealth TF-CBT program and identify potential strategies to improve implementation outcomes.

The objective of this study was to describe variation in implementation processes of an innovative telehealth TF-CBT training program, the Telehealth Outreach Program for Traumatic Stress (TOP-TS), and identify barriers and facilitators to program implementation, which can be utilized to develop implementation strategies for program sustainability.

2. Materials and Methods

This study was classified as quality improvement and did not require review by the Institutional Review Board. The Consolidated Criteria for Reporting Qualitative Research (COREQ) guided methods and results reporting [26].

2.1. Implementation Science Framework

The Exploration, Preparation, Implementation, Sustainment (EPIS) model was utilized to guide this study] after adaptation to the TF-CBT setting [27,28]. The EPIS model includes outer and inner contextual factors and bridging and innovation factors that affect implementation processes and outcomes. In the TF-CBT telehealth setting, outer factors are external to sites delivering TF-CBT (regulatory/legal standards, community demand, and funding), while inner factors are within sites (resources, leadership, and clinician and patient characteristics) and can serve as facilitators or barriers to implementation. Innovation factors are specific to the TF-CBT program (fit and complexity), while bridging factors link inner, outer, and innovation factors (collaborative engagement of the training site and clinical sites) (Figure 1).

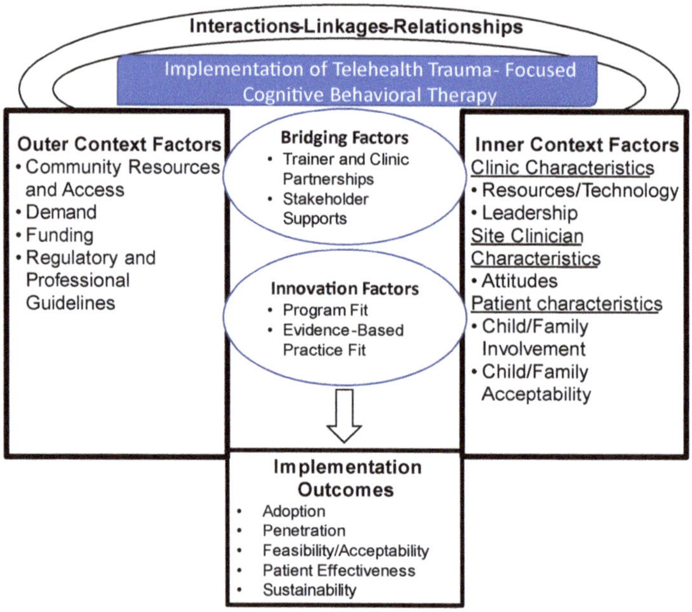

Figure 1. Framework for implementation of telehealth Trauma-Focused Cognitive Behavioral Therapy.

2.2. The Telehealth Outreach Program for Traumatic Stress (TOP-TS)

The TOP-TS was developed in 2015 by an interdisciplinary team of clinicians at a medical university. This program provides TF-CBT via telehealth modalities for underserved youths (racial/ethnic minorities, rural communities, and low socioeconomic status) in the United States and Puerto Rico. In addition to TF-CBT clinical services, the TOP-TS team provides education, training, and technical assistance and resources to mental health workforces delivering TF-CBT via telehealth in child advocacy centers, community mental health clinics, schools, hospitals, juvenile justice agencies, and other child-serving agencies targeting rural and underserved trauma-exposed youths and families in the US and Puerto Rico. A typical training program for instruction in the telehealth delivery of TF-CBT includes two live online sessions (average of 210 min each) completed via a live interactive webinar using videoconferencing software. Each training session includes an overview of TF-CBT treatment components, tips for telehealth treatment delivery, descriptions of additional resources available in shared online folders, and time for discussion. Follow-up consultation calls are available as an opportunity for participants to discuss challenges to TF-CBT delivery via telehealth post-training and implementation.

2.3. Participants

Study participants were mental health providers who attended TOP-TS live training sessions for delivering TF-CBT via telehealth within the prior two years. Participation in training within the past two years served as the cut-off for inclusion criteria to improve recall validity of participants specific to clinical experiences post-training. In addition, the TF-CBT telehealth training curriculum was developed during the explosion of telehealth services during the COVID-19 pandemic in 2020, with training sessions initiating in late 2020. Thus, when recruiting participants for the study (2022–2023), the majority of potential mental health care providers would have completed the program within the prior two years. An email invitation to complete an online self-report survey on telehealth utilization was sent to these providers. This email also asked participants if they would like to be contacted to complete a semi-structured interview, and these participants were then contacted to schedule the interview.

2.4. Data Collection

An 8-item quantitative and qualitative investigator-initiated self-report survey was developed to gain exploratory data on TF-CBT utilization via telehealth. Quantitative questions included the number and dates of training sessions attended, number of patients seen via telehealth in six months following training, and number of patients currently seen via telehealth. Qualitative questions were framed to identify potential facilitators and barriers to telehealth integration within sites. These open-ended questions asked clinicians to define advantageous components to launching and continuing the utilization of telehealth and provided space to report challenges to telehealth utilization in their practices. An additional question asked for the identification and description of any needed resources or support for initial and ongoing telehealth implementation [Supplementary Materials]. The survey was pilot tested with two providers who had completed the TF-CBT telehealth training over two years prior (and thus were not eligible for the study), and verbiage was edited based on their feedback. The survey email invitation was sent to 102 mental health providers who were potential participants, and then the same survey was also sent to all interview participants after they completed an interview (if they had not previously completed the survey). The survey link opened via a webpage to a Redcap database. The 8 questions were all located on one screen, and participants scrolled down to answer all questions. Average time for completion was 8–12 min. There were no missing data as each question required a response and no identifying information was collected in the survey responses. The survey remained open from 15 July 2022 to 27 April 2023. Reminder emails for survey completion were sent four times over this time frame. All survey respondents received a USD 20 gift card for completion.

A comprehensive semi-structured interview guide with standardized questions and probes was created based on initial exploratory survey results and the identified contextual factors relevant to the telehealth TF-CBT program in the adapted EPIS model. Interview questions corresponded to the outer, inner, bridging, and innovation factors in the EPIS model with additional probing questions created based on exploratory survey results. Two post-graduate trained female interviewers (RV, MHA; EJ, PhD) not involved in the delivery of the TF-CBT program completed individual interviews via telephone in April 2023. Verbal consent from participants was provided prior to beginning interviews, and interview participants received a USD 25 gift card for participation. Interviews lasted between 21 and 32 min, and field notes were taken during and immediately following each interview. Theme saturation was sought with several methods. The interviews included a set of participants with a range of experience and utilization levels with telehealth TF-CBT methods. This allowed for comprehensive coverage of EPIS domains and a wider range of understanding of factors affecting implementation. Data collection methods during the interviews supported probing, which permitted participant reports of additional factors affecting implementation. Lastly, ongoing monitoring of field notes after each interview supported theme saturation after interview completion [29].

2.5. Data Analysis

Interviews were transcribed verbatim, and NVIVO software (http://www.lumivero.com/ accessed on 10 January 2023). [30] was utilized for data analysis. NVIVO software enhances organization for the qualitative coding process as it permits users to efficiently code data, classify and sort themes, and share files across platforms. A combined inductive and deductive template analysis approach was utilized [31,32] with an initial codebook developed from the adapted EPIS model [27,28]. The initial codebook included codes based on operational definitions of EPIS domains of outer, inner, bridging, and innovation factors as well as codes for implementation outcomes and strategies.

Two coders independently applied the codebook to two interview transcripts and then met to discuss coding discrepancies. After discussion, two additional codes were created, and two codes were collapsed based on clarifying definitions in the EPIS model. The codebook was then utilized by the two coders independently to code the rest of the interview transcripts, with regular meetings between the coders taking place each time two additional transcripts were coded.

3. Results

3.1. Survey

Of the initial survey request, 10 surveys were completed, and 5 additional surveys were completed later by the interview participants. Thirteen participants (87%) that completed the survey reported currently seeing patients via telehealth with an average of 8 current telehealth patients (range of 2–40 current telehealth patients).

The participants' open-ended responses identified facilitators to telehealth utilization for TF-CBT post-training, which included access to training materials, insurance reimbursement, tablets made available for patients, shorter treatment sessions, ability to screen share, flexibility for scheduling, technology support, an existing telehealth platform, and supportive leadership. The open-ended responses identified barriers to telehealth utilization for TF-CBT, which included a lack of patient technology and connectivity issues, lack of space for telehealth equipment, internet connections, summer/non-routine schedules for children, patient resistance to online modalities, and patient distraction/confidentiality concerns. Suggested resources to improve telehealth utilization included resources for teenagers, resources for children with disabilities, assistance with insurance verification, stronger internet connection, technology assistance (help with internet connection and supplies—such as loaned tablets, ear buds, and hot spots), and supply boxes to mail items to patients.

3.2. Interviews

Eight female mental health provider clinicians completed interviews, and of these participants, six reported actively performing telehealth visits for TF-CBT. Five participants worked as clinicians in a child advocacy center, two worked for non-profit outpatient mental health facilities, and one worked for private mental health practice. The clinicians had been working in their current roles and facilities for a range of one year to eight years.

Interview Results—Barriers and Facilitators to TF-CBT Implementation

Table 1 displays the barriers and facilitators to the implementation of TF-CBT via telehealth as reported by the interview participants.

Table 1. Exemplary quotations: barriers and facilitators to TF-CBT implementation via telehealth.

External Factors		
Code	**Definition**	**Quotations**
Community Resources/Access	Patient and family barriers to accessing physician offices (for in-person counseling visits) and resources needed for telehealth visits	"I think because of our population. . .it is a rural area and it's very spread out, so we have a lot of transportation barriers. . .If they did have transportation, getting gas money to come to sessions, that was a barrier." (Clinician 7) "We get to access communities we couldn't access if we didn't have telehealth, like the Spanish-speaking community. We don't find a lot of bilingual clinicians across the state, so just having ability to connect with them via telehealth. . .breaks that barrier of them not getting services." (Clinician 2) "I do face one challenge. . .is their access to just the technology portion, access to devices where they can connect to telehealth services. And of course, everyone has a phone, but not everyone has access to internet from home." (Clinician 2) "So sometimes the connections work. . .they don't always work well, or just noise or distraction. . .and trying to get them into a quiet place." (Clinician 1)

Table 1. *Cont.*

External Factors		
Code	**Definition**	**Quotations**
Regulatory and Professional Guidelines	Policies related to telehealth, including reimbursement policies	"So our site, with our funding and so forth, preferred to have in person, and just with reimbursements. If it has to be telehealth, it has to be a video call on a certain platform. So they prefer in person, but sometimes there is a reason or an ability to do telehealth." (Clinician 1)
Bridging Factors		
Trainer and Clinic Partnerships	Operational style telehealth training team, strategies for support provision, and involvement of clinicians in training and implementation processes	"The trainers were excellent. . .very knowledgeable. They were top in their field, and really had a lot of good insights, even clinically some tools of what to do, how to help kids, how to get them to open up. . .how to continue to focus on the TF-CBT. They were very skilled and very helpful." (Clinician 1) "I liked that I could always access [trainers], especially once I start seeing clients, and just for their knowledge base within the systems already." (Clinician 4) ". . . just their experience. . .They've been doing it a lot. . .have great experience with different things that worked and didn't work and what pitfalls can happen. . ." (Clinician 6) "I also like that they went through a trauma narrative. . .we're going to write it together, so they can see it as it's being written, just like they would in the office. So really trying to mirror an office experience to what they're getting in telehealth." (Clinician 4) "They were always happy and willing for us to email them and ask questions. The consultation calls were really helpful, so we could problem solve together and talk about cases that we were having issues with. . ." (Clinician 5) "The [consultation calls] were helpful, because I was able to connect with other clinicians, and in a sense offer me some normalizing, that a lot of my challenges were also faced by other clinicians. And then sharing resources, sharing ways of doing things among each other, and obtaining guidance from the trainers on how to implement certain services." (Clinician 2) "I think it was good. And then having the length of time was really good. And then having the calls afterwards so if we had questions and being able to build on what we have learned over the course of them working through the practice skills of TF-CBT. And providing and showing different resources that were available to us, maybe that we hadn't had time to play around with, was very helpful. And them being able to bounce ideas off of each other about what was working for us, what wasn't working for us, and getting feedback from our peers." (Clinician 3)
Innovation Factors		
Program Fit	Degree to which telehealth training and TF- CBT program (content and complexities) match and fit goals, values, and tasks of clinic and staff	"It was very clear, many resources, many ideas, ways to interact with people via telehealth, and many of those were very practical and useful with in person therapy as well." (Clinician 1) "I think it's still going to continue to be needed, be used. And it helps many people that live far, especially in rural areas, or even city areas, where transportation and time is different. Our culture is people want things quick, fast, close, convenient kind of thing, and it fits that." (Clinician 1) "I thought it was great, it followed our practice of care. It gave us an outline for safety, like for those steps in creating what needed to happen to create the [program]; how we can get in touch with people and what was needed and required to provide the services." (Clinician 6)

Table 1. *Cont.*

Code	Definition	Quotations
External Factors		
Evidence-Based Practice Fit	Degree to which TF-CBT practices are feasible in site settings and perceptions about advantages and complexity of child trauma care delivered over telehealth	"With older kiddos, I had all sorts of great success, definitely. . .the treatment we provide has been just as successful as if it was face to face. I have families I've been able to engage very well through telehealth, and I have never met them in person. It's all been through video calls." (Clinician 2) ". . .doesn't necessarily work with the little ones. We have tried unsuccessfully. So I'm going to say in the five to seven age range, it's really hard for a child to connect fully on a video call. So that has been a barrier for me. . .So I'd rather see those children in person." (Clinician 2) "So far I've not seen any younger kiddos. But. . .I'm a people person as I like to have a person in front of me. I've struggled with initial building rapport. . .it feels a little less personal. I don't know if it's just me or if the kiddo's. . .maybe picked it up from me, or if they feel it as well. . ." (Clinician 3) ". . .I think that was and is my biggest concern with dealing with trauma with kids. I want to make sure that the rapport is there before we move into the heavy stuff. And I think it's harder through telehealth to build that rapport." (Clinician 3) "No, not totally successful. I think there have been some gains for my clients, but for the most part that connection is missing. And the ability to build trust that you need to be able to do, like the trauma narrative, is less than it would be if it was in person. . ." (Clinician 8) "But the connection piece I think, is the biggest piece. I think that it's easier to do things together when you're in the room together. . ." (Clinician 8) "In case for some reason they are needing additional support than what I can give them virtually. . ." (Clinician 4)
Inner Factors		
Resources/Technology	Level of resources and technology dedicated to adoption and ongoing telehealth operations; includes resources provided by training team	"I'm hoping as soon as we can get technology secured that I can go ahead and move forward with trying it with a client. . .I just need technology so I can try it." (Clinician 4) "Because it's not always a set place. But I've got to just make sure I get into a quiet room, clean background, and that I'm not distracted." (Clinician 1) "I like some of the protocols they had for emergencies. Make sure you know where the house is, address, location, what room the kid's in, that a parent is there, which is smart if you're doing exclusive telehealth, and dealing with someone in trauma. That just seems to be a very smart protocol that I wouldn't necessarily have thought of." (Clinician 1) "It was just so helpful, especially because I provide a lot of services in Spanish. . .they even provided a folder with resources in Spanish language. . .that was incredibly helpful for me and the other bilingual clinician. . .we didn't have that much in our agency for Spanish only." (Clinician 2)
Leadership	For implementation of TF-CBT telehealth program: leader commitment, involvement, and accountability	"I did talk with her. . .and she thought it would be a great idea to do [the training], since it is something that we're looking to build and increase, just so that we can see more of the clients that we're missing because of not being able to see everybody in office." (Clinician 3) "Oh, absolutely! The director. . .is very supportive. She's from a clinical background and very supportive of any kind of mental health that needs to be done. And the executive director was a therapist when the agency started, she's very supportive as well. And the clinical director is also supportive. And so we have a lot of people in upper management that are supportive, and then lots of staff that are supported as well." (Clinician 8) "She's opening up more and trying to help us do [telehealth] even though she still likes in-person. . .She knows sometimes [in-person therapy] is not realistic." (Clinician 7)

Table 1. *Cont.*

External Factors		
Code	**Definition**	**Quotations**
Clinician Attitudes	Site staff (clinicians) readiness to participate in TF-CBT telehealth training and attitudes, knowledge of TF-CBT telehealth program; competence and beliefs in capabilities to achieve implementation goals	"…that engagement portion, and then feeling a part of it, I find that it's really important to be able to offer them something very similar to what they would have got if they were in person." (Clinician 4) "It's like a definite backup option, so there's no reason to really not do therapy." (Clinician 8) "I think there's a time and a place for it. My preference is in person, just being able to see and be with them in person….and with our funding and so forth, preferred to have in person, and just with reimbursements. (Clinician 1) "I think there's willingness, but I think there's also a little bit of hesitation on the way that the client is going to respond. I think most of my coworkers prefer the face to face option." (Clinician 2) "At first, it [TF-CBT telehealth] wasn't something they were even looking at. And then I went through this training…then they became more open to the idea of offering telehealth, because they had wanted everything in person…. having those resources was very eye-opening for them, and opened the door to the idea of offering telehealth" (Clinician 4)
Child/Family Involvement	Degree to which family members and children are supportive and involved in TF-CBT telehealth program; includes involvement barriers and strategies to make program work more smoothly/be more feasible for families	"The fact that they show up, which means that there's some parental support, to making sure that they have the equipment ready, and that they're on time, and that it's a priority." (Clinician 5) "So [parent involvement] seems good, for the most part. The follow-up sometimes is via text or something else with them after, just kind of summing it up. It doesn't mean you can always get the parents after the call, or even at the beginning of the call. You know, it just, the phone passes off really quickly…trying to incorporate and keep parents involved is important, and that's a little bit of a struggle." (Clinician 1) "I have found that if I have the proper resources with activities for them, then they're more engaged, if it involves games, if it involves sort of virtual activities, where they can participate. Then they get to be more involved." (Clinician 2) "…as far as my teenagers, and even fifth graders, some of them, it is really easy to do [telehealth] with them. The attention span was longer…" (Clinician 7) "I wish I could have a little bit more involvement, but this is the nature of the beast anyway, because even with in-person, trying to get them the buy-in for them to participate, that can be a struggle. I guess it doesn't make really a difference if it was telehealth or not, whether or not they choose or how much they want to participate, the parent or guardian." (Clinician 7) "…explaining the model, and getting some buy-in from the parents, and helping them understand what the model is going to look like, and that we're going to do these things over telehealth…" (Clinician 5) "…and just kind of selling it. A lot of parents…when they hear I have to be home when they're doing the service or because it's …in the house. But then someone has to be there, or I have to be there, then it's not as inviting I think sometimes. But I think selling it more might help." (Clinician 6) "I don't think that children under the age of 8 or 9 or 10 should really be on telehealth because they have a hard time focusing. A lot of times parents will leave them alone in the room with their device…And their ability to participate on telehealth is really important. So there are kiddos who experience trauma but also experience ADHD, probably not going to recommend that they do telehealth because they're not going to focus. It's hard enough to work with them in a room." (Clinician 8)
Child/Family Acceptability	Perceived child/family value about health and well-being; degree to which program is satisfactory to children/families in participating sites; also includes strategies to make program more acceptable for families	"I think they appreciate it, because it does allow us to see kids and not keep them on a waitlist because of not having those evening [appointments] open. We're able to get them in much sooner by offering telehealth option…with the cost of gas it's much more time and cost-saving as well, because they're not having to drive an hour to come in for a session and then drive an hour home. So it's saving them that way." (Clinician 3) "The kids seem to like it… 50 min is long to keep their attention. Sometimes you get that personal feel with the kids. They'll show you their room or their house, maybe some artwork that they're working on…So that's kind of fun. Sometimes we do origami…like a simple little folding kind of pattern, making a little boat or something that has a little story to it. So it seems like they like that." (Clinician 1) "And then also the kids can be much more at ease because they're in a place that they know and they're already comfortable with." (Clinician 3) "And I think for the adolescent group, some of them actually prefer to meet via telehealth more than in person, because they're in the comfort of their own home, or they can be in their space, in their room…they just enjoy that comfort of home. And I have seen them for a long time." (Clinician 2) "My teenagers love it…look forward to it. I don't have a lot of absenteeism with them…" (Clinician 7)

3.3. Outer Factors

Community Resources/Access and Demand: The clinician participants described significant challenges for children living in rural areas to access crucial TF-CBT services, including a lack of available parent transportation, the inability of parents to stay for in-person therapy visits with their child due to scheduling conflicts, and lack of parent or family prioritization for therapy visits. In addition, the clinicians noted that language barriers make it difficult for some patients to receive timely in-person therapy due to wait times for available interpreters. The site clinicians described TF-CBT delivered via telehealth as a means to overcome these access barriers and meet the demand for this therapy in rural communities. However, the participants noted that offering therapy via telehealth also presents new access challenges including some families lacking stable Wi-Fi connections and electronic devices in homes to conduct telehealth visits. Additionally, background noise and other distractions were noted as an obstacle to the delivery of TF-CBT via telehealth in patients' homes.

Funding and Regulatory/Professional Guidelines: Regulatory policies related to funding, telehealth reimbursement, and professional practice were noted as ongoing barriers to the implementation of TF-CBT via telehealth, as there have been limitations from insurance companies on reimbursements for certain telehealth services. In addition, some clinical sites lack supplies needed for comprehensive telehealth operations, such as electronic tablets. Some clinicians reported that they had received grant funding for needed supplies, while others were considering grant proposals in the upcoming year to fund these resources. A lack of clear protocols to ensure HIPAA compliance and sound consent procedures when completing telehealth visits were also noted as ongoing complexities for telehealth visits.

3.4. Bridging Factors

Trainer and Clinic Partnerships: The collaborative and supportive nature of the experienced TF-CBT training team was described as vital to the telehealth training program. Trainers were noted to have a wealth of experience with TF-CBT telehealth delivery, as the participants stated that they were "insightful, knowledgeable, and top in their field" when sharing their expertise of effective care delivery across different populations. The comprehensive format of the training was also seen as beneficial as clinicians appreciated the resources provided in online shared folders, which included protocols and templates, therapy worksheets and games, videos for therapy sessions, and innovative therapy modalities. The training also provided hands-on examples of care delivery via telehealth. The participants valued the ability to contact the trainers via phone or email after the training sessions ended and valued ongoing communication and support provided as clinicians began and progressed with patient telehealth visits.

All participants agreed that the training program was an appropriate length of time, and they appreciated the condensed format which allowed for completion within a few months. The participants appreciated the format of consultation calls, which were provided as a post-training resource in which clinicians could join live online group sessions with trainers and other clinicians around the country that had recently completed the training. During the calls, the trainers provided additional updated resources for the delivery of TF-CBT via telehealth while allowing time for attendees to share experiences with patient telehealth visits. These calls allowed the clinicians to receive ongoing support and insights from the trainers and their peers.

Stakeholder Supports: In addition to the TF-CBT training team, the participants discussed other stakeholders that were key to the implementation of TF-CBT via telehealth. The steps of initiating and processing referrals needed for trauma-related counseling for children were described by varied processes, originating from child protective services, law enforcement agencies, other juvenile protective organizations, and family advocates. Family advocates work directly with families to assist with referrals for trauma care, discussions with the family to determine preferences for in-person or telehealth visits, scheduling, and identifying interpreters. School administrators and counselors were identified as key potential collaborators so clinicians could provide TF-CBT via telehealth during the school day to children, although medical and academic regulations and guidelines related to youths have been barriers to providing this care in schools. These intermediary organizations and staff were often noted as having a direct impact on volumes of children seen by the agency for TF-CBT.

3.5. Innovation Factors

Program Fit: The TF-CBT telehealth training program was described as an excellent fit for sites as the training met patient needs and site goals for providing TF-CBT care for rural communities. Although some participants reported that they had completed the training over a year prior, they continued to use the resources and knowledge learned and predicted continued utilization of the training content in the future.

Evidence-Based Practice Fit: Conversely, although the training was perceived as an excellent fit for site goals, the degree to which the TF-CBT methods were feasible via telehealth varied based on individual patient needs. Telehealth visits with teenage children were described as practical and very successful in providing TF-CBT as it was easier to engage older children via telehealth. However, telehealth sessions were deemed difficult to conduct with younger children and children with learning disabilities due to a lack of engagement with the screen modality and other complexities with this population. In addition, the clinicians reported a lack of 'connection' with patients when interacting through a screen and taking a longer time to create and build sustained rapport with their patients through telehealth. Several clinicians stated that the narrative component of TF-CBT is difficult to complete effectively via telehealth. There was also concern about children's need for more intensive trauma counseling care beyond what can be offered virtually via telehealth.

3.6. Inner Factors

Resources/Technology: A primary barrier to conducting telehealth visits was the availability of technology at sites, including laptops and tablets. Another challenge was identifying a quiet clean space with a professional background to conduct telehealth visits. Otherwise, resources were not identified as barriers for clinicians to conduct telehealth visits as the comprehensive training program provided the materials needed.

Resources were shared during the training and then stored as electronic documents in online shared folders so participants could access them at later dates. These documents included checklists for determining candidates for telehealth, protocols for emergencies, confidentiality and HIPAA compliance, templates for consent forms, check-in sheets to ensure an adult was present during visits, therapy worksheets, games and videos for utilization in therapy sessions, and online resources related to the conduct of TF-CBT components. Resources were also provided in Spanish. During the training sessions, the clinicians learned other essential concepts for conducting TF-CBT via telehealth including the importance of screen sharing, guidance on performing individual components of TF-CBT, such as a trauma narrative, cultural implications, and tips for how to build rapport and ensure children stay engaged. Introducing an innovative virtual relaxation room and other relaxation and coping skills were additional beneficial skills shared.

Leadership and Clinician Attitudes: There were mixed perceptions of leadership support within clinics for offering TF-CBT via telehealth to patients. Some sites reported initial and growing support over time from clinical and executive directors to offer telehealth services, as evidenced by encouragement to complete the telehealth training and the purchase of new equipment needed to offer telehealth services. Others felt that while their supervisors would support telehealth if needed, their preference was to provide in-person therapy visits. Similarly, site clinicians also had mixed preferences for offering TF-CBT via telehealth or in person. Some clinicians favored providing TF-CBT via telehealth and were committed to providing comparable services via telehealth as they do in person. Alternatively, some clinicians preferred in-person counseling visits because of reimbursement challenges with telehealth visits and the uncertainty of potential patient responses to the telehealth format. One clinician reported that team members and leadership at her site were initially not interested in offering TF-CBT via telehealth, but after she completed training and demonstrated the resources to the team, they became supportive and receptive to offering TF-CBT via telehealth.

Child/Family Involvement: There were varied observations of parent and child involvement with participation in TF-CBT via telehealth. Higher levels of family involvement were indirectly evident when younger children were present for telehealth appointments as a family member had set up the equipment for them at home and ensured they were logged in at the correct time. Some family members were cognizant to follow up with therapists, even via text, after telehealth visits. However, similar to in-person therapy visits, low parent and family involvement was also an ongoing challenge due to competing family demands and priorities. Explaining the telehealth model to parents was important to help them understand the format and potential benefits to their child. When family members were not present at home for the telehealth visits and children were left alone, therapists reported struggles with maintaining attention and engagement with the child. The training provided tips and games to introduce to children that had low engagement via telehealth modalities (children that turned off their screens or refused to speak), hence allowing them to overcome these challenges and make progress in treatment.

Child/Family Acceptability: The interviewees reported that the majority of families and patients appreciated the ability to conduct TF-CBT visits via telehealth. While participating in telehealth entails adjustment to a novel format, parents and family members appreciated that telehealth allows for appointments to be made sooner and saves them time and gas money from driving to appointments. Although at times, it was difficult to maintain the engagement of younger children for the entire telehealth visits, this population typically liked these visits because they felt comfortable in their own rooms and spaces which, at times, helped build a personal connection between the therapist and child as the child was able to demonstrate and share their room, art work, or other valued treasures via the screen. Teenagers typically favored the telehealth format as it allowed them flexibility to be on their own schedule and help with their younger siblings at home, as needed. One therapist described that she preferred meeting with all patients in person for the first visit to evaluate their preferences for visit format and determine feasibility for the telehealth format.

3.6.1. Interview Results—Implementation Outcomes and Potential Implementation Strategies for TF-CBT via Telehealth

Table 2 displays descriptions of implementation outcomes and potential implementation strategies for TF-CBT via telehealth, as reported by the interview participants.

Table 2. Exemplary quotations: implementation outcomes and strategies for TF-CBT via telehealth.

Implementation Outcomes		
Code	**Definition**	**Quotations**
Adoption	Description of 'initial decision' steps within organization to take on TF-CBT telehealth training and program	"It seems like most of my clients, I've met with at least one time, in person visit, is kind of our office protocol. Try to meet with them, do the initial assessment, and then evaluate where their needs are. And thinking of the process, it seemed like it went well initially, and that [telehealth] would be convenient for them, it would be a good thing for them, trying to see if it was a good fit." (Clinician 1) "So being able to offer telehealth was a big draw for us. [A co-therapist] has been doing [telehealth] because of COVID, without having training and kind of muddling along. She's going to take the training soon, just because I've sung the praises of how much I've learned from it and how much I've enjoyed it." (Clinician 3)

Table 2. *Cont.*

Implementation Outcomes		
Code	**Definition**	**Quotations**
Trauma-Based Care Penetration	Delivery and completion of telehealth program in site setting and integrated within existing care (completion of telehealth visit, follow-up visits)	"For me personally, when I'm doing intakes for my clients, I look at age, diagnosis, and at their ability to tolerate being on telehealth." (Clinician 8) "Every referral that comes in gets asked if they would like to consider telehealth." (Clinician 3) "I don't do as much as I used to. I used to do a lot. . .right after we got out of quarantine and people started returning to school, and a lot of things were done virtually. Now, I could say out of five of my clients, I only do one telehealth, and that's because she's in a different locality. She's 45 min away. So that's the only way we're able to do sessions." (Clinician 7)
Feasibility/ Acceptability	Clinician and site team perceptions of telehealth training and program, including extent to which training and program can be successfully conducted in site and degree to which program is agreeable or satisfactory	"I feel in some cases it's been very successful, and it accesses those that have a difficult time coming, or distance, possible language barriers. I'm also fluent in Spanish, and so I provide therapy in Spanish. We live in a rural area, so sometimes it was very effective when we were able to do our calls on a platform. . .and have a videoconferencing. It seemed very easy for the client to do." (Clinician 1) "I think it really has exceeded my expectations, because of the access to resources that I didn't have before. I think that has been key." (Clinician 2) "[Consultation calls] were helpful, because I was able to connect with other clinicians, and in a sense offer me some normalizing, that a lot of my challenges were also faced by other clinicians. And then the sharing, again, sharing resources, sharing ways of doing things among each other, and obtaining guidance from the trainers on how to implement certain services." (Clinician 2) "I thought the training was fantastic. I learned a lot of things that I hadn't thought about in starting telehealth, in general, but with TF-CBT. And being so new with TF-CBT. . .[it was] a priority for me to be able to see TF-CBT at work in the telehealth realm. Because, doing it in person and doing it through a computer, it is different. So that really appealed to me because we are in such a rural area, so that really was a draw for me to be able to take [training]. . .and grow my knowledge of TF-CBT in that aspect." (Clinician 3)
Patient Effectiveness Outcomes	Change in patient outcomes resulting from program	"But I think that it's doable and effective. . .We met our goals. They're doing better. They've been able to stay at school, or their emotional regulation skills are better. . .parents report their kids were doing better, so I think that that reflects to the model and delivery of telehealth." (Clinician 5) ". . .the treatment that we provide [via telehealth] has been just as successful as if it was face to face." (Clinician 2)
Sustainability	Extent to which newly implemented practice will be maintained within site's ongoing operations	"As we're going two years into it now. . .our director has been more open to getting us tools we need to be able to do [telehealth] properly. Just recently she spent TF funding to purchase us headsets, really nice headsets for our sessions. She upgraded some of our laptops and computers so that we could do our sessions. Some of them didn't have the proper camera or they were outdated. . .then upgraded our systems, like our internet, so it could support it. So she's opening up more and trying to help us, do [telehealth], even though she still likes the in-person." (Clinician 7)

Table 2. *Cont.*

Implementation Outcomes		
Code	**Definition**	**Quotations**
Implementation Strategies		
Education	MUSC training and education of site stakeholders about telehealth	"I would like to see a little bit more of. . .how different it is to provide services to communities, specific communities. . .not only Spanish-speaking, but also children with developmental disabilities, or children with ADHD or other conditions. Those kids won't stay on a video call the whole session. . ." (Clinician 2) "The only other thing that, at least for me, that would be helpful, is a lot of the resources in the [online folder] seem to be geared towards the younger kids. Maybe. . .having some things that are more for the teenagers." (Clinician 3) ". . .I feel at some point it would be nice to retake the telehealth training to get updated on new technology that might be helpful, or a new way of presenting something." (Clinician 4) "Every now and then, to maybe have a check-in consultation call to just see what new problems have arisen a year later. Like what are we seeing now that things have changed post-COVID, or what new things and resources are out there that we could now get from our trainers? Because I'm sure there's new ones." (Clinician 5)
Technical assistance	MUSC helping with technology and other set up and implementation issues	"We do have IT support that are off site. But as far as during sessions, if there's a problem we usually troubleshoot it ourselves. And then if we can't fix it then we would get our IT person involved." (Clinician 3) "We do have an IT person in the agency as a whole, but it's not to help us with telehealth services. It's more for general IT needs. . .But I think the clinicians do their own. When we got the iPads, we set up our own iPads that we were going to give to our clients." (Clinician 2) "I think just a little more help with the technology side of using the resources, sharing screens, some of that. Not everyone is familiar with that, including myself. . ..But there are great resources they have. I've seen them. But just knowing how to use them a little bit more." (Clinician 1)

Adoption: In terms of initial telehealth adoption, multiple clinicians described the COVID-19 pandemic as the prior impetus for incorporating virtual care into their practice. For those that had already been providing care via telehealth due to the pandemic, the TF-CBT telehealth training was described as a resource to make this care more effective, as it was noted that staff were "muddling along" with telehealth modalities prior to training. Others noted the gap in access for rural residents as an important factor influencing their initial adoption of delivering TF-CBT via telehealth.

Penetration: The extent to which telehealth had been incorporated into routine practice at each site after training varied and was dependent on individual clinic patient characteristics and also changing patient preferences. Some interviewees noted that their practice offers telehealth as an option to all referred patients, while others stated that telehealth is offered based on intake assessments and whether clinicians believe a patient can be effectively treated via telehealth. Multiple clinicians noted that the number of telehealth patients they see has decreased since the earlier days of the COVID-19 pandemic, in part due to patients' changing preferences. Despite this varied penetration of delivering TF-CBT via telehealth, for patients that received telehealth, the clinicians noted TF-CBT as highly effective in addressing trauma, "just as successful as if it was face to face".

Feasibility/Acceptability: The TF-CBT training program was described by all interviewees as highly beneficial regardless of the extent to which they were currently providing TF-CBT virtually. The interviewees cited potential increased access for patients as a major reason for the program's acceptability. The interviewees regularly discussed two features of the training program they found particularly beneficial: the online resources made available after training that included protocols, checklists, and other tools and the ongoing consultation calls with other peers and training program leaders for case discussions and problem-solving strategies.

Sustainability: Finally, the site clinicians generally predicted sustaining efforts to provide TF-CBT via telehealth when appropriate. Multiple interviewees noted investments that their organizations were making to sustain telehealth efforts, including purchasing new equipment, supporting ongoing telehealth training, developing educational materials for patients and partner organizations, and pursuing funding to support the program. While generally, practices seemed interested in continuing to provide telehealth as an option, some sites noted that it was not a major priority among their organizations partly due to limited reimbursement and funds for such activity.

3.6.2. Interview Results—Implementation Strategies (Table 2)

Education: When discussing the TF-CBT training program, many interviewees shared feedback on potential opportunities to enhance education and resources to further aid in the implementation of TF-CBT via telehealth. Many comments were related to the benefit and value of the expanded content provided in the online resources and training itself. Specifically, clinicians expressed a desire for support for tailoring this intervention to individual populations, including children with developmental disabilities or ADHD and those from other cultural backgrounds. Similarly, one respondent noted that the resources provided in the online folder seemed to target a younger audience and that creating more age-diverse materials might better support the use of these resources with teenagers. Others noted a desire for additional training on delivering other evidence-based training sessions via telehealth, such as problematic sexual behavior cognitive behavior therapy or eye movement desensitization and reprocessing. Finally, some expressed interest in content related to more policy and programmatic aspects of delivering TF-CBT via telehealth, such as education on models for loaning out technology to patients.

Many interviewees also mentioned interest in receiving continued support due to the 'ever-advancing' nature of telehealth and supportive technologies. Ideas included a refresher course, participation in peer collaboration calls, periodic 'check-in calls' with trainers, and regular email updates from the training team on new resources available.

Technical Assistance: For the most part, the interviewees did not note a need for ongoing technology support for the delivery of telehealth. A few discussed having information technology (IT) staff either on-site or remote who were devoted to IT needs. Others noted that most clinicians have been able to navigate IT issues that come up on their own, only escalating to IT staff when needed. One interviewee, however, noted that more help with technology aspects of telehealth, including sharing screens and accessing online resources, would be beneficial.

4. Discussion

Childhood trauma, specifically in underserved populations, is prevalent and associated with long-term detrimental outcomes [1,2,6]. There are documented disparities in access to mental health care [10–12], and the delivery of mental health care services via telehealth, specifically TF-CBT, has demonstrated improved access to care and patient outcomes in vulnerable populations [16,19,20,22]. However, there are challenges related to the implementation of tele-mental health care [22,24,33]. An innovative TF-CBT training program focused on telehealth delivery was developed to overcome these challenges and improve the implementation of this modality. This study utilized implementation science principles to explore the implementation processes and outcomes of TF-CBT delivery via telehealth in a variety of settings after clinicians' completion of the training program.

This study identified that a key facilitator of the successful implementation of TF-CBT via telehealth in clinics was the availability of applicable resources and support provided by the training team. Participants benefited from education provided by the training team during live training sessions and ongoing consultation calls, as well as online folders of resources that could be utilized in future clinical patient visits via telehealth. This valuable type of resource support is consistent with a report by Conradi et al., which described a process of rapidly transitioning mental health services from the in-person format to telehealth during the COVID-19 pandemic [33]. In this environment, site leaders facilitated multifaceted training which included education on conducting practice initiatives via telehealth and leveraging resources such as protocol documents and checklists via online folders, contributing to an overall smoother transition process for this clinic [33]. Similarly, Appleton et al. found that ongoing support through technical assistance or ongoing consultation tended to be strongly aligned with the successful implementation of tele-mental health [34]. Related to this concept is the benefit of leadership support to facilitate tele-mental health services. The advantage of supportive leadership was evident in our study through site leader encouragement for clinicians to participate in TF-CBT training and through leaders' provision of technology and supplies needed for transitions to the telehealth format; the benefits of leadership support for the implementation of tele-mental health has also been discussed in prior studies in the literature [21,33]. The presence of strong leadership has been demonstrated to improve the adoption of evidence-based practices in general mental health services [35,36], thus emphasizing the benefit of leadership support in the implementation of tele-mental health.

One of the primary barriers to the implementation of tele-mental health services in our study was a lack of availability of technology and internet connectivity issues at patients' homes. Patient engagement was also discussed as a challenge by multiple participants as it was difficult to interact and engage with patients via a telehealth screen; it was concluded that some patients had needs that may be more favorably served with in-person treatment services. These barriers of technology and connectivity in patient homes, as well as the assessment that the delivery of mental health services via telehealth may be ideal for specific populations, are consistent with previous reports from the literature [24,33,37], some of which identified that young children with attentional difficulties and risk concerns [24,33] may be treated more effectively with in-person therapy.

Despite the implementation barriers to telehealth TF-CBT that were noted in our study, the participants had favorable impressions of the delivery and long-term sustainability of TF-CBT via telehealth as it meets patient demand and can increase access to quality mental health care for vulnerable populations. Thus, strategies for telehealth TF-CBT can be created to enhance the implementation of this critical innovation [38–40].

Based on feedback from the clinician participants in our study, ongoing training and education would be valuable resources for the implementation and sustainment of TF-CBT via telehealth. This long-term education and support of stakeholders could include ongoing scheduled consultation calls, strategically planned every six months for all training participants, and continued leveraging of resources. The calls could include updates on new resources and protocols for clinical practice and technology and offer continued collaboration with other providers to share clinical experiences. The online folder of resources can continually be updated with new clinical protocols and resources to meet dynamic health care needs, as well as strategies for identifying ideal formats for mental health service delivery for potential patients when deciding between in-person versus telehealth modalities. Importantly, the training program would ensure all stakeholders receive timely communication (emails, shared folder notifications, etc.) for announcements of newly scheduled calls and training sessions and updated available materials.

As the importance and benefit of leadership in the implementation of new tele-mental health innovations is evident, the training program can include facilitation on developing stakeholder interrelationships with focus on the identification of a leader at clinical sites who will champion and support the delivery of TF-CBT via telehealth. This process can include continued focused contact with site leaders to highlight the value of TF-CBT via telehealth in meeting the health priorities of their clinic and the population being served. Continued communication and involvement with TF-CBT telehealth intermediary contacts such as referring organizations and family advocates is also key to continued stakeholder engagement.

The training program can also be adapted and tailored to a variety of patient needs and contexts to maximize effectiveness for diverse populations. Due to the sensitive nature of TF-CBT, adaptability is a vital component of TF-CBT delivery via telehealth. Some clinician participants requested additional resources for utilization with older children (age-appropriate for teenagers) and children with development disabilities, as well as cultural implications related to TF-CBT delivery. By continuing to adapt and tailor resources, the training program can facilitate the expansion of TF-CBT via telehealth to a broader and more diverse population.

Addressing the barriers to the delivery of TF-CBT via telehealth presented by limited connectivity or a lack of technology in patient homes should be addressed; of interest is that technology and connectivity barriers have increasingly become a focus among programmatic and policy leaders [41,42]. The federal government has invested funding to enhance access to high-speed internet and has multiple initiatives targeting individual patient access to internet and technology, such as the Affordable Connectivity and Lifeline programs [43,44]. Moreover, many philanthropic and industry-led initiatives have adopted digital health equity as a funding priority, creating partnerships and grantmaking opportunities to enhance access to digital health and other services among local communities [45,46]. Leveraging free internet at libraries, community centers, and schools is another emerging practice to support enhanced telehealth access [42,47]. Incorporating information on these programs, funding opportunities, and promising practices in TF-CBT telehealth training and online resources may better equip providers to help their patients navigate the digital divide.

Lastly, the training program can highlight methods to engage patients in participation with TF-CBT by demonstrating the value and convenience of this treatment for families. Patient perceptions of the telehealth format were discussed as a barrier to implementation, similar to prior studies that documented patient resistance to online modalities for the delivery of medical treatment [48]. Innovative direct marketing strategies to deliver the purpose and benefits of this program to patients can help alleviate this obstacle to telehealth modalities. In addition, resources focused on engaging young children during the telehealth visit would be advantageous to clinicians to overcome distractions experienced with telehealth in this population, especially considering that engaging young children in telemental health is often perceived among clinicians to be a barrier to care [49].

This study had a few limitations as it did not include parents or children to understand their direct perceptions on the delivery of TF-CBT via telehealth. In addition, the timing and relevance of this training was influenced by the COVID-19 pandemic. While many telehealth payment flexibilities have become permanent, there is still uncertainty regarding the long-term role of telehealth in the provision of health care. Thus, perceptions regarding its utility and challenges in implementation are likely to evolve as polices are further solidified. Lastly, five of eight interview participants worked within child advocacy centers, which may limit the generalizability of the results. However, the other three interview participants worked in different environments, and all eight participants expressed varied ranges of time periods for their current work roles and varied utilization of TF-CBT via telehealth, thus demonstrating diverse experiences and perceptions. Lastly, despite the survey remaining open for 9 months (July 2022–April 2023) and four reminder emails being sent during this time frame, there was a low response rate, most likely due to hectic and busy clinician schedules. Despite the limitations, this study utilized implementation science principles to describe moderators to the implementation of TF-CBT via telehealth after the completion of the training program, which were used for the identification of implementation strategies to maximize the implementation and sustainment of TF-CBT via telehealth. Future research can include larger sample sizes to increase the generalizability of the results as well as studies to test the effectiveness of strategies to improve intervention outcomes.

5. Conclusions

TF-CBT via telehealth can decrease access to care barriers for trauma-affected vulnerable populations and improve patient outcomes. The COVID-19 pandemic created an immediate need to launch telehealth programs to protect the public. However, many mental health clinics lacked the necessary training, tools, and support to implement a telehealth program. Our implementation study showed that leadership and staff buy in, community need, offering practical training resources, live training sessions, ongoing consultation, and funding to assist with access to technology (tablets and internet) were key facilitators in the successful implementation of TF-CBT via telehealth. A lack of access to technology and privacy, reimbursement challenges, and difficulties with engaging younger children or those with developmental disabilities were key barriers. Providing training, technical assistance, and tailored support in the delivery of TF-CBT via telehealth is a promising implementation strategy that can help increase access to quality mental health care for underserved populations.

Supplementary Materials: The following supporting information can be downloaded at: https://www.mdpi.com/article/10.3390/healthcare12212110/s1.

Author Contributions: Conceptualization, R.O.-A., K.K., D.F. and R.S.; methodology, R.O.-A., R.S., E.J., R.K. and K.K.; software, E.J. and R.K.; validation, E.J., R.K., R.O.-A. and R.S.; formal analysis, E.J. and R.K.; investigation, R.O.-A. and R.S.; resources, R.O.-A., R.S., K.K. and D.F.; data curation, E.J.; writing—original draft preparation, E.J., R.K. and R.S.; writing—review and editing, E.J., R.K., R.S., R.V., D.F., R.O.-A. and K.K.; project administration, R.V., R.O.-A., R.S., D.F. and K.K.; funding acquisition, D.F., K.K., R.O.-A. and R.S. All authors have read and agreed to the published version of the manuscript.

Funding: This research was made possible by the Health Resources and Services Administration (HRSA) of the US Department of Health and Human Services (HHS) as part of the National Telehealth Centers of Excellence Award (U66RH31458). The contents are those of the author(s) and do not necessarily represent the official views of nor endorsements by the HRSA, HHS, or the US Government.

Institutional Review Board Statement: Ethical review and approval were waived for this study because the Institutional Review Board classified this study as quality improvement.

Informed Consent Statement: Verbal informed consent was obtained from all subjects involved in the interviews in this study.

Data Availability Statement: The interview data are unavailable due to privacy concerns.

Conflicts of Interest: The authors declare no conflicts of interest. The funders had no role in the design of the study; in the collection, analyses, or interpretation of data; in the writing of the manuscript; or in the decision to publish the results.

References

1. Finkelhor, D.; Turner, H.A.; Shattuck, A.; Hamby, S.L. Violence, crime, and abuse exposure in a national sample of children and youth: An update. *JAMA Pediatr.* **2013**, *167*, 614–621. [CrossRef] [PubMed]
2. Kilpatrick, D.G.; Ruggiero, K.J.; Acierno, R.; Saunders, B.E.; Resnick, H.S.; Best, C.L. Violence and risk of PTSD, major depression, substance abuse/dependence, and comorbidity: Results from the National Survey of Adolescents. *J. Consult. Clin. Psychol.* **2003**, *71*, 692. [CrossRef] [PubMed]
3. Bethell, C.D.; Newacheck, P.; Hawes, E.; Halfon, N. Adverse childhood experiences: Assessing the impact on health and school engagement and the mitigating role of resilience. *Health Aff.* **2014**, *33*, 2106–2115. [CrossRef] [PubMed]
4. Fairbank, J.A.; Fairbank, D.W. Epidemiology of child traumatic stress. *Curr. Psychiatry Rep.* **2009**, *11*, 289–295. [CrossRef] [PubMed]
5. Kessler, R.C. Posttraumatic stress disorder: The burden to the individual and to society. *J. Clin. Psychiatry* **2000**, *61*, 4–14.
6. Alexander, A.A.; Harrelson, M.E. Assessment of childhood trauma in rural settings. In *Identifying, Treating, and Preventing Childhood Trauma in Rural Communities*; Advances in Psychology, Mental Health, and Behavioral Studies (APMHBS); Information Science Reference/IGI Global: Hershey, PA, USA, 2016; pp. 121–135.
7. Comer, J.S.; Barlow, D.H. The occasional case against broad dissemination and implementation: Retaining a role for specialty care in the delivery of psychological treatments. *Am. Psychol.* **2014**, *69*, 1–18. [CrossRef]

8. Merikangas, K.R.; Nakamura, E.F.; Kessler, R.C. Epidemiology of mental disorders in children and adolescents. *Dialogues Clin. Neurosci.* **2009**, *11*, 7–20. [CrossRef]
9. Whitney, D.G.; Peterson, M.D. US national and state-level prevalence of mental health disorders and disparities of mental health care use in children. *JAMA Pediatr.* **2019**, *173*, 389–391. [CrossRef]
10. Alegria, M.; Vallas, M.; Pumariega, A.J. Racial and ethnic disparities in pediatric mental health. *Child Adolesc. Psychiatr. Clin.* **2010**, *19*, 759–774. [CrossRef]
11. Merikangas, K.R.; He, J.-p.; Burstein, M.; Swendsen, J.; Avenevoli, S.; Case, B.; Georgiades, K.; Heaton, L.; Swanson, S.; Olfson, M. Service utilization for lifetime mental disorders in US adolescents: Results of the National Comorbidity Survey–Adolescent Supplement (NCS-A). *J. Am. Acad. Child Adolesc. Psychiatry* **2011**, *50*, 32–45. [CrossRef]
12. Rodgers, C.R.; Flores, M.W.; Bassey, O.; Augenblick, J.M.; Lê Cook, B. Racial/ethnic disparity trends in children's mental health care access and expenditures from 2010–2017: Disparities remain despite sweeping policy reform. *J. Am. Acad. Child Adolesc. Psychiatry* **2022**, *61*, 915–925. [CrossRef] [PubMed]
13. Gloff, N.E.; LeNoue, S.R.; Novins, D.K.; Myers, K. Telemental health for children and adolescents. *Int. Rev. Psychiatry* **2015**, *27*, 513–524. [CrossRef] [PubMed]
14. Myers, K.; Comer, J.S. The case for telemental health for improving the accessibility and quality of children's mental health services. *J. Child Adolesc. Psychopharmacol.* **2016**, *26*, 186–191. [CrossRef] [PubMed]
15. Myers, K.; Nelson, E.-L.; Rabinowitz, T.; Hilty, D.; Baker, D.; Barnwell, S.S.; Boyce, G.; Bufka, L.F.; Cain, S.; Chui, L. American telemedicine association practice guidelines for telemental health with children and adolescents. *Telemed. E-Health* **2017**, *23*, 779–804. [CrossRef] [PubMed]
16. Stewart, R.W.; Orengo-Aguayo, R.; Young, J.; Wallace, M.M.; Cohen, J.A.; Mannarino, A.P.; de Arellano, M.A. Feasibility and effectiveness of a telehealth service delivery model for treating childhood posttraumatic stress: A community-based, open pilot trial of trauma-focused cognitive–behavioral therapy. *J. Psychother. Integr.* **2020**, *30*, 274. [CrossRef]
17. Cohen, J.A.; Mannarino, A.P.; Deblinger, E. *Treating Trauma and Traumatic Grief in Children and Adolescents, Second Edition*; Guilford Publications: New York, NY, USA, 2017.
18. de Arellano, M.A.; Lyman, D.R.; Jobe-Shields, L.; George, P.; Dougherty, R.H.; Daniels, A.S.; Ghose, S.S.; Huang, L.; Delphin-Rittmon, M.E. Trauma-focused cognitive-behavioral therapy for children and adolescents: Assessing the evidence. *Psychiatr. Serv.* **2014**, *65*, 591–602. [CrossRef]
19. Stewart, R.W.; Orengo-Aguayo, R.E.; Cohen, J.A.; Mannarino, A.P.; de Arellano, M.A. A pilot study of trauma-focused cognitive–behavioral therapy delivered via telehealth technology. *Child Maltreatment* **2017**, *22*, 324–333. [CrossRef]
20. Stewart, R.W.; Orengo-Aguayo, R.E.; Gilmore, A.K.; de Arellano, M. Addressing barriers to care among Hispanic youth: Telehealth delivery of trauma-focused cognitive behavioral therapy. *Behav. Ther.* **2017**, *40*, 112.
21. Orengo-Aguayo, R.; Stewart, R.W.; Villalobos, B.T.; Hernandez Rodriguez, J.; Dueweke, A.R.; de Arellano, M.A.; Young, J. Listen, don't tell: Partnership and adaptation to implement trauma-focused cognitive behavioral therapy in low-resourced settings. *Am. Psychol.* **2020**, *75*, 1158. [CrossRef]
22. Stewart, R.W.; Orengo-Aguayo, R.; Wallace, M.; Metzger, I.W.; Rheingold, A.A. Leveraging technology and cultural adaptations to increase access and engagement among trauma-exposed African American youth: Exploratory study of school-based telehealth delivery of trauma-focused cognitive behavioral therapy. *J. Interpers. Violence* **2021**, *36*, 7090–7109. [CrossRef]
23. Gurm, K.; Wampold, B.E.; Piatt, C.; Jagodzinski, R.; Caperton, D.D.; Babins-Wagner, R. Effectiveness of telemental health during the COVID-19 pandemic: A propensity score noninferiority analysis of outcomes. *Psychotherapy* **2023**, *60*, 231–236. [CrossRef]
24. Lipschitz, J.M.; Connolly, S.L.; Van Boxtel, R.; Potter, J.R.; Nixon, N.; Bidargaddi, N. Provider perspectives on telemental health implementation: Lessons learned during the COVID-19 pandemic and paths forward. *Psychol. Serv.* **2022**, *20* (Suppl. S2), 11–19. [CrossRef] [PubMed]
25. Brownson, R.C.; Colditz, G.A.; Proctor, E.K. *Dissemination and Implementation Research in Health: Translating Science to Practice*; Oxford University Press: Oxford, UK, 2017.
26. Tong, A.; Sainsbury, P.; Craig, J. Consolidated criteria for reporting qualitative research (COREQ): A 32-item checklist for interviews and focus groups. *Int. J. Qual. Health Care* **2007**, *19*, 349–357. [CrossRef] [PubMed]
27. Aarons, G.A.; Green, A.E.; Willging, C.E.; Ehrhart, M.G.; Roesch, S.C.; Hecht, D.B.; Chaffin, M.J. Mixed-method study of a conceptual model of evidence-based intervention sustainment across multiple public-sector service settings. *Implement. Sci.* **2014**, *9*, 183. [CrossRef] [PubMed]
28. Aarons, G.A.; Hurlburt, M.; Horwitz, S.M. Advancing a conceptual model of evidence-based practice implementation in public service sectors. *Adm. Policy Ment. Health* **2011**, *38*, 4–23. [CrossRef] [PubMed]
29. Saunders, B.; Sim, J.; Kingstone, T.; Baker, S.; Waterfield, J.; Bartlam, B.; Burroughs, H.; Jinks, C. Saturation in qualitative research: Exploring its conceptualization and operationalization. *Qual. Quant.* **2018**, *52*, 1893–1907. [CrossRef]
30. NVivo Software. *NVivo Qualitative Software*; Lumivero: Denver, CO, USA, 2023. Available online: http://www.lumivero.com/ (accessed on 10 January 2023).
31. Brooks, J.; McCluskey, S.; Turley, E.; King, N. The Utility of Template Analysis in Qualitative Psychology Research. *Qual. Res. Psychol.* **2015**, *12*, 202–222. [CrossRef]
32. Crabtree, B.F.; Miller, W.L. Using Codes and Code Manuals: A Template Organizing Style of Interpretation. In *Doing Qualitative Research*, 2nd ed.; Sage Publications: Thousand Oaks, CA, USA, 1999; pp. 163–177.

33. Conradi, L.; Hazen, A.; Covert, J. The fast and the furious: The rapid implementation of tele-mental health practices within a children's advocacy center. *Glob. Implement. Res. Appl.* **2022**, *2*, 305–320. [CrossRef]
34. Appleton, R.; Barnett, P.; Vera San Juan, N.; Tuudah, E.; Lyons, N.; Parker, J.; Roxburgh, E.; Spyridonidis, S.; Tamworth, M.; Worden, M.; et al. Implementation strategies for telemental health: A systematic review. *BMC Health Serv. Res.* **2023**, *23*, 78. [CrossRef]
35. Aarons, G.A. Transformational and transactional leadership: Association with attitudes toward evidence-based practice. *Psychiatr. Serv.* **2006**, *57*, 1162–1169. [CrossRef]
36. Corrigan, P.W.; Garman, A.N. Transformational and transactional leadership skills for mental health teams. *Commun. Ment. Health J.* **1999**, *35*, 301–312. [CrossRef] [PubMed]
37. Siegel, A.; Zuo, Y.; Moghaddamcharkari, N.; McIntyre, R.S.; Rosenblat, J.D. Barriers, benefits and interventions for improving the delivery of telemental health services during the coronavirus disease 2019 pandemic: A systematic review. *Curr. Opin. Psychiatry* **2021**, *34*, 434. [CrossRef] [PubMed]
38. Powell, B.J.; Waltz, T.J.; Chinman, M.J.; Damschroder, L.J.; Smith, J.L.; Matthieu, M.M.; Proctor, E.K.; Kirchner, J.E. A refined compilation of implementation strategies: Results from the Expert Recommendations for Implementing Change (ERIC) project. *Implement. Sci.* **2015**, *10*, 1–14. [CrossRef] [PubMed]
39. Powell, B.J.; Fernandez, M.E.; Williams, N.J.; Aarons, G.A.; Beidas, R.S.; Lewis, C.C.; McHugh, S.M.; Weiner, B.J. Enhancing the impact of implementation strategies in healthcare: A research agenda. *Front. Public Health* **2019**, *7*, 3. [CrossRef]
40. Kirchner, J.E.; Smith, J.L.; Powell, B.J.; Waltz, T.J.; Proctor, E.K. Getting a clinical innovation into practice: An introduction to implementation strategies. *Psychiatry Res.* **2020**, *283*, 112467. [CrossRef]
41. Marzouk, S.; Velasquez, D.E.; Joseph, N.; Martin, A. Broadband for better health—Ensuring internet access for all. *BMJ* **2023**, *382*, 1673. [CrossRef]
42. Health Resources and Services Administration. Improving Access to Telehealth. Available online: https://telehealth.hhs.gov/providers/health-equity-in-telehealth/improving-access-to-telehealth (accessed on 15 November 2023).
43. The White House. Fact Sheet: Biden-Harris Administration Announces Over $40 Billion to Connect Everyone in America to Affordable, Reliable, High-Speed Internet. Available online: https://www.whitehouse.gov/briefing-room/statements-releases/2023/06/26/fact-sheet-biden-harris-administration-announces-over-40-billion-to-connect-everyone-in-america-to-affordable-reliable-high-speed-internet/ (accessed on 15 November 2023).
44. Affordable Connectivity Program. Universal Service Administration Company. Available online: https://www.affordableconnectivity.gov/ (accessed on 15 November 2023).
45. Durocher, K.; Boparai, N.; Jankowicz, D.; Strudwick, G. Identifying technology industry-led initiatives to address digital health equity. *Digit. Health* **2021**, *7*, 20552076211056156. [CrossRef]
46. McBeath, R.; Pathways to Digital Equity. How Communities Can Reach Their Broadband Goals and How Philanthropy Can Help. Benton Institute for Broadband and Society. 2022. Available online: https://www.benton.org/sites/default/files/pathways.pdf (accessed on 1 March 2024).
47. Chiricuzio, S. Public Libraries Tackle Telehealth Challenges. *Libr. J.* **2022**. Available online: https://www.libraryjournal.com/story/Public-Libraries-Tackle-Telehealth-Challenges#:~:text=Integrating%20telehealth%20into%20libraries%20will%20require%20cooperation,health%20systems,%20community-based%20organizations,%20and%20healthcare%20workers (accessed on 1 March 2024).
48. Almathami, H.K.Y.; Win, K.T.; Vlahu-Gjorgievska, E. Barriers and facilitators that influence telemedicine-based, real-time, online consultation at patients' homes: Systematic literature review. *J. Med. Internet Res.* **2020**, *22*, e16407. [CrossRef]
49. AlRasheed, R.; Woodard, G.S.; Nguyen, J.; Daniels, A.; Park, N.; Berliner, L.; Dorsey, S. Transitioning to telehealth for COVID-19 and beyond: Perspectives of community mental health clinicians. *J. Behav. Health Serv. Res.* **2022**, *49*, 524–530. [CrossRef]

healthcare

MDPI

Article

Telehealth Perceived Benefits and Self-Efficacy Do Not Mediate the Effects of Demographic, Health, and Social Determinants on Telehealth Use of Low-Income African American and Latino Residents of Public Housing in Los Angeles

Sharon Cobb [1], Attallah Dillard [1], Ehsan Yaghmaei [2], Mohsen Bazargan [3,4] and Shervin Assari [3,4,*]

1 Mervyn M. Dymally College of Nursing (MMDCON), Charles R. Drew University of Medicine and Science (CDU), Los Angeles, CA 90059, USA; sharoncobb1@cdrewu.edu (S.C.); atalahdillard@cdrewu.edu (A.D.)
2 Department of Family Medicine, Charles R. Drew University of Medicine and Science (CDU), Los Angeles, CA 90059, USA; ehsanyaghmaei@cdrewu.edu
3 Department of Internal Medicine, Charles R. Drew University of Medicine and Science (CDU), Los Angeles, CA 90059, USA; mohsenbazargan@cdrewu.edu
4 Department of Public Health, Charles R. Drew University of Medicine and Science (CDU), Los Angeles, CA 90059, USA
* Correspondence: assari@umich.edu

Abstract: Background: Marginalized low-income racial and ethnic minority residents of public housing represent an intersectional population with multiple health needs and low healthcare utilization. Telehealth has been proposed as a solution to address healthcare access disparities, yet the role of telehealth attitudes, including perceived benefits and self-efficacy, in influencing telehealth use of this population remains unknown. Objective: This study investigates whether two domains of telehealth attitudes, namely self-efficacy and perceived benefits (expectancy), mediate the relationship between demographic, health, and social determinants of telehealth use among low-income racial and ethnic minority residents of public housing in Los Angeles. Methods: This cross-sectional study analyzed data collected from low-income racial and ethnic minority residents of public housing in Los Angeles. Measures included demographic factors (age and gender), social determinants of health (e.g., education, language, and primacy care provider), health (chronic illnesses and physical mobility), telehealth attitudes (perceived benefits and self-efficacy), and telehealth use frequency. Mediation analysis was conducted to test whether telehealth attitudes explained the association between demographic, social, and health determinants of telehealth use. Results: The findings revealed that neither of the two domains of telehealth attitudes, including perceived benefits and self-efficacy, were significantly associated with telehealth use. As such, these attitude domains did not operate as mediators of the relationship between demographic, health, and social determinants of telehealth use. Conclusion: The study results suggest that structural barriers, rather than individual attitudes, primarily drive telehealth use disparities among this intersectional population. Interventions aimed at increasing telehealth adoption should prioritize addressing systemic inequities rather than focusing solely on changing individual attitudes. These findings underscore the importance of structural solutions to promote equitable telehealth access in marginalized communities.

Keywords: telehealth; social determinants of health; racial and ethnic minorities; public housing; intersectionality; health disparities; mediation analysis

1. Background

Racial and ethnic minority residents of public housing represent the intersection of three distinct social and contextual dimensions [1]: low-income status, racial and ethnic minority identity, and residency in public housing. Each of these factors independently shapes individuals' experiences, resources, and access to healthcare, including telehealth [2]. However, their intersection creates unique conditions that cannot be fully understood by examining any single factor in isolation [3–6]. This aligns with the intersectionality theory and framework [7,8], which emphasizes how overlapping social identities and systemic inequalities create compounded effects. Despite the growing importance of telehealth, limited research has focused on the attitudes and usage patterns of this intersectional population, leaving a significant gap in understanding how these combined identities influence telehealth utilization and the potential barriers they face. This gap underscores the need for targeted studies and interventions to address the specific challenges and opportunities within this community.

Racial and ethnic minority residents of public housing often exhibit lower rates of healthcare utilization despite experiencing multiple chronic health conditions and complexing health needs [9–11]. Structural barriers such as financial constraints, limited access to transportation, and systemic discrimination in healthcare settings contribute to their reduced healthcare use [12,13]. Commonly centralized in urban residential cities, public housing areas have faced social and racialized patterns of residential segregation for decades, leading to systemic socioeconomic disparities [14–16]. Therefore, availability and access to health care facilities and providers may be increasingly lower in communities surrounding public housing areas [17,18]. Residents in public housing may be unlikely to find a primary or specialty provider within the local community, such as mental health or cardiology [19–21]. The mismatch between their elevated unmet health needs and lower healthcare utilization usage highlights the urgency of addressing the systemic and structural inequities that impede their ability to access and benefit from healthcare, including emerging modalities like telehealth.

Racial and ethnic minorities, specifically African Americans and Latinos, in low-income areas are likely to live in under-resourced and underserved areas and face extreme disparities in their healthcare seeking behaviors and encounters [22]. African Americans and Latinos exhibit low levels of healthcare utilization, including mental health [23]. Additionally, African American and Latinos may delay their care, which resulted in a study of 33 Latinas discussing treatment seeking behaviors of urinary incontinence [24]. Research shows minorities are more likely to rate printed materials as their preferred source of health communication compared to smartphones and tablets [25]. Yet, minorities who utilize the internet for health information are likely to have a higher education level and worse health status [26,27], despite its positive benefits for this group [28].

Telehealth presents a promising solution to address the healthcare access challenges faced by racial and ethnic minority residents of public housing [29]. By reducing logistical barriers such as transportation and providing more flexible options for care, telehealth has the potential to bridge the gap between their multiple health needs and low healthcare utilization. However, the effectiveness of telehealth adoption within this population may be influenced by their attitudes toward this modality [30]. Additionally, marginalized minorities are more likely to utilize telehealth via smartphone as compared to a computer [31]. The Health Belief Model [32,33] suggests that perceived benefits of telehealth, such as convenience and accessibility, could play a critical role in shaping behavior. Similarly, the Theory of Reasoned Action [34,35] highlights the importance of perceived self-efficacy in adopting telehealth services, where individuals' confidence in their ability to use and benefit from the technology may influence their engagement. While these theoretical frameworks provide valuable insights, it remains unclear whether these associations are observed among this intersectional population.

Perceived benefits of telehealth can encompass improved patient health, positive feelings of empowerment and support, efficient communication, and greater patient education [36,37]. Telehealth self-efficacy is focused on the individual's belief that they have the ability to perform the necessary actions to overcome barriers toward telehealth use and adoption and increase confidence [38–42]. More research is needed to understand whether and how telehealth attitudes, including perceived benefits [43–46] and self-efficacy [47–50], influence actual telehealth use in this group of public housing residents.

Informed by the Health Belief Model and the Theory of Reasoned Action, the overall aim of this study is to investigate whether telehealth perceived benefits and self-efficacy mediate the relationship between social determinants of health and telehealth utilization among African American and Latino public housing residents in Los Angeles. As a secondary aim, this study seeks to examine the gap in empirical evidence on how social, economic, and contextual factors influence telehealth utilization. Ultimately, the findings of this research will inform interventions and policies to enhance equitable access to telehealth services for marginalized communities.

2. Methods

2.1. Study Design

This cross-sectional study utilized a structured, face to face survey for data collection among African American and Latino residents of public housing areas in Los Angeles.

2.2. Participants

A total of 252 African American and Latino adults residing in four public housing areas located in South Los Angeles, California, were included in this study. Data collection spanned between August 2023 and January 2024. Out of 14 public housing sites managed by the Housing Authority of the City of Los Angeles (HACLA), 4 sites were selected, comprising a total of 2306 housing units. HACLA, one of the oldest public housing authorities in the United States, primarily oversees multiple government-controlled and affordable housing units in the Los Angeles region. As the issuer of housing for low-income individuals, HACLA currently accommodates 118,554 individuals across 6058 units. The average family income of those served by HACLA is substantially less than both the county and national averages (USD 24,881, compared to USD 68,044 and USD 62,843, respectively). Notably, more than 75% of HACLA residents self-identify as Latino, while 22% identify as African American/Black. The four selected housing sites are located within Service Planning Area (SPA) 6 of Los Angeles County, a region that is home to over one million residents and is marked by pronounced health disparities compared to other areas within the county.

2.3. Sampling

Participants were recruited through nonrandom sampling. Eligibility criteria including residency in SPA 6, self-identification as Latino or African American, and the ability to complete the interview in either English or Spanish. Adults aged 18 years or older were invited to participate, with eligibility for public housing determined based on income, age, disability status, and U.S. citizenship or immigration status.

2.4. Ethics

All participants provided written informed consent, and the study protocol received approval from the Institutional Review Board (IRB) at Charles R. Drew University of

Medicine and Science. The survey collected detailed data on demographic characteristics, socioeconomic status, access to and utilization of healthcare services, health behaviors, and overall health status.

2.5. Measurement

A range of demographic, socioeconomic, and health-related data were collected from the participants. Basic demographic information included age and gender. *Age* was treated as a continuous variable ranging from 18 to 77 years. *Gender*, based on self-identification, was categorized as a dichotomous variable: (1) Female and (2) Male.

2.5.1. Socioeconomic Status

We measured their socioeconomic status by the following variables: *Educational Level*, assessed by self-report based on the highest level of education completed, which was categorized into five levels: (1) 8th grade or less, (2) some high school, no diploma, (3) high school graduate or GED equivalent, (4) associate degree or some college, and (5) baccalaureate degree or higher.

Primary verbal language, which was measured as a dichotomous variable: (1) English, and (2) Spanish.

Chronic Conditions: participants reported if they have been diagnosed with any of the following conditions: cancer, chronic obstructive pulmonary disease (COPD), diabetes mellitus, cardiovascular diseases, hypertension, sleep disorders, and stroke. The number of chronic conditions was measured on a scale from 0 to 8.

Physical mobility was assessed using four items from the health-related quality of life survey (SF-12), which evaluated the extent to which participants' health restricted their physical mobility. Participants were asked if their health limited them in moderate activities (e.g., moving a table, pushing a vacuum cleaner, bowling, or playing golf) and climbing several stairs, and, if so, to what extent. Participants also reported how often their physical health caused them to accomplish less than they desired and if there were limitations with their daily activities over the past four weeks. A total "Physical Mobility Limitation" score was calculated by summing these four items, with scores ranging from 4 to 12; higher scores indicated fewer limitations in physical mobility. The Cronbach's alpha reliability coefficient for this 4-item scale was 0.820.

Participants were asked if they have a regular doctor or healthcare provider for primary care. This variable was dichotomous, with responses categorized as follows: (0) no and (1) yes.

2.5.2. Telehealth

Telehealth utilization: Telehealth usage incorporated participants using one of the following devices to communicate virtually with their provider for a medical visit: computer, smartphone or telephone, or tablet. We assessed two aspects of attitudes toward telehealth utilization by utilizing questions and statements from previously established surveys on telehealth perceptions. Specifically, we incorporated items from recognized resources to measure responses to True/False statements concerning self-efficacy and perceived benefits of telehealth. The aggregated responses produced quantitative scores with higher scores indicating a more positive attitude toward telehealth [8,9]. The Cronbach's alpha reliability coefficients for both of these domains were above 0.70. The outcome was the frequency of telehealth use in the past 12 months. The specific question read as "How many times have you used telehealth in the past 12 months?".

Telehealth perceived benefits: Telehealth perceived benefits refer to an individual's recognition of the advantages of using telehealth services, such as increased accessibility, convenience, reduced travel time, and cost savings. Patients and providers who perceive telehealth as beneficial are more likely to adopt and utilize it for routine and specialized care. Additionally, perceived benefits extend beyond logistical convenience to include improved health monitoring, timely interventions, and better management of chronic conditions, particularly for individuals in remote or underserved areas.

Telehealth self-efficacy: Telehealth self-efficacy describes an individual's confidence in their ability to effectively use telehealth technology for healthcare needs. This construct encompasses skills such as navigating telehealth platforms, troubleshooting technical issues, and communicating effectively with healthcare providers in a virtual setting. Higher self-efficacy is associated with greater engagement in telehealth services, as individuals who feel competent in using these tools are more likely to participate in virtual consultations, follow medical advice, and integrate telehealth into their routine healthcare management.

2.6. Statistical Analysis

Our analysis comprised three sections. First, we conducted a descriptive analysis of all participants. Second, we used Pearson correlation coefficients to examine the bivariate association between all study variables including social determinants of health, telehealth perceived benefits and self-efficacy, and telehealth utilization within the past year and all other independent variables. Third, we employed a structural equation model (SEM) to evaluate the association between social determinants of health, telehealth attitudes, and the frequency of telehealth visit attendance. The analysis included demographic factors (age and gender), socioeconomic status (education), language, physical mobility, number of chronic conditions, and having a regular doctor or healthcare provider as predictors, positive attitude towards telehealth care utilization as mediators, and telehealth use as the outcome.

3. Results

Table 1 presents the characteristics of the study sample. This study comprised 252 African American and Latino individuals aged between 18 and 77 years (mean = 45 ± 15). Approximately 75% of the participants were female. Regarding educational attainment, 39% of participants reported never completing high school, 22% completed high school, 26% graduated from high school or attained a GED, and the remaining 12% held an associate degree or had some college education. Furthermore, 82% of the participants had a regular doctor/healthcare provider for primary care, and 74% indicated Spanish as their preferred language. At least 19% reported one chronic condition, whereas 15% had two chronic conditions, and 18% had three or more chronic conditions. The average physical mobility limitation score was 9 with a standard deviation of 2, indicating a lower level of physical mobility limitation within the sample. Regarding the use of telehealth services in the past 12 months, the data indicate that the majority of participants have not used telehealth services. With regard to telehealth utilization, 53% reported no telehealth usage within the past year, 20% participated once, 15% completed a telehealth visit twice, and 12% reported at least three telehealth visits.

Table 1. Descriptive statistics for demographic variables (n = 252).

	N (%)
Gender	
Male	64 (25)
Female	188 (75)

Table 1. *Cont.*

	N (%)
Education	
8th grade or less	99 (39)
Some high school, no diploma	56 (22)
Graduated from high school or have a GED equivalent	66 (26)
Associate degree or some college/Bachelor's Degree	31 (12)
Language	
English	65 (26)
Spanish	187 (74)
Primary Care Provider	
No	45 (18)
Yes	207 (82)
Chronic Conditions	
0	122 (48)
1	47 (19)
2	39 (15)
3 or more	44 (18)
How many times have you used telehealth in the past 12 months?	
0	133 (53)
1	50 (20)
2	37 (15)
3	19 (7)
4 or more	13 (5)
	Mean (SD)
Age (Yrs)	45 (15)
Physical Mobility	9 (2)
Attitude Toward Telehealth Care Utilization (Self-Efficacy)	2.151 (0.11)
Attitude Toward Telehealth Care Utilization (Expectancy)	2.381 (0.12)
Number of Chronic Conditions (scale of 0–8)	1 (2)

Table 2 shows bivariate correlations between the use of telehealth services in the past 12 months and other study variables. Findings revealed that age and education were not correlated with telehealth utilization. However, gender ($r = -0.138$; $p < 0.05$), language ($r = -0.151$; $p < 0.05$), physical mobility limitation ($r = -0.220$; $p < 0.001$), and number of chronic diseases ($r = 0.196$; $p < 0.001$) were associated with telehealth utilization. In addition, having a primary care provider ($r = 0.196$; $p < 0.001$) was significantly associated with telehealth utilization.

Table 2. Bivariate correlations between telehealth utilization and other study variables.

	1	2	3	4	5	6	7	8	9	10
1. Age	1.00									
2. Gender	−0.08	1.00								
3. Education	−0.49 **	0.08	1.00							
4. Language	0.32 **	−0.14 *	−0.51 **	1.00						

Table 2. *Cont.*

	1	2	3	4	5	6	7	8	9	10
5. Physical Mobility Limitation	−0.25 **	0.01	0.21 **	0.03	1.00					
6. Number of Chronic conditions	0.34 **	−0.05	−0.13 *	0.05	−0.39 **	1.00				
7. Primary Care Provider	0.09	−0.11	−0.01	−0.04	−0.15 **	0.18 **	1.00			
8. Attitude Telehealth Care Utilization (Expectancy)	0.01	−0.07	0.07	−0.13 *	−0.04	0.04	0.08	1.00		
9. Attitude Telehealth Care Utilization (Self-Efficacy)	−0.02	−0.02	0.18 *	−0.16 **	0.01	−0.03	0.05	0.76 **	1.00	
10. Telehealth Care Utilization (Frequency)	0.04	−0.14 *	0.03	−0.15 *	−0.22 **	0.20 **	0.20 **	0.25 **	0.24 **	1.00

Note: ** Correlation is significant at the 0.01 level (two-tailed), and * correlation is significant at the 0.05 level (two-tailed).

The structural equation model results (Table 3, Figure 1) showed that telehealth expectancy was not significantly associated with telehealth utilization (B = 0.102, SE = 0.090, 95% CI = −0.075 to 0.280, p = 0.258). Similarly, telehealth self-efficacy did not demonstrate a significant relationship with telehealth utilization (B = 0.142, SE = 0.091, 95% CI = −0.036 to 0.320, p = 0.118). Among the covariates, age (B = −0.028, SE = 0.071, 95% CI = −0.168 to 0.111, p = 0.691) and education (B = −0.028, SE = 0.076, 95% CI = −0.177 to 0.121, p = 0.712) were not significant predictors of telehealth utilization. Gender, however, was significantly associated with telehealth use, with men reporting lower telehealth utilization compared to women (B = −0.128, SE = 0.059, 95% CI = −0.243 to −0.013, p = 0.029). Language preference also showed significance, with Spanish speakers reporting less frequent telehealth use (B = −0.135, SE = 0.069, 95% CI = −0.270 to 0.000, p = 0.050). Having a regular provider was positively associated with telehealth utilization (B = 0.121, SE = 0.059, 95% CI = 0.005 to 0.237, p = 0.041), and chronic disease status approached significance (B = 0.125, SE = 0.066, 95% CI = −0.004 to 0.254, p = 0.058). Physical fitness was inversely related to telehealth utilization (B = −0.149, SE = 0.065, 95% CI = −0.276 to −0.022, p = 0.021).

Table 3. Summary of the structural equation model with telehealth frequency as the outcome.

	B	SE	95%	CI	p
Telehealth Expectancy					
Age (Yr)	0.060	0.076	−0.089	0.208	0.432
Gender (Men)	−0.080	0.063	−0.203	0.043	0.201
Education	0.048	0.080	−0.109	0.205	0.548
Language (Spanish)	−0.132	0.074	−0.276	0.013	0.074
Regular Doctor	0.056	0.064	−0.069	0.180	0.381
Chronic Disease	0.016	0.071	−0.123	0.154	0.826
Physical Fitness	−0.012	0.070	−0.149	0.125	0.867
Intercept	1.678	0.584	0.533	2.823	0.004
Telehealth Self-Efficacy					
Age (Yr)	0.104	0.075	−0.043	0.251	0.164
Gender (Men)	−0.038	0.062	−0.160	0.084	0.545
Education	0.172	0.079	0.018	0.326	0.029
Language (Spanish)	−0.112	0.073	−0.254	0.031	0.126
Regular Doctor	0.046	0.063	−0.077	0.170	0.463
Chronic Disease	−0.047	0.070	−0.184	0.090	0.504
Physical Fitness	−0.005	0.069	−0.140	0.131	0.947
Intercept	1.153	0.581	0.013	2.292	0.047

Table 3. *Cont.*

	B	SE	95%	CI	*p*
Telehealth Utilization (Frequency)					
Telehealth Expectancy	0.102	0.090	−0.075	0.280	0.258
Telehealth Self-Efficacy	0.142	0.091	−0.036	0.320	0.118
Age	−0.028	0.071	−0.168	0.111	0.691
Gender (Men)	−0.128	0.059	−0.243	−0.013	0.029
Education	−0.028	0.076	−0.177	0.121	0.712
Language (Spanish)	−0.135	0.069	−0.270	0.000	0.050
Regular Doctor	0.121	0.059	0.005	0.237	0.041
Chronic Disease	0.125	0.066	−0.004	0.254	0.058
Physical Fitness	−0.149	0.065	−0.276	−0.022	0.021
Intercept	1.748	0.547	0.676	2.820	0.001

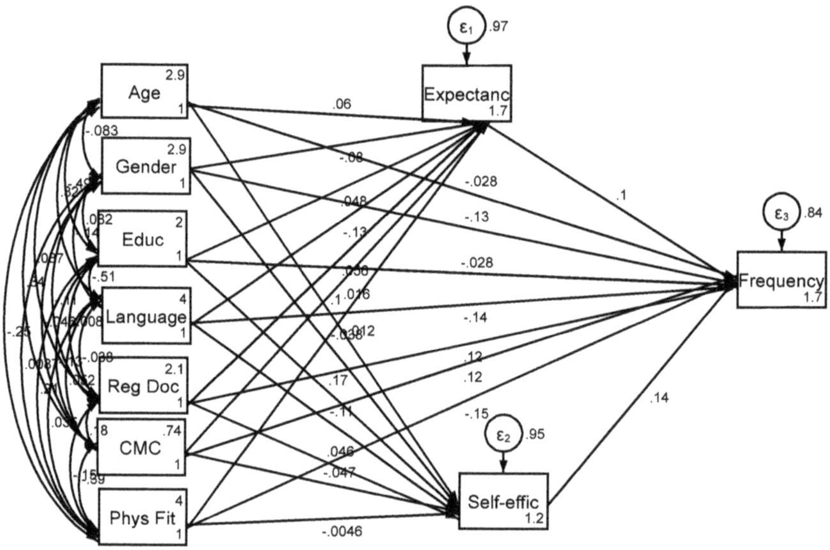

Figure 1. Summary of the structural equation model with telehealth frequency as the outcome. Note: CMC: chronic medical condition; Reg Doc: having a regular provider; Educ: own educational attainment; Language (Spanish); Gender: male gender; Physical Fit (SF12 Score); Expectanc: telehealth expectancy (expected benefits); Frequency: telehealth utilization frequency; Self-effic: self-efficacy to use telehealth.

The results indicate that education significantly predicted telehealth self-efficacy, with higher levels of education associated with greater self-efficacy (B = 0.172, SE = 0.079, 95% CI = 0.018 to 0.326, p = 0.029). None of the other predictors, including age (B = 0.104, SE = 0.075, 95% CI = −0.043 to 0.251, p = 0.164), gender (B = −0.038, SE = 0.062, 95% CI = −0.160 to 0.084, p = 0.545), language preference (Spanish speakers: B = −0.112, SE = 0.073, 95% CI = −0.254 to 0.031, p = 0.126), having a regular doctor (B = 0.046, SE = 0.063, 95% CI = −0.077 to 0.170, p = 0.463), chronic disease (B = −0.047, SE = 0.070, 95% CI = −0.184 to 0.090, p = 0.504), or physical fitness (B = −0.005, SE = 0.069, 95% CI = −0.140 to 0.131, p = 0.947), significantly predicted self-efficacy.

For telehealth expectancy, none of the predictors showed significant associations. Age (B = 0.060, SE = 0.076, 95% CI = −0.089 to 0.208, p = 0.432), gender (B = −0.080, SE = 0.063, 95% CI = −0.203 to 0.043, p = 0.201), education (B = 0.048, SE = 0.080, 95% CI = −0.109 to 0.205, p = 0.548), language preference (Spanish speakers: B = −0.132, SE = 0.074, 95% CI = −0.276 to 0.013, p = 0.074), having a regular doctor (B = 0.056, SE = 0.064, 95% CI = −0.069 to 0.180, p = 0.381), chronic disease (B = 0.016, SE = 0.071, 95% CI = −0.123 to 0.154, p = 0.826), and physical fitness (B = −0.012, SE = 0.070, 95% CI = −0.149 to 0.125, p = 0.867) were not significant predictors of expectancy.

4. Discussion

This study examined the associations between socioeconomic status, health factors, telehealth perceived beliefs and self-efficacy, and telehealth utilization among African American residents within Los Angeles public housing areas.

4.1. Highlights from the Study

The findings revealed that telehealth attitudes, specifically perceived beliefs and self-efficacy, did not mediate the relationship with telehealth utilization. Instead, sociodemographic and health factors, such as gender, language preference, access to a regular doctor, and physical fitness, emerged as significant predictors of telehealth use. Additionally, education was the only significant predictor of telehealth self-efficacy, while no factors were significantly associated with telehealth perceived beliefs.

The absence of an effect of education on telehealth expectancy or utilization (frequency) can be explained by the theory of Marginalization-Related Diminished Returns (MDRs) [51]. According to this theory, factors such as limited resources in the social context, low-quality education, segregation, and other aspects of social marginalization weaken the real-life impact of socioeconomic status (SES) indicators, such as education, for underserved populations [52].

The results highlight the role of demographic, socioeconomic, and health factors in telehealth utilization. Women were more likely to use telehealth services, consistent with prior research suggesting gendered patterns in healthcare-seeking behavior [53–57]. Across studies and settings, women show more frequent healthcare use [53–57]. Language preference also played a significant role, with Spanish speakers reporting lower telehealth use. Not being able to speak English fluently in an English-speaking country is shown to be a barrier against health care use [58–61]. This finding underscores the need for culturally and linguistically tailored telehealth interventions to reduce barriers for non-English-speaking populations [62–64]. Furthermore, access to a regular doctor was positively associated with telehealth use, suggesting that existing relationships with healthcare providers may facilitate telehealth adoption [65–68]. Conversely, better physical fitness was linked to lower telehealth utilization, potentially reflecting a lower perceived need for medical care among healthier individuals.

One of the major findings of this study was that both telehealth attitudes have very limited predictive value for telehealth care utilization. While telehealth attitudes, including expectancy and self-efficacy, are often theorized to influence behavior, our findings suggest these attitudes did not significantly predict telehealth use in this intersectional population. This discrepancy may reflect the dominance of structural and systemic barriers in shaping telehealth behaviors, overshadowing the potential role of individual attitudes. The lack of significant predictors for telehealth expectancy further suggests that structural inequities may limit the extent to which individuals perceive benefits from telehealth services. On the other hand, the significant association between education and telehealth self-efficacy aligns with existing theories, such as the Health Belief Model and the Theory of Reasoned Action, which emphasize the role of education in shaping confidence and the perceived ability to engage with health technologies.

4.2. Implications

The findings have significant implications for addressing healthcare disparities through telehealth. Interventions should prioritize dismantling structural barriers, such as social segregation and improving language access and increasing provider availability. For instance, expanding access to bilingual telehealth platforms and fostering trust-based relationships between under-resourced populations and healthcare providers could play a pivotal role in enhancing telehealth adoption. Additionally, targeted efforts to engage men and individuals with limited access to regular care are essential to ensuring equitable telehealth use. Interventions that overly emphasize improving individual-level attributes, such as attitudes toward telehealth, are unlikely to bring about meaningful behavioral change. Effective solutions must go beyond individual attitudes and address systemic and structural factors to achieve lasting impact.

4.3. Study Limitations

This study has several limitations that should be acknowledged. First, the cross-sectional design limits the ability to draw causal inferences about the relationships between social determinants, telehealth attitudes, and telehealth use. While the findings provide valuable insights, they only capture a snapshot in time, leaving the temporal dynamics and causal pathways unexplored. Second, this study was conducted in Los Angeles using a non-random, convenience sample, which limits the generalizability of the results to other regions or populations. The unique socioeconomic, cultural, and healthcare landscape of Los Angeles may have influenced the findings, and different results could emerge in other cities or rural areas. Third, the study sample was not representative of all low-income racial and ethnic minority residents of public housing, further constraining the broader applicability of the results. Additionally, key contextual factors, such as neighborhood characteristics, access to public transportation, and broader systemic inequities, were not included in the analysis but could play a critical role in shaping telehealth utilization.

4.4. Future Research

Future research should address these limitations by employing longitudinal designs to better understand the dynamic and evolving nature of telehealth adoption over time. Tracking changes in telehealth attitudes and utilization in response to policy shifts, technological advancements, or targeted interventions could provide deeper insights into causal relationships. Moreover, qualitative studies are essential to explore the nuanced experiences and barriers faced by this intersectional population, adding depth to the quantitative findings and uncovering factors that may not be captured by surveys or structured data collection. Larger and more representative sample sizes should also be prioritized to enhance the generalizability of findings. Expanding the scope of research to include additional variables such as neighborhood characteristics, access to public transportation, and mental health indicators (e.g., depression) could provide a more comprehensive understanding of the factors influencing telehealth use. Furthermore, incorporating measures of discrimination and mistrust—common barriers in healthcare access for marginalized populations—would help to elucidate their potential impact on telehealth attitudes and behavior. By addressing these gaps, future studies can build on the present findings to inform more effective policies and interventions aimed at promoting equitable telehealth adoption among underserved communities.

5. Conclusions

In conclusion, this study underscores the importance of addressing structural barriers to increase telehealth use among low-income racial and ethnic minority residents of public housing. While telehealth attitudes, such as expectancy and self-efficacy, were not significant predictors of utilization, demographic and systemic factors played a more prominent role. These findings suggest that structural interventions, rather than solely focusing on individual attitudes, are necessary to bridge telehealth disparities and promote equitable access to healthcare in underserved communities.

Author Contributions: Conceptualization, M.B.; Methodology, S.C., A.D., M.B. and S.A.; Software, E.Y.; Formal analysis, A.D. and E.Y.; Investigation, S.C.; Resources, S.C.; Data curation, S.C., A.D. and S.A.; Writing—original draft, S.A.; Writing—review and editing, S.C., E.Y., M.B., A.D. and S.A.; Funding acquisition, M.B. All authors have read and agreed to the published version of the manuscript.

Funding: Drs. Sharon Cobb and Attallah Dillard, scholars in the Clinical Research Education and Career Development (CRECD) program at Charles R. Drew University of Medicine and Science, received support for their research-related efforts through the NIMHD/NIH Award number R25 MD007610 (PI = Mohsen Bazargan). Some of Dr. Ehsan Yaghmaei support comes from CRECD (statistical support for CRECD scholars). Dr. Assari contribution to this work was in-Kind and not supported by CRECD or NIH funds.

Institutional Review Board Statement: The study protocol received approval from the Institutional Review Board (IRB) at Charles R. Drew University of Medicine and Science (IRB Approval Number: 1746099, approval date: 22 April 2021).

Informed Consent Statement: Informed consent was obtained from all subjects involved in this study.

Data Availability Statement: The original contributions presented in this study are included in this article. Further inquiries can be directed to the corresponding authors.

Acknowledgments: The researchers wish to acknowledge the participants as well as the Housing Authority of the City of Los Angeles (HACLA) who made this study possible.

Conflicts of Interest: The authors declare no conflicts of interest.

References

1. Aratani, Y. Public housing revisited: Racial differences, housing assistance, and socioeconomic attainment among low-income families. *Soc. Sci. Res.* **2010**, *39*, 1108–1125. [CrossRef]
2. Fauth, R.C.; Leventhal, T.; Brooks-Gunn, J. Short-term effects of moving from public housing in poor to middle-class neighborhoods on low-income, minority adults' outcomes. *Soc. Sci. Med.* **2004**, *59*, 2271–2284. [CrossRef]
3. Carter, W.H.; Schill, M.H.; Wachter, S.M. Polarisation, public housing and racial minorities in US cities. *Urban Stud.* **1998**, *35*, 1889–1911. [CrossRef]
4. Murdie, R.A. 'Blacks in near-ghettos?' black visible minority population in metropolitan Toronto housing authority public housing units. *Hous. Stud.* **1994**, *9*, 435–457. [CrossRef]
5. DeLuca, S.; Garboden, P.M.; Rosenblatt, P. Segregating shelter: How housing policies shape the residential locations of low-income minority families. *Annals Am. Acad. Political Soc. Sci.* **2013**, *647*, 268–299. [CrossRef]
6. Jahoda, M.; West, P.S. Race relations in public housing. *J. Soc. Issues* **1951**, *7*, 132–139. [CrossRef]
7. Bowleg, L. The problem with the phrase women and minorities: Intersectionality—An important theoretical framework for public health. *Am. J. Public Health* **2012**, *102*, 1267–1273. [CrossRef]
8. Atewologun, D. *Intersectionality Theory and Practice*; Oxford University Press: Oxford, UK, 2018; pp. 1–20.
9. Dutton, D.B. Explaining the low use of health services by the poor: Costs, attitudes, or delivery systems? *Am. Sociol. Rev.* **1978**, *43*, 348–368. [CrossRef]
10. Price, J.H.; Desmond, S.M.; Snyder, F.F.; Kimmel, S.R. Health Care and Poor Patients. *J. Fam. Pract.* **1988**, *27*, 615–621.
11. Kirby, J.B. Poor people, poor places and access to health care in the United States. *Soc. Forces* **2008**, *87*, 325–355. [CrossRef]

12. Preker, A.S.; Carrin, G.; Dror, D.; Jakab, M.; Hsiao, W.; Arhin-Tenkorang, D. Rich-poor differences in health care financing. In *Health Financing for Poor People–Resource Mobilization and Risk Sharing*; The World Bank: Washington, DC, USA, 2004; pp. 3–52.
13. Carder, P.; Luhr, G.; Kohon, J. Differential Health and Social Needs of Older Adults Waitlisted for Public Housing or Housing Choice Vouchers. *J Aging Soc Policy* **2016**, *28*, 246–260. [CrossRef] [PubMed]
14. Fagan, J.; Davies, G.; Carlis, A. Race and selective enforcement in public housing. *J. Empir. Leg. Stud.* **2012**, *9*, 697–728. [CrossRef]
15. Goetz, E.G. Where have all the towers gone? The dismantling of public housing in US cities. *J. Urban Aff.* **2011**, *33*, 267–287. [CrossRef]
16. Holloway, S.R.; McNulty, T.L. Contingent urban geographies of violent crime: Racial segregation and the impact of public housing in Atlanta. *Urban Geogr.* **2003**, *24*, 187–211. [CrossRef]
17. Haley, D.F.; Linton, S.; Luo, R.; Hunter-Jones, J.; Adimora, A.A.; Wingood, G.M.; Bonney, L.; Ross, Z.; Cooper, H.L. Public Housing Relocations and Relationships of Changes in Neighborhood Disadvantage and Transportation Access to Unmet Need for Medical Care. *J. Health Care Poor Underserved* **2017**, *28*, 315–328. [CrossRef]
18. Yamamoto, T.; Hanazato, M.; Hikichi, H.; Kondo, K.; Osaka, K.; Kawachi, I.; Aida, J. Change in Geographic Accessibility to Dental Clinics Affects Access to Care. *J. Dent. Res.* **2023**, *102*, 719–726. [CrossRef]
19. Hodgkinson, S.; Godoy, L.; Beers, L.S.; Lewin, A. Improving Mental Health Access for Low-Income Children and Families in the Primary Care Setting. *Pediatrics* **2017**, *139*, e20151175. [CrossRef]
20. Lascher, S.; Tasir-Rodriguez, W.; Moon, G.; Irizzary, M.; Baney, M.; Kellogg, F.R. Government public housing health needs assessment: Focus on race, ethnicity, and the older adult: Background, methods, and demographics. *Care Manag. J.* **2013**, *14*, 118–124. [CrossRef]
21. Foster, B.; Ledgerwood, D.M.; Struble, C.A.; Fodor, M.C.; Jordan, P.; Krishnan, A.C.; Turner, B.; Pearson, C.; Twiner, M.J.; Levy, P.D. Public Housing Resident Perspectives on Smoking, Barriers for Smoking Cessation, and Changes in Smoking Mandates. *Inquiry* **2022**, *59*, 469580221092814. [CrossRef]
22. Wang, X.; Seyler, B.C.; Chen, T.; Jian, W.; Fu, H.; Di, B.; Yip, W.; Pan, J. Disparity in healthcare seeking behaviors between impoverished and non-impoverished populations with implications for healthcare resource optimization. *Humanit. Soc. Sci. Commun.* **2024**, *11*, 1208. [CrossRef]
23. Gearing, R.E.; Washburn, M.; Brewer, K.B.; Yu, M.; Bjugstad, A.; Torres, L.R. Predictors of Help-Seeking for Mental Health Treatment Among Latinos. *J. Racial Ethn. Health Disparities* **2023**, *10*, 1869–1877. [CrossRef] [PubMed]
24. Siddiqui, N.Y.; Ammarell, N.; Wu, J.M.; Sandoval, J.S.; Bosworth, H.B. Urinary Incontinence and Health-Seeking Behavior Among White, Black, and Latina Women. *Female Pelvic Med. Reconstr. Surg.* **2016**, *22*, 340–345. [CrossRef]
25. Powe, B.D. Health Information Seeking Among Rural African Americans, Caucasians, and Hispanics: It Is Built, Did They Come? *Nurs. Clin. N. Am.* **2015**, *50*, 531–543. [CrossRef]
26. Lee, Y.J.; Boden-Albala, B.; Larson, E.; Wilcox, A.; Bakken, S. Online health information seeking behaviors of Hispanics in New York City: A community-based cross-sectional study. *J. Med. Internet Res.* **2014**, *16*, e176. [CrossRef]
27. Bjarnadottir, R.I.; Millery, M.; Fleck, E.; Bakken, S. Correlates of online health information-seeking behaviors in a low-income Hispanic community. *Inf. Health Soc. Care* **2016**, *41*, 341–349. [CrossRef]
28. Sherman, L.D.; Goidel, K.; Bergeron, C.D.; Smith, M.L. Web-Based Health Information Seeking Among African American and Hispanic Men Living With Chronic Conditions: Cross-sectional Survey Study. *J. Med. Internet Res.* **2021**, *23*, e26180. [CrossRef]
29. Jezewski, E.; Miller, A.; Eusebio, M.; Potter, J. Targeted telehealth education increases interest in using telehealth among a diverse group of low-income older adults. *Int. J. Environ. Res. Public Health* **2022**, *19*, 13349. [CrossRef]
30. Luo, J.; Ahmad, S.F.; Alyaemeni, A.; Ou, Y.; Irshad, M.; Alyafi-Alzahri, R.; Alsanie, G.; Unnisa, S.T. Role of perceived ease of use, usefulness, and financial strength on the adoption of health information systems: The moderating role of hospital size. *Humanit. Soc. Sci. Commun.* **2024**, *11*, 516. [CrossRef]
31. Broffman, L.; Harrison, S.; Zhao, M.; Goldman, A.; Patnaik, I.; Zhou, M. The Relationship Between Broadband Speeds, Device Type, Demographic Characteristics, and Care-Seeking Via Telehealth. *Telemed. J. E Health* **2023**, *29*, 425–431. [CrossRef]
32. Hsieh, H.; Tsai, C. An Empirical Study to Explore the Adoption of Telehealth: Health Belief Model Perspective. *J. Eng. Sci. Technol. Rev.* **2013**, *6*, 1–5. [CrossRef]
33. Chuang, B.-K.; Tsai, C.-H.; Hsieh, H.-L.; Tumurtulga, T. Applying health belief model to explore the adoption of telecare. In Proceedings of the 2013 IEEE/ACIS 12th International Conference on Computer and Information Science (ICIS), Niigata, Japan, 16–20 June 2013; pp. 269–272.
34. Hsieh, H.-L.; Lai, J.-M.; Chuang, B.-K.; Tsai, C.-H. Determinants of telehealth continuance intention: A multi-perspective framework. *Healthcare* **2022**, *10*, 2038. [CrossRef] [PubMed]
35. Wedell, L.E. Theoretical Exploration of the Association Between Telehealth Use and Intention to Use Teledentistry. Master's Thesis, University of Minnesota, Minneapolis, MN, USA, 2024.

36. Dryden, E.M.; Kennedy, M.A.; Conti, J.; Boudreau, J.H.; Anwar, C.P.; Nearing, K.; Pimentel, C.B.; Hung, W.W.; Moo, L.R. Perceived benefits of geriatric specialty telemedicine among rural patients and caregivers. *Health Serv. Res.* **2023**, *58* (Suppl. S1), 26–35. [CrossRef] [PubMed]
37. Serrano, L.P.; Maita, K.C.; Avila, F.R.; Torres-Guzman, R.A.; Garcia, J.P.; Eldaly, A.S.; Haider, C.R.; Felton, C.L.; Paulson, M.R.; Maniaci, M.J.; et al. Benefits and Challenges of Remote Patient Monitoring as Perceived by Health Care Practitioners: A Systematic Review. *Perm. J.* **2023**, *27*, 100–111. [CrossRef] [PubMed]
38. Yuen, K.F.; Chua, J.Y.; Li, X.; Wang, X. The determinants of users' intention to adopt telehealth: Health belief, perceived value and self-determination perspectives. *J. Retail. Consum. Serv.* **2023**, *73*, 103346. [CrossRef]
39. Glanz, K.E.; Lewis, F.M.E.; Rimer, B.K. *Health Behavior and Health Education: Theory, Research, and Practice*; Jossey-Bass/Wiley: Hoboken, NJ, USA, 1990.
40. Glanz, K.; Rimer, B.K.; Viswanath, K. *Theory, Research, and Practice in Health Behavior and Health Education*; John Wiley & Sons: Hoboken, NJ, USA, 2008.
41. Mason, J.; Woodward, M. Self-efficacy as a mediator between psychologists' technology affinity and telehealth satisfaction. *Aust. Psychol.* **2024**, 1–13. [CrossRef]
42. Rikhy, R.S.; Dela Cruz, J.; Rattan, A.; Bibi, A.; Rangrej, S. The Self-Efficacy of Physicians to Communicate With Patients via Telemedicine in Lieu of Face-to-Face Visits in Light of the COVID-19 Pandemic: An Observational Study. *Cureus* **2022**, *14*, e25739. [CrossRef]
43. Finkelstein, S.M.; Speedie, S.M.; Zhou, X.; Potthoff, S.; Ratner, E.R. Perception, satisfaction and utilization of the VALUE home telehealth service. *J. Telemed. Telecare* **2011**, *17*, 288–292. [CrossRef]
44. Gajarawala, S.N.; Pelkowski, J.N. Telehealth benefits and barriers. *J. Nurse Pract.* **2021**, *17*, 218–221. [CrossRef]
45. Wardlow, L.; Roberts, C.; Archbald-Pannone, L.; Collaborative for Telehealth and Aging. Perceptions and uses of telehealth in the care of older adults. *Telemed. E-Health* **2023**, *29*, 1143–1151. [CrossRef]
46. Kabir, H.; Hasan, M.K.; Jamil, S.; Chowdhury, S.R.; Mitra, D.K. Knowledge, perceived benefits, perceived concerns, and predisposition to use telehealth services in Bangladesh: A cross-sectional survey. *BMC Digit. Health* **2024**, *2*, 61. [CrossRef]
47. Ciere, Y.; Cartwright, M.; Newman, S.P. A systematic review of the mediating role of knowledge, self-efficacy and self-care behaviour in telehealth patients with heart failure. *J. Telemed. Telecare* **2012**, *18*, 384–391. [CrossRef] [PubMed]
48. Lek, J.J.; Cham, K.M.; Merolli, M. Evaluating perceived technology self-efficacy and telehealth acceptance in optometry students. *Clin. Exp. Optom.* **2024**, 1–12. [CrossRef] [PubMed]
49. Söylemez, B.A.; Özgül, E.; Küçükgüçlü, Ö.; Yener, G. Telehealth applications used for self-efficacy levels of family caregivers for individuals with dementia: A systematic review and Meta-analysis. *Geriatr. Nurs.* **2023**, *49*, 178–192. [CrossRef]
50. van Houwelingen, T.; Ettema, R.G.; Bleijenberg, N.; van Os-Medendorp, H.; Kort, H.S.; Ten Cate, O. Educational intervention to increase nurses' knowledge, self-efficacy and usage of telehealth: A multi-setting pretest-posttest study. *Nurse Educ. Pract.* **2021**, *51*, 102924. [CrossRef]
51. Assari, S. Health Disparities due to Diminished Return among Black Americans: Public Policy Solutions. *Soc. Issues Policy Rev.* **2018**, *12*, 112–145. [CrossRef]
52. Assari, S. Unequal Gain of Equal Resources across Racial Groups. *Int. J. Health Policy Manag.* **2018**, *7*, 1–9. [CrossRef]
53. Liu, L.; Wang, C.; Yang, S.; Lo, K.; Yang, X. Gender Differences in Healthcare-Seeking Behaviors in China's Ageing Population: An Empirical Study of Shanghai. *Research Square* **2020**. [CrossRef]
54. Kana, S.; Arjyal, A.; Wallace, L.; Nwameme, A.; Mbachu, C.; Islam, F.; Huque, S.; Salma, U.; Shrestha, G.; Elsey, H. *Influence of Changing Gender and Social Norms on Health Seeking Behaviour and Health Systems in Cities*; CHORUS: Wellington, New Zealand, 2023.
55. Onah, M.N.; Horton, S. Male-female differences in households' resource allocation and decision to seek healthcare in south-eastern Nigeria: Results from a mixed methods study. *Soc. Sci. Med.* **2018**, *204*, 84–91. [CrossRef]
56. Cameron, K.A.; Song, J.; Manheim, L.M.; Dunlop, D.D. Gender disparities in health and healthcare use among older adults. *J. Women's Health* **2010**, *19*, 1643–1650. [CrossRef]
57. Bertakis, K.D.; Azari, R.; Helms, L.J.; Callahan, E.J.; Robbins, J.A. Gender differences in the utilization of health care services. *J. Fam. Pract.* **2000**, *49*, 147–152.
58. Cheng, E.M.; Chen, A.; Cunningham, W. Primary language and receipt of recommended health care among Hispanics in the United States. *J. Gen. Intern. Med.* **2007**, *22*, 283–288. [CrossRef] [PubMed]
59. Timmins, C.L. The impact of language barriers on the health care of Latinos in the United States: A review of the literature and guidelines for practice. *J. Midwifery Women's Health* **2002**, *47*, 80–96. [CrossRef] [PubMed]
60. Diamond, L.C.; Tuot, D.S.; Karliner, L.S. The use of Spanish language skills by physicians and nurses: Policy implications for teaching and testing. *J. Gen. Intern. Med.* **2012**, *27*, 117–123. [CrossRef] [PubMed]
61. DuBard, C.A.; Gizlice, Z. Language spoken and differences in health status, access to care, and receipt of preventive services among US Hispanics. *Am. J. Public Health* **2008**, *98*, 2021–2028. [CrossRef]

62. Al-Amer, R.; Ramjan, L.; Glew, P.; Darwish, M.; Salamonson, Y. Translation of interviews from a source language to a target language: Examining issues in cross-cultural health care research. *J. Clin. Nurs.* **2015**, *24*, 1151–1162. [CrossRef]
63. Gil-Salmerón, A.; Katsas, K.; Riza, E.; Karnaki, P.; Linos, A. Access to healthcare for migrant patients in Europe: Healthcare discrimination and translation services. *Int. J. Environ. Res. Public Health* **2021**, *18*, 7901. [CrossRef]
64. Matías-Carrelo, L.E.; Chávez, L.M.; Negrón, G.; Canino, G.; Aguilar-Gaxiola, S.; Hoppe, S. The Spanish translation and cultural adaptation of five mental health outcome measures. *Cult. Med. Psychiatry* **2003**, *27*, 291–313. [CrossRef]
65. Beal, A.; Hernandez, S. Patient reports of the quality of care in community health centers: The importance of having a regular provider. *J. Health Care Poor Underserved* **2010**, *21*, 591–605. [CrossRef]
66. Lambrew, J.M.; Defriese, G.H.; Carey, T.S.; Ricketts, T.C.; Biddle, A.K. The effects of having a regular doctor on access to primary care. *Med. Care* **1996**, *34*, 138–151. [CrossRef]
67. Ettner, S.L. The relationship between continuity of care and the health behaviors of patients: Does having a usual physician make a difference? *Med. Care* **1999**, *37*, 547–555. [CrossRef]
68. Mahmood, A.; Mosalpuria, K.; Wyant, D.K.; Bhuyan, S.S. Association between having a regular health provider and access to services linked to electronic health records. *Hosp. Top.* **2019**, *97*, 1–10. [CrossRef]

healthcare

MDPI

Review

Mapping Research Trends on the Implications of Telemedicine for Healthcare Professionals: A Comprehensive Bibliometric Analysis

Chiara Bernuzzi *, Maria Adele Piccardo and Chiara Guglielmetti

Department of Economics, Management and Quantitative Methods (DEMM), University of Milan, Via Conservatorio, 7, 20122 Milan, Italy; mariaadele.piccardo@unimi.it (M.A.P.); chiara.guglielmetti@unimi.it (C.G.)
* Correspondence: chiara.bernuzzi@unimi.it

Abstract: Background/Objectives: The digital transformation in healthcare is reshaping care delivery by enhancing patient care and flexibility. However, it also poses potential challenges to healthcare professionals' wellbeing and work practices. To date, research on the implications of telemedicine for healthcare professionals remains limited and inconclusive. This study aims to provide a comprehensive overview of this research field using a quantitative, bibliometric approach. **Methods:** Articles were systematically selected from Web of Science and Scopus databases, focusing on empirical, peer-reviewed articles written in English, involving healthcare professionals and focusing on telemedicine. **Results:** The dataset consists of 160 papers. The analysis reveals a significant increase in publications starting from 2012, with a notable surge in 2020, reflecting the impact of the COVID-19 pandemic. The University of New Mexico and the Cleveland Clinic Foundation, both in the United States, were identified as the institutions with the highest number of published articles. Most studies were published in clinical-focused journals (e.g., Journal of Medical Internet Research and BMC Health Services Research), emphasizing the field's dominant orientation. The intellectual structure reveals that wellbeing, work practices, and communications between patients and professionals are central themes. **Conclusions:** This bibliometric analysis provides scholars with a clearer understanding of the intellectual structure of research on the implications of telemedicine for healthcare professionals, addressing key gaps left by previous reviews. While telemedicine offers numerous advantages, such as enhanced access to care and greater flexibility, it also raises challenges related to healthcare professionals' wellbeing, work practices, and communication with patients. Both contextual factors (e.g., digital skills training) and individual characteristics (e.g., attitudes toward telemedicine) play a significant role in shaping healthcare professionals' experiences with telemedicine. By identifying influential contributors and thematic patterns, this study offers a foundation for future research and informs the development of targeted interventions to sustain healthcare professionals in digitally mediated care environments.

Keywords: telemedicine; healthcare professionals; wellbeing; work outcomes; bibliometric analysis

1. Introduction

In recent years, telemedicine has become a key component of healthcare delivery by offering innovative solutions for patient care, especially in remote and underserved areas [1]. Telemedicine involves the use of digital communication and information technologies by medical professionals to deliver essential healthcare services, enabling the exchange of accurate information necessary for diagnosis, treatment, and prevention, regardless of time and location constraints [2]. This term encompasses a wide array of applications, such as remote consultations, distance health monitoring, and telerehabilitation [3]. It has the potential to improve access to care, streamline services, and enhance patient outcomes [4]. The relevance of telemedicine has surged particularly in the context of the COVID-19 pandemic, during which it enabled the provision of care at a distance, avoiding physical contact between patients and healthcare providers [5,6]. Telemedicine is now recognized not only for its capacity to enhance access to care, but also for its transformative effects on healthcare practice. To date, much of the research in this field has focused on technological advancements and on the effects of telemedicine on patient care [7]. However, healthcare professionals (i.e., individuals in the medical field, including physicians, nurses, and allied healthcare professionals responsible for delivering healthcare services to patients; HCPs [8]) are the ones implementing and managing these technology-driven services. This suggests the need to understand how telemedicine impacts HCPs, to ensure its successful and sustainable integration into healthcare systems.

Previous research has shown that the introduction of new technologies in the workplace often leads to changes and challenges [9], which can affect workers' wellbeing. In the healthcare sector, digitalization represents both an opportunity and a burden [10]. On the one hand, it offers benefits such as greater flexibility [11], increased autonomy, and improved patient care [7]; on the other hand, it may exacerbate issues such as higher workload [12] and the erosion of traditional patient–professional relationships [11]. Telemedicine, therefore, is a double-edged sword: while it can optimize healthcare delivery, it also presents significant challenges for HCPs [13]. Despite a growing body of research examining HCPs' acceptance of telemedicine tools [14,15], studies specifically addressing the implications of telemedicine on HCPs' wellbeing remain scarce and fragmented, often producing mixed or context-specific results [16,17]. This represents a critical gap, as HCPs play a fundamental role in ensuring high-quality, safe, and sustainable healthcare. Indeed, prior studies have shown that distress and fatigue among physicians are associated with an increased risk of medical errors [18]. Although scholarly interest in telemedicine has intensified—particularly in the wake of the COVID-19 pandemic—most research has primarily focused on technological advancements, clinical applications, and patient outcomes, with considerably less attention given to HCPs' perspectives. Even when reviews are available, they tend to concentrate on specific types of telemedicine services (e.g., video consultations [19]) or on HCPs' attitudes and digital competencies [14,20–22], while largely overlooking the implications for wellbeing and work practices. To our knowledge, no previous study has employed bibliometric analysis to systematically map the scientific literature on the implications of telemedicine for HCPs, identify influential contributors, and uncover thematic patterns and knowledge gaps. Such an approach is essential not only to conceptually organizing the field, but also to highlighting underexplored areas and guiding future research directions.

To address these gaps, this study presents a bibliometric analysis aimed at providing a structured overview of the scientific literature on the implications of telemedicine for HCPs. The objectives of this analysis are threefold: (1) to map the evolution and distribution of scholarly production in this area, identifying key contributors (authors, institutions, countries, and journals); (2) to explore the conceptual structure of this field by identifying major research themes and emerging topics related to HCPs' experience with telemedicine; and (3) to highlight underexplored areas and provide suggestions for future research directions that could better support HCPs in digitally mediated care environments.

In line with these objectives, the following research questions guide this analysis:

(RQ1) Which journal(s), institution(s), and country(s) have the most publications in this research field?

(RQ2) What are the most researched themes and emerging topics related to HCPs' experiences with telemedicine?

(RQ3) What are the relevant future directions for research in this field?

Through this comprehensive approach, we aim to provide a foundation for a more nuanced understanding of the challenges posed by telemedicine adoption among HCPs.

2. Materials and Methods

Bibliometric analysis is widely recognized as a robust and systematic tool for evaluating the scientific output of a research field [23]. Unlike other review methods, such as systematic or scoping reviews, bibliometric analysis adopts a macro-level perspective that enables researchers to trace the evolution of a field's intellectual, social, and conceptual structures over time [23,24]. By grounding the review process in the statistical measurement of scientific production, scholars, and activity, this method ensures a systematic, transparent, and reproducible approach to knowledge mapping [25].

Crucially, bibliometric analysis relies on objective and replicable procedures, thereby minimizing interpretive bias and enhancing methodological rigor compared to more narrative or qualitative approaches [23,26]. In a moment of rapid growth and transformation in telemedicine, this approach provides strategic insights that traditional literature reviews may not fully capture. As telemedicine continues to reshape healthcare delivery, bibliometric methods offer a structured and data-driven overview of research trends and knowledge diffusion patterns, supporting scholars in navigating the complexity of this evolving field.

By offering a comprehensive and structured perspective, bibliometric analysis offers a solid foundation for the development of innovative research directions and the advancement of scholarly discussion [27].

The following sections detail the data collection and analysis processes, in accordance with the methodological guidelines proposed by Aria and Cuccurullo [25] and the guidelines for reporting bibliometric reviews in biomedical literature (BIBLIO) [28].

2.1. Data Collection

Documents were retrieved from two primary databases: Web of Science (WoS) and Scopus. These databases were selected for their comprehensive coverage of journals and articles with detailed metadata [29]. Regarding WoS, only articles indexed in the Science Citation Index Expanded (SCI Expanded), the Social Science Citation Index (SSCI) and the Emerging Sources Citation Index (ESCI) were considered. To capture a wide range of studies focusing on HCPs' perspectives regarding the adoption of telemedicine tools, a search strategy was developed using the following keywords: physician* OR doctor* OR clinician* OR "healthcare manager*" OR "healthcare professional*" OR "healthcare worker*" OR "healthcare personnel" OR "health personnel" OR "health manager*" OR "health professional*" OR "health worker*" OR "medical staff" OR professional* OR nurse* AND telemedicine OR telehealth OR ehealth OR telemonitoring OR telecare AND wellbeing OR "professional wellbeing" OR "work-related stress" OR "job stress" OR "occupational stress" OR "work environment" OR workplace. The keywords were carefully selected to balance inclusivity and specificity, aiming to capture relevant studies while minimizing irrelevant results. In Scopus, the search focused on titles, abstracts, and keywords, while in WoS, the search was conducted based on the topic (TS). The search was further refined by language (English) and document type (article). No time restrictions were applied to ensure the inclusion of all relevant articles and to capture the field's evolution from its initial stage. The search string retrieved a total of 841 articles, with 601 from Scopus and 240 from WoS.

2.2. Inclusion and Exclusion Criteria

Only empirical, peer-reviewed articles written in English, involving samples of HCPs (e.g., doctors, nurses) and focusing on telemedicine as a research topic, published up to 2023, were included in the analysis. Conceptual papers, conference proceedings, dissertations, protocols, review articles, and studies not focused on HCPs or telemedicine were excluded due to their limited contribution to the research questions and conceptual mapping. Similarly, studies addressing digital training/interventions for workers outside the healthcare context, or those mentioning telemedicine only incidentally, were also excluded. No restrictions were applied concerning the journal's impact factor or the country of origin of the studies, to ensure a broad and inclusive overview of the empirical literature available in the field.

2.3. Screening Process

Following the completion of the semi-automated filtering process using database tools, a total of 841 articles were identified and subsequently checked for duplicates. After this step, 655 unique articles remained for further evaluation based on the established inclusion and exclusion criteria. In line with the Preferred Reporting Items for Systematic Reviews and Meta-Analyses (PRISMA) [30], two independent reviewers screened the titles and abstracts to assess their relevance to the research objectives. In cases of discrepancies between the reviewers, group discussions and detailed re-examinations of the studies were conducted until consensus was reached. Only articles unanimously deemed relevant were retained, leading to a refined dataset of 204 documents. A similar strategy was adopted during the final screening phase, in which the full text of the selected articles was reviewed to ensure compliance with the eligibility criteria [25]. As a result, 44 additional articles were excluded, leaving a final dataset of 160 articles. The screening process is illustrated in Figure 1.

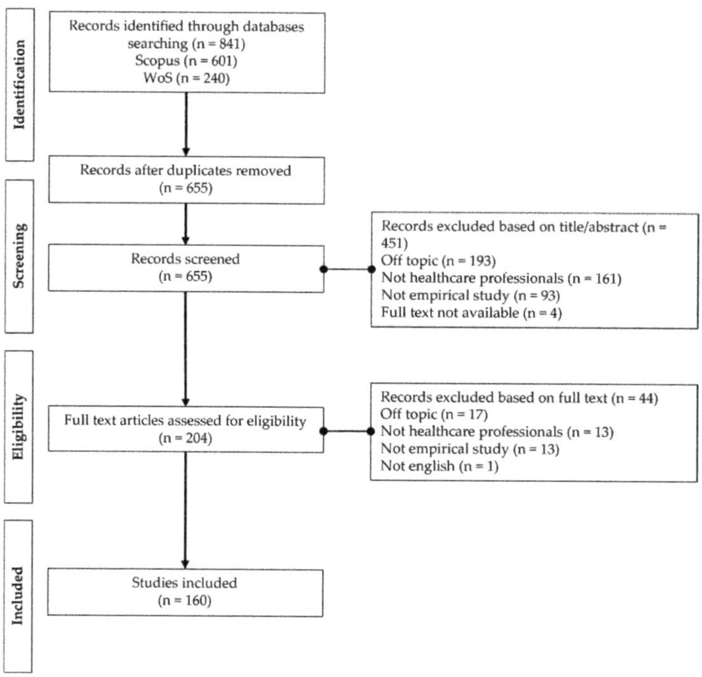

Figure 1. Flow diagram of records identified, screened, and included in the bibliometric analysis, according to PRISMA guidelines.

2.4. Data Analysis

A bibliometric analysis was conducted using the Bibliometrix R-package (version 4.1.4, available at https://www.bibliometrix.org/home/index.php/layout/biblioshiny, accessed on 12 October 2024), a free and open source software that provides tools for quantitative bibliometric research [25]. Metadata (e.g., authors, citations, keywords) from the 160 selected articles were exported as a plain text file for subsequent analysis.

This study includes a performance analysis aimed at examining the characteristics of the sample and evaluating the influence of scientific output, including metrics such as the number of publications, citation rates, and the contributions of the different countries. These metrics are commonly used in bibliometric research to assess scientific productivity (e.g., number of publications), impact (e.g., citations), and the geographical and institutional distribution of knowledge. Their inclusion allows for a comprehensive overview of the research field [23]. Additionally, the most frequently used terms related to HCPs' perspectives on telemedicine were analyzed. This was followed by co-word and thematic analyses to explore and map the intellectual structure of the research domain [31]. Specifically, co-word analysis assumes that the co-occurrence of keywords reflects the underlying themes within documents, thus allowing for the detection and visual representation of topic clusters in the field [26]. Thematic analysis was then applied to identify the main research themes and measure their relevance in relation to the development of the overall field [32].

3. Results

3.1. Data Description

This bibliometric analysis included a total of 160 articles published between 2001 and 2023. These articles were distributed across 119 different sources. In total, the analysis identified 483 unique authors from 43 different countries (Table 1).

Table 1. Overview of the contributions.

	Dataset Features	
General information	Timespan	2001:2023
	Journals	119
	Documents	160
	Annual growth rate (%)	14.46
	Average citations per document	14.03
	Average citations per year per doc	3.83
	References	4895
Document contents	Author's keywords	600
Authors	Authors	905

3.2. Global Publication Trends

The annual scientific production exhibited notable fluctuations in the number of published works. Initially, the field showed modest activity, with only 2 publications in 2001. However, several years passed without significant output, indicating that interest in telemedicine, especially concerning the point of view of HCPs, was in its early stages. From 2012 onwards, there was a steady increase in publications, peaking in 2020. Specifically, the number of publications rose from fewer than 10 per year between 2001 and 2019, to more than 14 per year starting in 2020. The upward trend continued, with 37 articles published in 2023, suggesting growing recognition of the importance of considering HCPs' perspectives on telemedicine adoption. Figure 2 illustrates the publication trend.

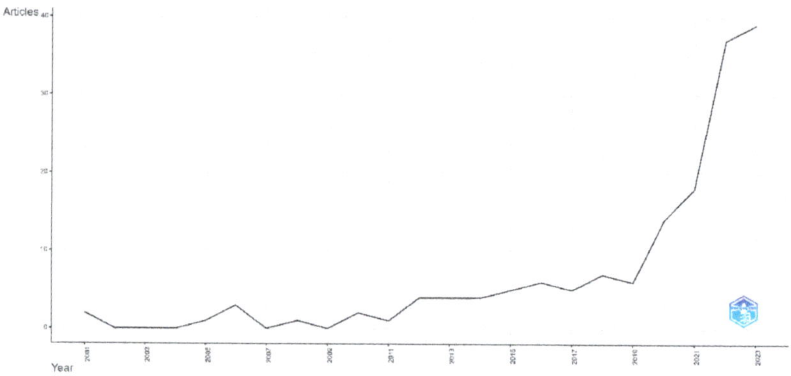

Figure 2. Annual scientific production.

3.3. Most Relevant Journals, Articles, Countries and Affiliations

An analysis of the sources revealed a small subset of journals that dominate the literature in this field (Table 2). Notably, journals such as the Journal of Medical Internet Research and BMC Health Services Research were identified as leading platforms for disseminating research on telemedicine from the HCPs' perspective. The main disciplinary focus of each journal was identified using Scopus classification. Interestingly, all journals were in the health or medical domain, with no journals in psychology or humanities.

Table 2. Most relevant journals.

	n	Highest Percentile (Source: Scopus)
Journal of Medical Internet Research	10	Health Informatics
BMC Health Services Research	7	Health Policy
International Journal of Environmental Research And Public Health	6	/
BMC Medical Informatics And Decision Making	4	/
BMJ Open	3	General Medicine
Plos One	3	Multidisciplinary
Telemedicine Reports	3	Medicine (miscellaneous)
Australian Journal of Primary Health	2	/
Frontiers in Digital Health	2	/
Health Informatics Journal	2	Health Informatics

N = number of published articles.

Table 3 presents the ten most cited articles. The most frequently cited article was published by Hennemann and colleagues [33], followed by the one written by Katzman and colleagues [34] and Villani and colleagues [35].

The geographical distribution of research output indicates the leading role of certain countries in advancing telemedicine research from the perspective of HCPs (Figure 3). The United States emerged as the most prolific contributor, with the highest number of publications (n = 138). Other major contributors included Australia (n = 54), United Kingdom (n = 34), and European countries such as Sweden (n = 33) and Finland (n = 23).

Focusing on affiliations, the University of New Mexico (n = 10) and the Cleveland Clinic Foundation (n = 8), both based in the United States, emerged as the most productive institutions. Ranked third was Linköping University (n = 6) in Sweden, where e-health is one of the key areas of research activity (Figure 4).

Table 3. Top manuscript by citation.

Ranking	Article	Number of Citations	Number of Citations per Year
1	Hennemann et al. [33]	123	15.38
2	Katzman et al. [34]	94	8.55
3	Villani et al. [35]	85	7.08
4	Maguire et al. [36]	81	8.1
5	Moeckli et al. [37]	71	1.39
6	Vehko et al. [38]	67	11.16
7	Srinivasan et al. [39]	62	12.4
8	Bolier et al. [40]	61	5.54
9	Grünloh et al. [41]	55	6.11
10	Ruiz Morilla et al. [42]	54	6.75

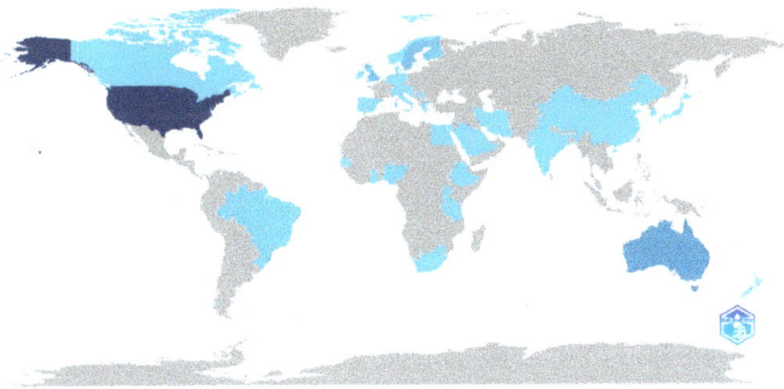

Figure 3. Scientific production by country. Different shades of blue indicate different productivity rates: dark blue = high productivity; grey = no articles.

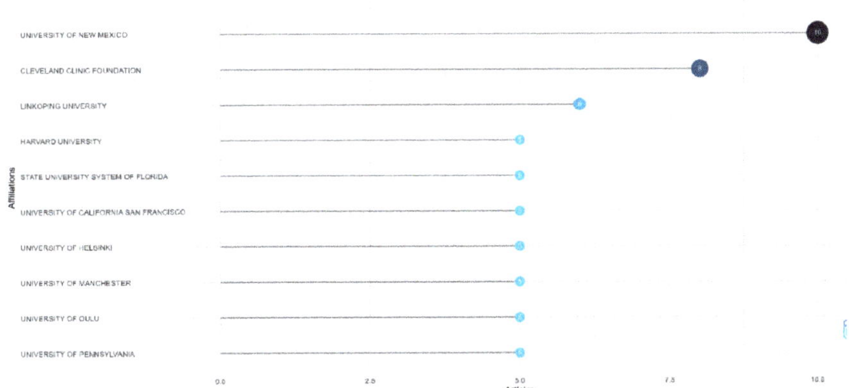

Figure 4. Most relevant affiliations. Different shades of blue represent varying productivity levels: dark blue indicates high productivity, while light blue indicates low productivity.

3.4. Most Relevant Words and Frequency over Time

An analysis of authors' keywords offered valuable insights into the dominant terms in the scientific literature. Notably, terms such as "COVID-19" and "ICT" were among the most frequently occurring words, underscoring their centrality to the discourse. Other frequent keywords included "mental health", "smartphone", and "wellbeing" (Figure 5).

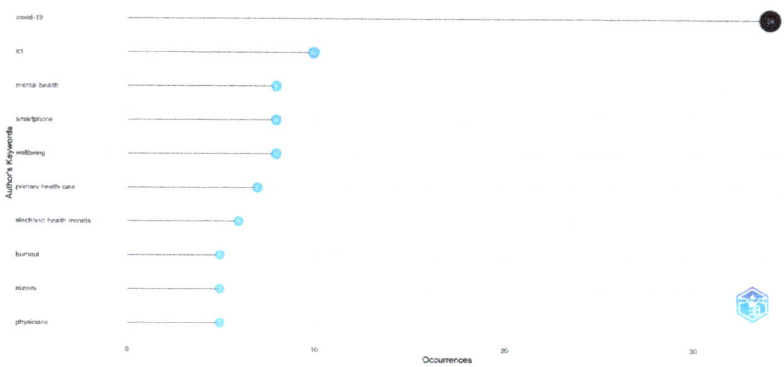

Figure 5. Words frequency. Different shades of blue represent varying frequency levels: dark blue indicates high frequency, while light blue indicates low frequency.

3.5. Co-Word Analysis

A co-word analysis was conducted to identify the cognitive structure and conceptual linkages within the selected research domain [43]. To simplify the analysis, keywords related to the overarching term "telemedicine" were removed from the search query. Additionally, broad terms (e.g., factors) and those referring to research methodologies (e.g., qualitative research, cross-sectional studies) were excluded. Keyword spelling was standardized (e.g., singular/plural forms, hyphenation). Using the author's keywords as the unit of analysis, this approach identifies terms (nodes) that frequently co-occur in literature and assesses their relationships. The size of each node reflects the keyword occurrence (i.e., betweenness degree; B), while the thickness of the connecting lines indicates the strength of co-occurrence (i.e., centrality degree; C). A total of 49 nodes and 9 clusters were identified.

Figure 6 shows that the "COVID-19" cluster emerged as the most relevant area (B = 510.02 and C = 0.01), with a strong connection with "Mental health". This cluster also includes terms such as "Burnout" and "Psychiatry". The "Wellbeing" cluster was the second most relevant (B = 217.84 and C = 0.01), showing several associations with the "COVID-19" cluster. It includes terms such as "ICT" (Information and Communication Technology), and "Primary health care". The "Healthcare delivery" cluster appeared as the third most relevant (B = 96.36 and C = 0.01), with links to the "Wellbeing" cluster. This cluster includes terms such as attitudes and attitudes of health personnel. Notably, the "Acceptability" cluster (B = 0 and C = 0.5), which includes terms such as "Feasibility" and "Implementation science", appeared disconnected from the other clusters.

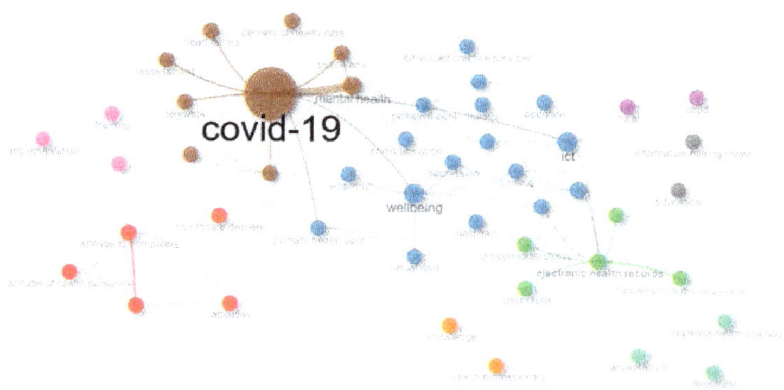

Figure 6. Co-word analysis.

3.6. Thematic Analysis

Using the approach outlined by Cobo and colleagues [32], a thematic map was created to highlight the key themes. The themes are positioned across four quadrants, defined by two factors: density and centrality. Density reflects the internal cohesion of a network, indicating how well-developed a theme is. Centrality, on the other hand, measures the extent to which a theme interacts with other themes, representing its importance in the overall development of the research area [32]. The intersection of the density and centrality axes produces four distinct quadrants, including different themes (i.e., motor themes, niche themes, emerging or declining themes and basic themes). In the thematic map, the size of each bubble reflects the frequency of word occurrences within each cluster, with larger bubbles representing more frequent themes [44].

Author's keywords were used as the unit of analysis, and the following parameters were configured: number of words set to 300, minimum frequency set to 2, and number of labels set to 1. A total of 22 clusters emerged (Figure 7).

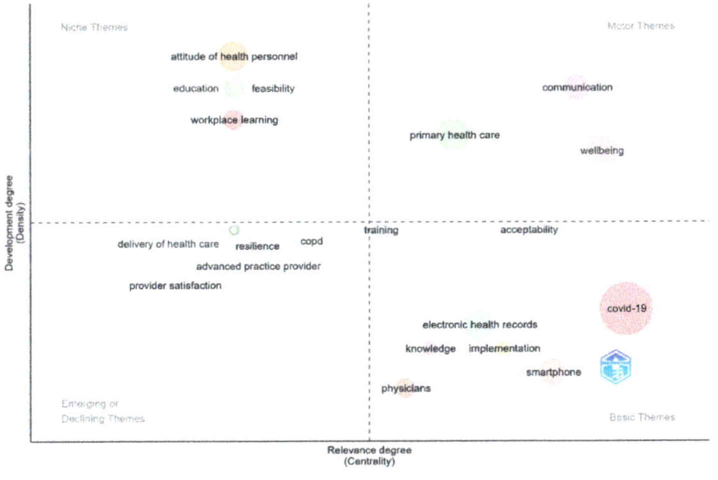

Figure 7. Thematic map.

The first quadrant includes "motor themes", characterized by high centrality and high density. These are well-established and crucial themes that shape the research field. Three motor themes were identified: "wellbeing", "primary healthcare", and "communication", with the first two having similar bubble sizes. The "wellbeing" cluster refers to research on the impact of telemedicine on the wellbeing of both HCPs' and patients. Studies have explored how telemedicine can affect HCPs' wellbeing [45], as well as how online mental health programs can support nurses' wellbeing [35,40]. Other research has investigated HCPs' perceptions of how ICT use may improve or hinder patients' wellbeing [46,47]. The "primary health care" cluster explores how telemedicine influences physicians' work in primary care. For instance, Fernemark and colleagues [48] conducted an in-depth analysis of job demands, job control, and social support for physicians using digital consultations. Additionally, Björndell and Premberg [49] demonstrated that video consultations can enhance physicians' work situations and wellbeing. Finally, "communication" emerged as a key theme, highlighting the importance of effective communication in telemedicine. Providing virtual care is challenging for physicians, who must reinforce their communication skills and their ability to manage misunderstandings [50,51]. Effective communication is also crucial for maintaining patient engagement [52].

The second quadrant highlights "niche themes", characterized by both low density and low centrality, suggesting that these themes are either underdeveloped or becoming less relevant over time. The largest bubble within this quadrant is "Attitude of health personnel", indicating that this is the most discussed area. This cluster focuses on how HCPs' attitudes toward telemedicine can influence its implementation. Specifically, studies have identified key factors that affect the acceptance and perceived usefulness of various telemedicine approaches [37,42]. Similarly, the "feasibility" cluster includes studies examining HCPs' opinions on the feasibility of different telemedicine methods [53,54]. The "education" cluster addresses the need for HCPs operating in digital environments to possess the knowledge, skills, and resources to provide optimal patient care through telemedicine. This cluster includes literature on identifying educational needs [55] and evaluating the effectiveness of telemedicine training programs [56]. The "workplace learning" cluster focuses on providing HCPs with training and interprofessional education programs to develop their skills. Closely related to telemedicine, workplace learning equips HCPs with the competencies needed to effectively use telemedicine tools, such as video consultations [57], while also fostering collaboration among professionals via telehealth [58].

The third quadrant includes "emerging or declining themes" which are underdeveloped and marginal. The "resilience" cluster—represented by a small bubble—encompasses research where digital health platforms were used to implement programs aimed at improving the resilience (i.e., a personal resource that supports individuals in managing stress and recover from adversities [59]) and wellbeing of HCPs [60,61]. This highlights that telemedicine services benefit not only patients but also HCPs, as digital platforms are used to improve their resilience and wellbeing. Moreover, "provider satisfaction" cluster includes articles aimed at investigating HCPs' satisfaction with telemedicine and virtual care delivery [62,63].

The fourth quadrant features "basic themes", which are characterized by high centrality and low density. These themes are central to the field but remain underdeveloped. The "COVID-19" cluster is represented by the largest bubble, signifying that it is the most prevalent theme in this quadrant. This cluster includes studies examining HCPs' experiences with the adoption of telemedicine services during the pandemic [64,65]. The "physicians" cluster focuses on this specific group of HCPs. Several studies have explored in depth the experiences of physicians with digitalization and its impact on their work environment [41,66]. Additionally, the "knowledge" cluster underscores the importance of assessing physicians' understanding of telemedicine services [67,68]. The "training" cluster focuses on academic research on interventions or programs designed to enhance HCPs' skills in using telemedicine. Articles in this cluster explore the effectiveness of training aimed at improving communication skills among nurses in telehealth [69] and enhancing the virtual clinical skills of clinicians [70]. The presence of the "acceptability" cluster highlights the importance of evaluating HCPs' willingness to use telemedicine and the variables that influence this predisposition. Studies in this cluster generally reveal high levels of acceptability, although specific concerns depend on the type of service. For instance, healthcare providers deemed telemedicine for medical abortion highly acceptable but expressed concerns about its safety and effectiveness [54]. In addition to users' acceptability, the "implementation" cluster emphasizes the need to consider organizational and contextual factors that may affect the adoption of telemedicine services, such as telehealth for abortion care [71] or video consultations [57].

4. Discussion

The present bibliometric analysis aimed to provide a comprehensive overview of the current state of research on the implications of telemedicine for HCPs. While previous reviews on the adoption of telemedicine among HCPs exist [19,20], to the best of our knowledge, this is the first study to apply a quantitative, bibliometric approach to this specific area of research. By employing this method, we were able to uncover key trends and thematic clusters that qualitative analyses might not fully capture, thus offering a more comprehensive understanding of the research landscape.

Our analysis revealed a marked increase in scientific publications beginning in 2012, likely fueled by technological advancements such as the widespread adoption of telemedicine platforms and improvements in digital infrastructure. However, the most significant peak in publications occurred from 2020 onward, underscoring the profound impact of the COVID-19 pandemic. This theme emerged consistently across various analyses within this bibliometric study, emphasizing the pivotal role of COVID-19. During this period, telemedicine emerged as a key tool for healthcare delivery amidst lockdowns and physical distancing measures [6,72,73]. Notably, the volume of articles published in 2023 remains substantial, indicating that telemedicine's relevance extends beyond the crisis and suggesting a shift toward more sustained and integrated adoption of these tools in HCPs' work. Interestingly, other bibliometric analyses focused on telemedicine—such as those examining patient's role [74] or specific healthcare areas [75]—have found similar surges in research output during the same period. This convergence across different aspects of telemedicine research points to a broader academic recognition of the field's relevance.

The predominance of health and medical journals, such as the Journal of Medical Internet Research and BMC Health Services Research, suggests that research on the implications of telemedicine for HCPs is predominantly housed within the clinical sector. Notably, contributions from psychology or the social sciences are scarce, representing a gap in the literature that could provide valuable insights into the psychological, social, and organizational dimensions of telemedicine adoption and use.

Geographically, our analysis aligns with previous studies showing that research in the telemedicine field is primarily concentrated in high-income countries [74,76]. The United States, Australia, and the United Kingdom emerge as key contributors, followed by some European countries. This prominence likely reflects the advanced healthcare systems and robust technological infrastructures in these nations, which facilitate the adoption of telemedicine [77]. These countries also tend to have innovation-driven cultures that prioritize the rapid diffusion of new technologies [76,78]. Notably, our analysis also identified contributions from non-Western countries, including Nigeria, Ethiopia, India, and Japan. Although these countries currently have lower publication volumes, their presence in the dataset highlights a growing global interest in the implications of telemedicine for HCPs.

The co-word analysis revealed that "COVID-19" and "wellbeing" are frequently studied together, indicating that the recent literature has largely centered on how telemedicine implementation during the pandemic influenced HCPs' wellbeing [64,65]. In contrast, there has been limited research examining "wellbeing" and "resilience", highlighting an underdeveloped area that merits further investigation, particularly in high-stress environments such as emergency care. Furthermore, thematic analysis identified "wellbeing" as a motor theme, revealing a strong connection with mental health concerns such as burnout and stress, especially during the COVID-19 pandemic. Some studies explored the potential of digital interventions in supporting professionals' psychological wellbeing—for instance, mobile-based mental health support or resilience training programs [35,40,60,61]. However, this theme remains underexplored, especially in relation to longitudinal effects or contextual moderators such as workload or organizational support. The analysis highlights a gap in understanding how telemedicine-induced stress might impact not only job satisfaction, but also quality of care, reinforcing the need for targeted strategies to protect HCPs' mental health in digital environments.

The co-word and thematic analyses allowed for the development of a framework (Figure 8) that provides an integrative structure summarizing the main trends in the literature. This framework synthesizes the key themes into an organized structure, offering a comprehensive view of the field. It highlights underexplored areas such as the relationship between resilience and wellbeing and provides insights into future research and implementation strategies, helping to identify key factors that can improve HCPs' experiences and the effectiveness of healthcare delivery.

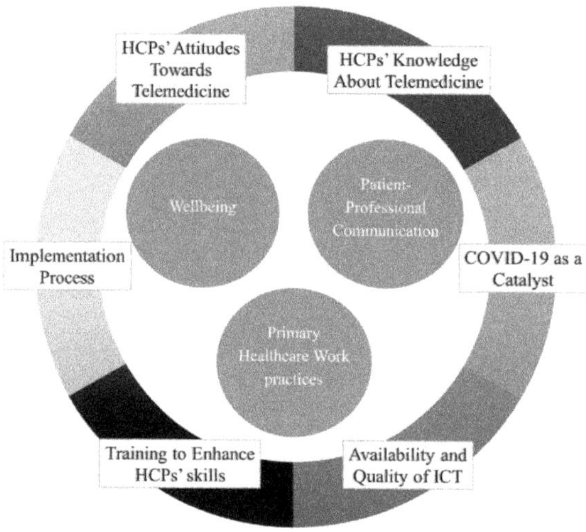

Figure 8. Integrative framework.

The intellectual structure of the field reveals three core themes: wellbeing, primary healthcare work practices, and patient–professional communication. These findings suggest that the wellbeing of HCPs is a central dimension in the study of telemedicine adoption. For instance, Werkmeister and colleagues [45] highlighted how constant connectivity and the blurring of boundaries between work and private life can deplete HCPs' psychological resources. Additional evidence suggests that the digitization of healthcare can lead to increased job demands, such as time pressure and cognitive overload associated with poor usability of digital platforms [12,38]. Similarly, Fernemark and colleagues [48] found that virtual care models can alter the balance between job demands, control, and support, with potential consequences for HCPs' wellbeing. Specific features of telemedicine may introduce new stressors that heighten the risk of burnout among HCPs [16]. These include not only the increased administrative burden and patients' difficulties in using the technology [7], but also the cognitive strain associated with managing complex virtual interactions. Notably, while telemedicine may reduce some administrative tasks, it can simultaneously intensify mental workload by requiring the continuous adaptation of work practices and communication strategies in a digital context.

Thus, in addition to its impact on wellbeing, the adoption of telemedicine has significantly transformed daily clinical practice, particularly in primary care, offering both opportunities and challenges. For instance, Björndell and Premberg [49] demonstrated that video consultations can enhance physicians' work situations by offering greater flexibility in managing patient appointments and reducing travel time, especially in rural areas. However, the shift to telemedicine can also lead to feelings of isolation from colleagues and reduce opportunities for in-person collaboration, which is often a key source of professional support in primary care settings. Similarly, communication between patients and HCPs in telemedicine settings presents significant challenges [50,51]. Ensuring effective communication is essential for improving the quality of telemedicine care, particularly in promoting patient engagement and enabling successful digital interactions [52]. This aligns with previous research highlighting the difficulties of web-based patient–professional communication [79] and reinforces the pivotal role of strong patient–professional communication in supporting medication adherence and achieving positive clinical outcomes [80].

Both contextual and personal factors shape these core themes and their interactions. Among the contextual factors, the emergence of "COVID-19" as a basic theme reflects the pandemic's role as a catalyst for telemedicine adoption, with a significant impact on HCPs' wellbeing. The pandemic intensified these issues, as HCPs were required to rapidly adapt to remote care settings, often without sufficient support or training [21]. The success of telemedicine hinges on the quality and availability of "ICT" infrastructure (including smartphones), which significantly affects both HCPs' experiences and patient outcomes. Furthermore, organizational policies and practices, such as providing HCPs with adequate "training" to develop both technical and soft skills, are essential for promoting the successful "implementation" of telemedicine. Additionally, training can help improve HCPs' knowledge and awareness of telemedicine, enabling them to better cope with the changes associated with its introduction.

Among personal factors, HCPs' "attitudes toward telemedicine" are crucial in determining its success and influencing their wellbeing. In addition to attitudes, the level of "knowledge" that HCPs possess about telemedicine services shapes their experiences and perceptions of care quality. A positive attitude and greater familiarity with telemedicine can foster successful adoption, while higher technical proficiency increases the likelihood that HCPs will advocate for improvements in ICT and training within their organizations.

These findings suggest that telemedicine is a double-edged sword. On the one hand, its flexibility and enhanced access to care have been celebrated as key benefits, especially during the pandemic. On the other hand, our findings confirm that these advantages are accompanied by significant trade-offs that may influence HCPs' wellbeing [48,81].

Existing models used to study telemedicine from the perspective of HCPs, such as the Technology Acceptance Model [82] and the Unified Theory of Acceptance and Use of Technology [83], primarily focus on individual cognitive factors (e.g., perceived usefulness, ease of use, or behavioral intention) influencing telemedicine acceptance and the intention to use it [14,22,84]. While these frameworks provide valuable insights into the adoption process, they overlook the broader impact of telemedicine on HCPs' wellbeing and daily clinical practice.

By contrast, the framework proposed in this study emphasizes wellbeing as a central dimension in the telemedicine experience. It integrates contextual (e.g., pandemic-related changes, infrastructure, organizational support) and personal factors (e.g., attitudes, knowledge), highlighting the complex interplay between technology use and professional sustainability. This broader perspective advances the field by reframing telemedicine as a complex organizational transformation rather than a mere technological intervention.

The main takeaway from this framework is that successful telemedicine implementation requires more than just technological readiness. The wellbeing of HCPs is not a side effect of telemedicine implementation, but a pivotal outcome that directly impacts sustainability and quality of care. Promoting HCPs' mental health should therefore be considered a strategic priority in any telemedicine integration program. In addition, resistance to change remains a significant challenge when introducing telemedicine services. This resistance can stem from various factors, such as uncertainty about new technologies, fear of increased workload, or concerns about diminished patient relationships [7,85]. Therefore, policymakers and healthcare leaders should foster a culture of adaptability, providing adequate training, and promoting the value of telemedicine to both professionals and patients. By integrating both technological and interpersonal aspects of telemedicine, they can ensure that the benefits of digital healthcare are maximized while minimizing its potential drawbacks for professionals.

Implications for Practice

While training in digital skills is essential, our findings suggest that technical preparation alone is not sufficient to support HCPs in the transition to telemedicine. Specifically, issues such as HCPs psychological wellbeing and digital communication skills emerged as key themes in the literature.

Several studies highlight the need for more holistic and multidimensional support strategies. For instance, some institutions have implemented digital mentorship programs and peer-support groups to foster mutual learning and reduce the sense of isolation often experienced in remote work environments [57]. Other promising practices include micro-training sessions focused on communication skills in virtual settings—such as teach-back techniques or emotional attunement in video consultations [69]—which can mitigate misunderstandings and enhance patient engagement. Therefore, healthcare leaders should invest in structured training programs that not only enhance digital competencies but also address concerns related to work overload, job satisfaction, and role clarity. In line with our thematic findings, the promotion of a supportive organizational culture—one that values flexibility, professional autonomy, and ongoing feedback—is essential in reducing resistance and increasing acceptance of digital tools.

Moreover, initiatives aimed at improving telemedicine adoption should be co-designed with healthcare staff, acknowledging their perspectives and fostering a sense of ownership. Clear communication about the purpose, benefits, and expected changes related to telemedicine use can also help mitigate perceived threats, such as the loss of relational quality with patients or increased administrative burden.

In addition to skill-based training, healthcare organizations should also invest in psycho-educational interventions that allow professionals to process the deeper shifts in their professional identity, role boundaries, and interpersonal dynamics brought about by telemedicine. Creating spaces for structured reflection (e.g., interprofessional debriefing sessions or facilitated workshops) can provide emotional relief and strengthen professionals' capacity to adapt constructively to digital change. These supportive interventions are particularly relevant in high-stress environments, where the adoption of telemedicine may otherwise exacerbate existing psychological burdens.

By integrating these organizational and relational aspects with technological innovation, healthcare institutions and policymakers can ensure that telemedicine becomes a sustainable and accepted part of clinical practice, rather than a source of additional strain or uncertainty for professionals.

5. Conclusions

This bibliometric analysis offers a comprehensive overview of the research landscape on the implications of telemedicine adoption among HCPs. The findings indicate a steady increase in scientific output starting in 2012, with a notable surge in publications from 2020 onward, reflecting the impact of the COVID-19 pandemic as a catalyst for telemedicine implementation. The findings of this bibliometric analysis enabled the development of a conceptual framework that synthesizes the core themes of the field. While telemedicine provides numerous advantages, such as improved access to care and increased flexibility, it also poses challenges for wellbeing, primary healthcare work practices, and communication between patients and professionals. Contextual and personal factors significantly influence how HCPs experience telemedicine. In summary, this study contributes to the literature by revealing that the wellbeing of HCPs is a core issue in telemedicine implementation—often neglected in prior research. Future strategies must balance technological benefits with the psychological needs of professionals to ensure effective and humane digital healthcare delivery. By uncovering key conceptual insights into the intellectual structure of this research field, this bibliometric analysis highlights not only well established themes but also underexplored areas, providing a foundation for future research directions.

6. Suggestions for Future Research

The findings of this bibliometric analysis identify key areas for future research on the implications of telemedicine for HCPs. The analysis of the main journals suggests the need for a more heterogeneous and multidisciplinary approach, incorporating perspectives from psychology and social sciences, which have been underrepresented in the current literature. Our findings underscore the close connection between telemedicine adoption and HCPs' wellbeing and work outcomes. Future research should delve deeper into this area, particularly through longitudinal studies that examine the long-term impact of telemedicine on HCPs, including how the use of these technologies influences their work practices, stress levels, and overall wellbeing.

Additionally, qualitative studies exploring how professional identity is reshaped in telemedicine contexts could provide valuable insights into the evolving roles and relationships between HCPs and patients. The shift from in-person to virtual care may alter professionals' perceptions of their roles and responsibilities [4]. Understanding these changes is essential to support HCPs in maintaining their professional identity in a rapidly digitalizing environment.

Themes related to resilience and provider satisfaction remain underdeveloped in the current literature. Future studies should investigate how telemedicine can be utilized to support HCPs' mental health and resilience, particularly in high-stress environments (e.g., first aid). Moreover, our analysis reveals that most research on telemedicine is concentrated in high-income countries, with limited representation from low-income countries. Future research should explore how telemedicine is implemented in resource-limited settings, where its impact on HCPs may differ significantly from that in high-income contexts.

Furthermore, this bibliometric analysis revealed a lack of research on the effects of telemedicine on collaboration within healthcare teams. Future studies should examine the dynamics of virtual teamwork, the development of collaborative skills in digital environments, and how telemedicine either facilitates or hinders effective interprofessional collaboration. As telemedicine becomes integrated into healthcare systems, it is crucial to explore the role of training in equipping HCPs with both the technical and soft skills necessary for successful telemedicine use. Future research should assess the effectiveness of training programs and identify best practices for skill development.

In addition, the role of organizational policies and support mechanisms in facilitating telemedicine adoption requires further exploration. Future research should explore ways in which organizations can effectively support HCPs through policies, training, and resources that improve telemedicine adoption, enhance job satisfaction, and reduce burnout. Organizational factors such as leadership, culture, and resource allocation should be examined in relation to the successful implementation of telemedicine.

Finally, while the present study provides a comprehensive overview of the intellectual and thematic landscape of the literature on telemedicine from the perspective of HCPs, it does not include a systematic classification of the reviewed studies in terms of epidemiological methods or study designs. Future research could build upon these findings by conducting a systematic review. Such an approach would offer deeper insights into the robustness of the existing evidence base and complement the bibliometric and content-driven perspective presented here.

Author Contributions: Conceptualization, C.B., M.A.P. and C.G.; Methodology, C.B. and M.A.P.; Software, C.B.; Validation, C.B., M.A.P. and C.G.; Formal Analysis, C.B.; Investigation, C.B.; Resources, C.B. and M.A.P.; Data Curation, C.B. and M.A.P.; Writing—Original Draft Preparation, C.B.; Writing—Review and Editing, C.B., M.A.P. and C.G.; Visualization, C.B. and M.A.P.; Supervision, C.G.; Project Administration, C.B. and C.G.; Funding Acquisition, C.G. All authors have read and agreed to the published version of the manuscript.

Funding: This research was funded by MUSA—Multilayered Urban Sustainability Action—project, funded by the European Union—NextGenerationEU, under the National Recovery and Resilience Plan (NRRP) Mission 4 Component 2 Investment Line 1.5: Strengthening of research structures and creation of R&D "innovation ecosystems", set up of "territorial leaders in R&D". Project code: ECS 000037.

Institutional Review Board Statement: Not applicable.

Informed Consent Statement: Not applicable.

Data Availability Statement: The data associated with this research may be available upon reasonable request.

Conflicts of Interest: The authors declare no conflicts of interest.

References

1. Weißenfeld, M.M.; Goetz, K.; Steinhäuser, J. Facilitators and Barriers for the Implementation of Telemedicine from a Local Government Point of View—A Cross-Sectional Survey in Germany. *BMC Health Serv. Res.* **2021**, *21*, 919. [CrossRef]
2. World Health Organization. *Telemedicine: Opportunities and Developments in Member States: Report on the Second Global Survey on eHealth*; World Health Organization: Geneva, Switzerland, 2010.
3. Tore, N.G.; Oskay, D.; Haznedaroglu, S. The Quality of Physiotherapy and Rehabilitation Program and the Effect of Telerehabilitation on Patients with Knee Osteoarthritis. *Clin. Rheumatol.* **2023**, *42*, 903–915. [CrossRef] [PubMed]
4. Ezeamii, V.C.; Okobi, O.E.; Wambai-Sani, H.; Perera, G.S.; Zaynieva, S.; Okonkwo, C.C.; Ohaiba, M.M.; William-Enemali, P.C.; Obodo, O.R.; Obiefuna, N.G. Revolutionizing Healthcare: How Telemedicine Is Improving Patient Outcomes and Expanding Access to Care. *Cureus* **2024**, *16*, e63881. [CrossRef] [PubMed]
5. Ohannessian, R.; Duong, T.A.; Odone, A. Global Telemedicine Implementation and Integration Within Health Systems to Fight the COVID-19 Pandemic: A Call to Action. *JMIR Public Health Surveill.* **2020**, *6*, e18810. [CrossRef] [PubMed]
6. Ghildiyal, N.; Bangari, M. Telemedicine. Zero Contagion Risk and Enabler of Healthcare Fire Sales. *Curr. Med. Res. Pract.* **2023**, *13*, 26–31. [CrossRef]
7. Bernuzzi, C.; Piccardo, M.A.; Marsilio, M.; Calcaterra, V.; Zuccotti, G.; Guglielmetti, C. Value Co-Creation in Telemedicine: A Qualitative Study of Pediatricians' Expectations Regarding Telehomecare Implementation in an Italian Pediatric Hospital. *J. Healthc. Leadersh.* **2024**, *16*, 485–500. [CrossRef]
8. World Health Organization. Transforming and Scaling up Health Professionals' Education and Training: World Health Organization Guidelines 2013. In *Transforming and Scaling up Health Professionals' Education and Training: World Health Organization Guidelines*; WHO: Geneva, Switzerland, 2013; p. 124.
9. Scholze, A.; Hecker, A. Digital Job Demands and Resources: Digitization in the Context of the Job Demands-Resources Model. *Int. J. Environ. Res. Public Health* **2023**, *20*, 6581. [CrossRef]
10. Qvarfordt, M.; Lagrosen, S. Healthcare Digitalisation and Its Association with Quality and Employee Health, a Mixed-Methods Study. *Int. J. Workplace Health Manag.* **2024**, *17*, 1–20. [CrossRef]

11. Breton, M.; Sullivan, E.E.; Deville-Stoetzel, N.; McKinstry, D.; DePuccio, M.; Sriharan, A.; Deslauriers, V.; Dong, A.; McAlearney, A.S. Telehealth Challenges during COVID-19 as Reported by Primary Healthcare Physicians in Quebec and Massachusetts. *BMC Fam. Pract.* **2021**, *22*, 192. [CrossRef]
12. Frennert, S.; Petersson, L.; Erlingsdottir, G. "More" Work for Nurses: The Ironies of EHealth. *BMC Health Serv. Res.* **2023**, *23*, 411. [CrossRef]
13. Galle, A.; Semaan, A.; Huysmans, E.; Audet, C.; Asefa, A.; Delvaux, T.; Afolabi, B.B.; El Ayadi, A.M.; Benova, L. A Double-Edged Sword—Telemedicine for Maternal Care during COVID-19: Findings from a Global Mixed-Methods Study of Healthcare Providers. *BMJ Glob. Health* **2021**, *6*, e004575. [CrossRef] [PubMed]
14. Garavand, A.; Aslani, N.; Nadri, H.; Abedini, S.; Dehghan, S. Acceptance of Telemedicine Technology among Physicians: A Systematic Review. *Inform. Med. Unlocked* **2022**, *30*, 100943. [CrossRef]
15. Abdelghany, I.K.; AlMatar, R.; Al-Haqan, A.; Abdullah, I.; Waheedi, S. Exploring Healthcare Providers' Perspectives on Virtual Care Delivery: Insights into Telemedicine Services. *BMC Health Serv. Res.* **2024**, *24*, 1. [CrossRef]
16. Boksa, V.; Pennathur, P. Assessing Contributing and Mediating Factors of Telemedicine on Healthcare Provider Burnout. *Health Policy Technol.* **2024**, *13*, 100942. [CrossRef]
17. Veiga, M.G.; Felizi, R.T.; Fernandes, C.E.; Oliveira, E. WhatsApp and Gynecologist-Patient Interaction: Development and Validation of a Questionnaire to Assess the Stress Perceived by the Doctor. *Rev. Bras. Ginecol. Obs./RBGO Gynecol. Obstet.* **2022**, *44*, 497–502. [CrossRef] [PubMed]
18. West, C.P. Association of Resident Fatigue and Distress With Perceived Medical Errors. *JAMA* **2009**, *302*, 1294. [CrossRef]
19. Baluszek, J.B.; Wiig, S.; Myrnes-Hansen, K.V.; Brønnick, K.K. Specialized Healthcare Practitioners' Challenges in Performing Video Consultations to Patients in Nordic Countries—A Systematic Review and Narrative Synthesis. *BMC Health Serv. Res.* **2022**, *22*, 1432. [CrossRef]
20. Chereka, A.A.; Mekonnen, G.B.; Yirsaw, A.N.; Mengistie, B.A.; Getachew, E.; Lakew, G.; Shibabaw, A.A.; Kitil, G.W. Attitudes towards Telemedicine Services and Associated Factors among Health Professionals in Ethiopia: A Systematic Review and Meta-Analysis. *BMC Health Serv. Res.* **2024**, *24*, 1505. [CrossRef]
21. Ftouni, R.; AlJardali, B.; Hamdanieh, M.; Ftouni, L.; Salem, N. Challenges of Telemedicine during the COVID-19 Pandemic: A Systematic Review. *BMC Med. Inform. Decis. Mak.* **2022**, *22*, 207. [CrossRef]
22. Rouidi, M.; Elouadi, A.; Hamdoune, A. Acceptance and Use of Telemedicine Technology by Health Professionals: Development of a Conceptual Model. *Digit. Health* **2022**, *8*, 205520762210816. [CrossRef]
23. Öztürk, O.; Kocaman, R.; Kanbach, D.K. How to Design Bibliometric Research: An Overview and a Framework Proposal. *Rev. Manag. Sci.* **2024**, *18*, 3333–3361. [CrossRef]
24. Donthu, N.; Kumar, S.; Mukherjee, D.; Pandey, N.; Lim, W.M. How to Conduct a Bibliometric Analysis: An Overview and Guidelines. *J. Bus. Res.* **2021**, *133*, 285–296. [CrossRef]
25. Aria, M.; Cuccurullo, C. Bibliometrix: An R-Tool for Comprehensive Science Mapping Analysis. *J. Informetr.* **2017**, *11*, 959–975. [CrossRef]
26. Fusco, F.; Marsilio, M.; Guglielmetti, C. Co-Production in Health Policy and Management: A Comprehensive Bibliometric Review. *BMC Health Serv. Res.* **2020**, *20*, 504. [CrossRef]
27. Mukherjee, D.; Lim, W.M.; Kumar, S.; Donthu, N. Guidelines for Advancing Theory and Practice through Bibliometric Research. *J. Bus. Res.* **2022**, *148*, 101–115. [CrossRef]
28. Montazeri, A.; Mohammadi, S.; M. Hesari, P.; Ghaemi, M.; Riazi, H.; Sheikhi-Mobarakeh, Z. Preliminary Guideline for Reporting Bibliometric Reviews of the Biomedical Literature (BIBLIO): A Minimum Requirements. *Syst. Rev.* **2023**, *12*, 239. [CrossRef]
29. Ball, R.; Tunger, D. Science Indicators Revisited—Science Citation Index versus SCOPUS: A Bibliometric Comparison of Both Citation Databases. *Inf. Serv. Use* **2007**, *26*, 293–301. [CrossRef]
30. Moher, D.; Liberati, A.; Tetzlaff, J.; Altman, D.G. Preferred Reporting Items for Systematic Reviews and Meta-Analyses: The PRISMA Statement. *PLoS Med.* **2009**, *6*, e1000097. [CrossRef]
31. Callon, M.; Courtial, J.P.; Laville, F. Co-Word Analysis as a Tool for Describing the Network of Interactions between Basic and Technological Research: The Case of Polymer Chemsitry. *Scientometrics* **1991**, *22*, 155–205. [CrossRef]
32. Cobo, M.J.; López-Herrera, A.G.; Herrera-Viedma, E.; Herrera, F. Science Mapping Software Tools: Review, Analysis, and Cooperative Study among Tools. *J. Am. Soc. Inf. Sci. Technol.* **2011**, *62*, 1382–1402. [CrossRef]
33. Hennemann, S.; Beutel, M.E.; Zwerenz, R. Ready for EHealth? Health Professionals' Acceptance and Adoption of EHealth Interventions in Inpatient Routine Care. *J. Health Commun.* **2017**, *22*, 274–284. [CrossRef] [PubMed]
34. Katzman, J.G.; Comerci, G.; Boyle, J.F.; Duhigg, D.; Shelley, B.; Olivas, C.; Daitz, B.; Carroll, C.; Som, D.; Monette, R.; et al. Innovative Telementoring for Pain Management: Project ECHO Pain. *J. Contin. Educ. Health Prof.* **2014**, *34*, 68–75. [CrossRef]
35. Villani, D.; Grassi, A.; Cognetta, C.; Toniolo, D.; Cipresso, P.; Riva, G. Self-Help Stress Management Training through Mobile Phones: An Experience with Oncology Nurses. *Psychol. Serv.* **2013**, *10*, 315–322. [CrossRef]

36. Maguire, R.; Ream, E.; Richardson, A.; Connaghan, J.; Johnston, B.; Kotronoulas, G.; Pedersen, V.; McPhelim, J.; Pattison, N.; Smith, A.; et al. Development of a Novel Remote Patient Monitoring System. *Cancer Nurs.* **2015**, *38*, E37–E47. [CrossRef]
37. Moeckli, J.; Cram, P.; Cunningham, C.; Reisinger, H.S. Staff Acceptance of a Telemedicine Intensive Care Unit Program: A Qualitative Study. *J. Crit. Care* **2013**, *28*, 890–901. [CrossRef] [PubMed]
38. Vehko, T.; Hyppönen, H.; Puttonen, S.; Kujala, S.; Ketola, E.; Tuukkanen, J.; Aalto, A.-M.; Heponiemi, T. Experienced Time Pressure and Stress: Electronic Health Records Usability and Information Technology Competence Play a Role. *BMC Med. Inform. Decis. Mak.* **2019**, *19*, 160. [CrossRef] [PubMed]
39. Srinivasan, M.; Asch, S.; Vilendrer, S.; Thomas, S.C.; Bajra, R.; Barman, L.; Edwards, L.M.; Filipowicz, H.; Giang, L.; Jee, O.; et al. Qualitative Assessment of Rapid System Transformation to Primary Care Video Visits at an Academic Medical Center. *Ann. Intern. Med.* **2020**, *173*, 527–535. [CrossRef]
40. Bolier, L.; Ketelaar, S.M.; Nieuwenhuijsen, K.; Smeets, O.; Gärtner, F.R.; Sluiter, J.K. Workplace Mental Health Promotion Online to Enhance Well-Being of Nurses and Allied Health Professionals: A Cluster-Randomized Controlled Trial. *Internet Interv.* **2014**, *1*, 196–204. [CrossRef]
41. Grünloh, C.; Cajander, Å.; Myreteg, G. "The Record Is Our Work Tool!"—Physicians' Framing of a Patient Portal in Sweden. *J. Med. Internet Res.* **2016**, *18*, e167. [CrossRef]
42. Ruiz Morilla, M.D.; Sans, M.; Casasa, A.; Giménez, N. Implementing Technology in Healthcare: Insights from Physicians. *BMC Med. Inform. Decis. Mak.* **2017**, *17*, 92. [CrossRef]
43. Escobar, O.R.; Leone, D.; Malafronte, P.; Mele, S. The Effect of Telemedicine on Patients' Wellbeing: A Systematic Review. *J. Innov. Econ. Manag.* **2021**, *35*, 9–31. [CrossRef]
44. Widyanty, W.; Oktasari, D.P.; Riyanto, S.; Nusraningrum, D.; Damayanti, S.; Sumaedi, S.; Bakti, I.G.M.Y.; Dinaseviani, A.; Prasetya, P.; Fahlevi, M. Employee Green Behavior: Mapping Knowledge Structures and Future Directions. *Cogent Bus. Manag.* **2025**, *12*, 2440814. [CrossRef]
45. Werkmeister, B.J.; Haase, A.M.; Fleming, T.; Officer, T.N. Experiences of the COVID-19 Lockdown and Telehealth in Aotearoa New Zealand: Lessons and Insights from Mental Health Clinicians. *Int. J. Environ. Res. Public Health* **2023**, *20*, 4791. [CrossRef]
46. Boe Danbjørg, D.; Wagner, L.; Rønde Kristensen, B.; Clemensen, J. Nurses' Experience of Using an Application to Support New Parents after Early Discharge: An Intervention Study. *Int. J. Telemed. Appl.* **2015**, *2015*, 1–10. [CrossRef]
47. Sävenstedt, S.; Sandman, P.O.; Zingmark, K. The Duality in Using Information and Communication Technology in Elder Care. *J. Adv. Nurs.* **2006**, *56*, 17–25. [CrossRef]
48. Fernemark, H.; Skagerström, J.; Seing, I.; Ericsson, C.; Nilsen, P. Digital Consultations in Swedish Primary Health Care: A Qualitative Study of Physicians' Job Control, Demand and Support. *BMC Fam. Pract.* **2020**, *21*, 241. [CrossRef]
49. Björndell, C.; Premberg, Å. Physicians' Experiences of Video Consultation with Patients at a Public Virtual Primary Care Clinic: A Qualitative Interview Study. *Scand. J. Prim. Health Care* **2021**, *39*, 67–76. [CrossRef]
50. Rothwell, E.; Ellington, L.; Planalp, S.; Crouch, B. Exploring Challenges to Telehealth Communication by Specialists in Poison Information. *Qual. Health Res.* **2012**, *22*, 67–75. [CrossRef] [PubMed]
51. Sigesmund, D.; Coe, J.B.; Khosa, D.; Moore, I.C. Veterinarians Are Reluctant to Recommend Virtual Consultations to a Fellow Veterinarian. *J. Am. Vet. Med. Assoc.* **2023**, *261*, 1820–1828. [CrossRef]
52. Brandt, C.J.; Isidora Søgaard, G.; Clemensen, J.; Søndergaard, J.; Bo Nielsen, J. Determinants of Successful Ehealth Coaching for Consumer Lifestyle Changes: Qualitative Interview Study among Health Care Professionals. *J. Med. Internet Res.* **2018**, *20*, e237. [CrossRef]
53. Amuasi, J.H.; Agbogbatey, M.K.; Sarfo, F.S.; Beyuo, A.; Duah, K.; Agasiya, P.; Arthur, A.; Appiah, L.; Nguah, S.B.; Bockarie, A.; et al. Feasibility, Acceptability, and Appropriateness of a Mobile Health Stroke Intervention among Ghanaian Health Workers. *J. Neurol. Sci.* **2022**, *439*, 120304. [CrossRef]
54. Piay-Fernández, N.; Stenbacka, E.; Jaramillo, M.C.; Guerrero, G.; Solano Rodríguez, A.A.; Montenegro, P.; Moreno, D.C.; Cleeve, A. Implementing Medical Abortion through Telemedicine in Colombia: A Qualitative Study. *Sex. Reprod. Health Matters* **2023**, *31*, 2236780. [CrossRef] [PubMed]
55. Lerret, S.M.; Nuccio, S.; Compton, A.; Keegan, M.; Rapala, K. Nurses' Experiences and Perspectives of the Telehealth Working Environment and Educational Needs. *J. Contin. Educ. Nurs.* **2023**, *54*, 501–508. [CrossRef] [PubMed]
56. Benwell, N.; Hird, K.; Thomas, N.; Furness, E.; Fear, M.; Sweetman, G. Effectiveness and Efficiency of Training in Digital Healthcare Packages: Training Doctors to Use Digital Medical Record Keeping Software. *Aust. Health Rev.* **2017**, *41*, 479–484. [CrossRef] [PubMed]
57. Eriksen, S.; Dahler, A.M.; Øye, C. The Informal Way to Success or Failure? Findings from a Comparative Case Study on Video Consultation Training and Implementation in Two Danish Hospitals. *BMC Health Serv. Res.* **2023**, *23*, 1135. [CrossRef]
58. Bautista, C.A.; Huang, I.; Stebbins, M.; Floren, L.C.; Wamsley, M.; Youmans, S.L.; Hsia, S.L. Development of an Interprofessional Rotation for Pharmacy and Medical Students to Perform Telehealth Outreach to Vulnerable Patients in the COVID-19 Pandemic. *J. Interprof. Care* **2020**, *34*, 694–697. [CrossRef]

59. Bernuzzi, C.; Sommovigo, V.; Setti, I. The Role of Resilience in the Work-Life Interface: A Systematic Review. *Work* **2022**, *73*, 1147–1165. [CrossRef]
60. DePierro, J.; Marin, D.B.; Sharma, V.; Costello, Z.; Starkweather, S.; Katz, C.L.; Lim, S.; Charney, D.S. Developments in the First Year of a Resilience-Focused Program for Health Care Workers. *Psychiatry Res.* **2021**, *306*, 114280. [CrossRef]
61. Lee, D.; Lee, W.J.; Choi, S.-H.; Jang, J.-H.; Kang, D.-H. Long-Term Beneficial Effects of an Online Mind-Body Training Program on Stress and Psychological Outcomes in Female Healthcare Providers. *Medicine* **2020**, *99*, e21027. [CrossRef]
62. Maniaci, M.J.; Maita, K.; Torres-Guzman, R.A.; Avila, F.R.; Garcia, J.P.; Eldaly, A.; Forte, A.J.; Matcha, G.; Pagan, R.; Paulson, M.R. Provider Evaluation of a Novel Virtual Hybrid Hospital at Home Model. *Int. J. Gen. Med.* **2022**, *15*, 1909–1918. [CrossRef]
63. Brault, M.E.; Laudermith, A.; Kroll-Desrosiers, A. Telemedicine During COVID-19 Response: A Welcome Shift for Younger Female Healthcare Workers. *J. Gen. Intern. Med.* **2023**, *38*, 627–632. [CrossRef] [PubMed]
64. Haines, K.J.; Sawyer, A.; McKinnon, C.; Donovan, A.; Michael, C.; Cimoli, C.; Gregory, M.; Berney, S.; Berlowitz, D.J. Barriers and Enablers to Telehealth Use by Physiotherapists during the COVID-19 Pandemic. *Physiotherapy* **2023**, *118*, 12–19. [CrossRef] [PubMed]
65. White, J.; Byles, J.; Walley, T. The Qualitative Experience of Telehealth Access and Clinical Encounters in Australian Healthcare during COVID-19: Implications for Policy. *Health Res. Policy Syst.* **2022**, *20*, 9. [CrossRef] [PubMed]
66. Saukkonen, P.; Elovainio, M.; Virtanen, L.; Kaihlanen, A.-M.; Nadav, J.; Lääveri, T.; Vänskä, J.; Viitanen, J.; Reponen, J.; Heponiemi, T. The Interplay of Work, Digital Health Usage, and the Perceived Effects of Digitalization on Physicians' Work: Network Analysis Approach. *J. Med. Internet Res.* **2022**, *24*, e38714. [CrossRef]
67. Elareed, H.R.; Elroby, F.A.; Adly, E.S.; Mohamed Lotfy, A.M. Knowledge and Moral Attitude toward Telemedicine among Egyptian Physicians. *J. Public Health (Bangkok)* **2023**, *33*, 933–940. [CrossRef]
68. George, P.P.; Edathotty, T.T.; Gopikrishnan, S.; Prasanth, P.S.; Mathew, S.; Mohammed Ameen, A.A. Knowledge, Awareness, and Attitude among Practicing Orthodontist on Teledentistry during COVID Pandemic in Kerala: A Cross-Sectional Survey. *J. Pharm. Bioallied Sci.* **2021**, *13*, S846–S850. [CrossRef]
69. Morony, S.; Weir, K.; Duncan, G.; Biggs, J.; Nutbeam, D.; Mccaffery, K.J. Enhancing Communication Skills for Telehealth: Development and Implementation of a Teach-Back Intervention for a National Maternal and Child Health Helpline in Australia. *BMC Health Serv. Res.* **2018**, *18*, 162. [CrossRef]
70. Phillips, Z.; Wong, L.; Crotty, K.; Horlick, M.; Johnston, R.; Altshuler, L.; Zabar, S.; Jay, M.; Dembitzer, A. Implementing an Experiential Telehealth Training and Needs Assessment for Residents and Faculty at a Veterans Affairs Primary Care Clinic. *J. Grad. Med. Educ.* **2023**, *15*, 456–462. [CrossRef]
71. Godfrey, E.M.; Fiastro, A.E.; Jacob-Files, E.A.; Coeytaux, F.M.; Wells, E.S.; Ruben, M.R.; Sanan, S.S.; Bennett, I.M. Factors Associated with Successful Implementation of Telehealth Abortion in 4 United States Clinical Practice Settings. *Contraception* **2021**, *104*, 82–91. [CrossRef]
72. Busso, M.; Gonzalez, M.P.; Scartascini, C. On the Demand for Telemedicine: Evidence from the COVID-19 Pandemic. *Health Econ.* **2022**, *31*, 1491–1505. [CrossRef]
73. Shaver, J. The State of Telehealth Before and After the COVID-19 Pandemic. *Prim. Care Clin. Off. Pract.* **2022**, *49*, 517–530. [CrossRef]
74. Bernuzzi, C. Exploring Patient Role From Compliance To Engagement In Telemedicine: A Comparative Bibliometric Analysis Across Psychology And Medicine. *Humanit. Soc. Sci. Commun.* **2025**, *under revision*.
75. Zeng, N.; Liu, M.-C.; Zhong, X.-Y.; Wang, S.-G.; Xia, Q.-D. Knowledge Mapping of Telemedicine in Urology in the Past 20 Years: A Bibliometric Analysis (2004–2024). *Digit. Health* **2024**, *10*, 20552076241287460. [CrossRef] [PubMed]
76. Waqas, A.; Teoh, S.H.; Lapão, L.V.; Messina, L.A.; Correia, J.C. Harnessing Telemedicine for the Provision of Health Care: Bibliometric and Scientometric Analysis. *J. Med. Internet Res.* **2020**, *22*, e18835. [CrossRef]
77. Fisk, M.; Livingstone, A.; Pit, S.W. Telehealth in the Context of COVID-19: Changing Perspectives in Australia, the United Kingdom, and the United States. *J. Med. Internet Res.* **2020**, *22*, e19264. [CrossRef]
78. Sampat, B.; Drummond, M. Another Special Relationship? Interactions between Health Technology Policies and Health Care Systems in the United States and the United Kingdom. *J. Health Polit. Policy Law.* **2011**, *36*, 119–139. [CrossRef]
79. Laukka, E.; Huhtakangas, M.; Heponiemi, T.; Kujala, S.; Kaihlanen, A.-M.; Gluschkoff, K.; Kanste, O. Health Care Professionals' Experiences of Patient-Professional Communication Over Patient Portals: Systematic Review of Qualitative Studies. *J. Med. Internet Res.* **2020**, *22*, e21623. [CrossRef]
80. Zeng, J.; Gao, Y.; Hou, C.; Liu, T. The Impact of Doctor–Patient Communication on Medication Adherence and Blood Pressure Control in Patients with Hypertension: A Systematic Review. *PeerJ* **2024**, *12*, e18527. [CrossRef] [PubMed]
81. Horwood, C.; Luthuli, S.; Mapumulo, S.; Haskins, L.; Jensen, C.; Pansegrouw, D.; McKerrow, N. Challenges of Using E-Health Technologies to Support Clinical Care in Rural Africa: A Longitudinal Mixed Methods Study Exploring Primary Health Care Nurses' Experiences of Using an Electronic Clinical Decision Support System (CDSS) in South Africa. *BMC Health Serv. Res.* **2023**, *23*, 30. [CrossRef]

82. Davis, F.D. Perceived Usefulness, Perceived Ease of Use, and User Acceptance of Information Technology. *MIS Q.* **1989**, *13*, 319. [CrossRef]
83. Venkatesh, V.; Morris, M.G.; Davis, G.B.; Davis, F.D. User Acceptance of Information Technology: Toward a Unified View. *MIS Q.* **2003**, *27*, 425. [CrossRef]
84. Shiferaw, K.B.; Mengiste, S.A.; Gullslett, M.K.; Zeleke, A.A.; Tilahun, B.; Tebeje, T.; Wondimu, R.; Desalegn, S.; Mehari, E.A. Healthcare Providers' Acceptance of Telemedicine and Preference of Modalities during COVID-19 Pandemics in a Low-Resource Setting: An Extended UTAUT Model. *PLoS ONE* **2021**, *16*, e0250220. [CrossRef] [PubMed]
85. Scott Kruse, C.; Karem, P.; Shifflett, K.; Vegi, L.; Ravi, K.; Brooks, M. Evaluating Barriers to Adopting Telemedicine Worldwide: A Systematic Review. *J. Telemed. Telecare* **2018**, *24*, 4–12. [CrossRef] [PubMed]

healthcare

MDPI

Article

Pharmacists' Interventions in Virtual Diabetes Clinics: Cost-Effectiveness Feasibility Study

Sinaa Al-Aqeel [1,*], Alaa Mutlaq [2], Njood Alkhalifa [1], Deem Alnassar [1], Rashed Alghanim [2], Wafa Algarni [2] and Sultanah Alshammari [2]

[1] Department of Clinical Pharmacy, College of Pharmacy, King Saud University, Riyadh 11451, Saudi Arabia
[2] General Administration of Pharmaceutical Care, Ministry of Health, Riyadh 11451, Saudi Arabia
* Correspondence: salageel@ksu.edu.sa

Abstract: Background: Telepharmacy, the provision of patient care services by pharmacists through the use of telecommunications technology, is associated with improved diabetes-related outcomes and access to healthcare. The primary aim of this study was to characterize pharmacists' interventions at a virtual pharmacist-led diabetes clinic (PLDC). The secondary aim was to assess the feasibility of conducting a future cost-effectiveness study of the PLDCs. **Methods:** This prospective observational feasibility study was conducted within a pharmacist-led clinic at Seha Virtual Hospital, Riyadh, Saudi Arabia. Two intern pharmacists collected data between 31 July 2024 and 31 January 2025. **Results:** Seventy-five patients (mean [SD] age 50.47 years [14.95]) attended the clinic. The majority were female (58.7%), had type 2 diabetes (86.6%), and were from outside Riyadh (97.3%). The communication with patients was carried out mainly via telephone (73, 97.3%). The mean consultation duration was 7.64 min (SD = 5.68). A total of 179 interventions were conducted, with a mean number of interventions per patient of 2.5 (median 3, min 0, max 5). The most common intervention was patient education and counseling about their disease and medications. While it was feasible to capture the details of pharmacist interventions and resource use data, incomplete data on patient outcomes presented a challenge. **Conclusions:** Our detailed documentation of pharmacist–patient encounters revealed the ability of pharmacists to identify and manage the problems of diabetes patients at virtual PLDCs. Our feasibility study identified a few challenges that need to be addressed when designing future cost-effectiveness studies.

Keywords: diabetes mellitus; telemedicine; telepharmacy; pharmaceutical services

1. Introduction

In 2021, approximately 529 million people were living with diabetes worldwide, and more than 1.31 billion people are projected to have diabetes by 2050 [1]. An estimated 37.8 million total diabetes-related years of life were lost and 41.4 million years lived with disability in 2021 [1]. The total cost of diagnosed diabetes in the U.S. was estimated to be nearly USD 412 billion in 2022 [2].

Pharmacists play an important role in diabetes care management and positively impact diabetes-related morbidity and mortality [3–10]. Telepharmacy is the provision of patient care services by pharmacists through the use of telecommunications technology [11]. Cao et al. [12] performed a systematic review on the effectiveness of telepharmacy for patients with diabetes and determined that telepharmacy was associated with a reduction in glycated hemoglobin (HbA1c) and the risk of hypoglycemia. Another systematic review [13] revealed that, compared with usual care, telepharmacy results in similar or better outcomes in patients with diabetes.

Although research on the effectiveness of telepharmacy has reported promising findings, its cost-effectiveness remains uncertain [14,15]. Given this evidence gap, policymakers lack the information required to make decisions on the funding and reimbursement of telepharmacy services. Cost-effectiveness, sustainability, and reimbursement agreement are significant challenges that e-health and telemedicine implementation face [16,17].

A key strategic objective of the Saudi Health Sector Transformation Program is to increase access to healthcare services. As evidence for telehealth effectiveness has accumulated [18,19], the Saudi Ministry of Health (MoH) has supported the use of innovations, e-health services, virtual care, and digital solutions to improve healthcare accessibility. The Seha Virtual Hospital (SVH), launched in February 2022, is a MoH hospital that facilitates access to specialized virtual healthcare for all regions of Saudi Arabia. It supports 170 hospitals around the Kingdom and offers more than 30 specialized clinics with a capacity of more than 400,000 patients annually [20]. One of these clinics is the pharmacist-led diabetes and internal medicine clinic, which started in November 2023.

Few Saudi studies have examined the effectiveness of face-to-face pharmacist-led diabetes clinic (PLDC) using a nonrandomized study design [21–23]. One study evaluated the cost-effectiveness of virtual integrated care clinics for patients with diabetes during the COVID-19 pandemic, with pharmacists being one member of the team, compared with a traditional care model before the pandemic [24]. Thus, local evidence on the effectiveness and cost-effectiveness of telepharmacy services for diabetes patients is lacking.

The primary aim of this study was to characterize pharmacists' interventions in a virtual PLDC. The secondary aim was to assess the feasibility of conducting a future cost-effectiveness study of the PLDCs through four objectives: estimating eligibility, recruitment, and follow-up rates; assessing the feasibility of collecting outcome and cost data; identifying barriers and facilitators for the service provision; and evaluation and refinement of the data collection form. The design of the feasibility study was in accordance with relevant guidelines [25,26].

2. Materials and Methods

2.1. Study Design

This was a prospective, observational, feasibility study. The observational nature of the study enabled us to characterize interventions using real-world processes and data without any changes to the pharmacist's routine patient management.

2.2. Setting and Participants

This study was conducted within a pharmacist-led diabetes and internal medicine clinic at SVH. Virtual care at the clinic was offered to patients one day a week, for four hours. Two senior clinical pharmacists alternated running the clinic each week. Clinical pharmacists in Saudi Arabia have postgraduate year 1 (PGY1) with 2 years of experience, postgraduate year 2 (PGY2), or a master's degree in Clinical Pharmacy with 2 years of experience. All diabetic patients referred to the clinic were eligible.

2.3. Data Collection

A Google Form-based data collection form was developed based on previous tools [27–29]. The form collected data on patient characteristics and problems as well as pharmacist interventions to address the identified problems. Our data collection form was developed using several previously published, comprehensive, and validated tools. It integrates principles from a tool designed to improve the characterization and consistent reporting of clinical pharmacy services [27], an internationally recognized system for classifying drug-related problems [30], and a comprehensive tool for assessing the clinical and economic impact of pharmacists' interventions [28]. Two intern pharmacists collected data between 31 July 2024 and 31 January 2025.

2.4. Outcome Measures

The outcomes of our study's primary aim were characteristics of patients referred to the clinic, types of drug-related problems, and the components of pharmacist interventions.

The outcome of our study's secondary aim, the feasibility study, was eligibility, recruitment, and attendance rates and the feasibility of collecting outcome and cost data. The eligibility rate was calculated as the number of eligible patients relative to those screened. The recruitment rate was estimated as the number of patients recruited per month. The attendance rate was calculated as the proportion of virtual consultations completed as scheduled. For the outcome measure, we assessed the feasibility of collecting HbA1c values before and after the intervention during the study period. For cost data, we assessed the feasibility of identifying resource items used during consultation and measuring the quantity of resources used (volumes).

The cost-effectiveness analysis adopted the perspective of the MoH SVH. The comparator to PLDC is usual care. We assumed that usual care involved no pharmacist intervention; hence, no additional costs for pharmacist time or patients' transportation were estimated. For the analysis, we planned to estimate the incremental cost-effectiveness ratio (ICER) by dividing the difference in costs by the difference in in HbA1c reduction observed.

2.5. Data Analysis

Variables are described as numbers with percentages (n, %) or means with standard deviations (SDs). As a feasibility study that did not aim to assess intervention effectiveness against statistical criteria, a power calculation was not conducted, but we aimed to recruit 70 participants in line with previous recommendations [26].

3. Results

3.1. Patient Characteristics

During the study period, 75 patients had virtual consultations. The mean patient age was 50.47 years (SD = 14.95). The majority of patients had type 2 diabetes (86.6%), were admitted to the clinic for the first time (65.3%), and were from outside Riyadh (97.3%) (Table 1).

Table 1. Patient characteristics.

	n	%
Age (years)		
<50	39	52.4
≥50	35	46.6
Sex		
Male	31	41.3%
Female	44	58.7%

Table 1. *Cont.*

	n	%
Appointment nature		
New	49	65.4%
Follow-up	26	34.6%
Region		
Riyadh	2	2.7%
Outside Riyadh	73	97.3%
Type of diabetes		
Type 1	10	13.4%
Type 2	65	86.6%

3.2. Characterization of Pharmacists' Activities and Interventions

We described the components of pharmacist interventions using the Descriptive Elements of Pharmacist Intervention Characterization Tool [27]. Contact between the pharmacist and patient occurred in a private and individual manner. The recipient of the intervention was the patient or a caregiver (n = 6). The workflow of the clinic is depicted in Figure 1. Patients were referred to the PLDC because of uncontrolled HbA1c, polypharmacy, the addition of new medicine, suspected nonadherence, and the ability to update the patient's medication list. These patients were provided with the service through a scheduled appointment via telephone (73, 97.3%) or video conference (2, 2.6%) based on the patient preference. For two patients, the consultation started as a video conference, but for technical reasons, it was changed to telephone. The pharmacist obtained information for patient assessment from a digital health records platform and from patients. To construct appropriate interventions, pharmacists started by updating the patients' medication list to assess the appropriateness of drug indications, contraindications, duplicated drug therapy, and medication interactions. Then, the pharmacists evaluated medication effectiveness (69, 92.0%) and safety (53, 70.6%) by evaluating patients' symptoms and fasting glucose and HbA1c levels. In 89% of the consultations (n = 67), the pharmacists assessed adherence by asking the patients if they took their medications, at what time, and if they adjusted doses according to blood glucose readings. On a few occasions (n = 13), the pharmacists asked the patients to take photographs of their medications or home blood glucose test readings and send them via WhatsApp.

According to a published tool [30] to classify drug-related problems and identify the causes of these problems, all patients lacked optimal treatment effects, as demonstrated by their uncontrolled HbA1c levels. Based on pharmacists' discussions with the patients, the cause of this problem was related to the patient's behavior, specifically inappropriate antidiabetic medication doses (too low, too high); not taking the medications at all; inappropriate timing or dosing intervals; and unhealthy lifestyles. Few patients had problems related to treatment safety, as demonstrated by duplicate therapy (n = 2) and medication side effects (n = 4).

In total, 179 interventions were conducted. The mean number of interventions per patient was 2.5 (median 3, min 0, max 5). The most common intervention was patient education and counseling about their disease and medications (Table 2).

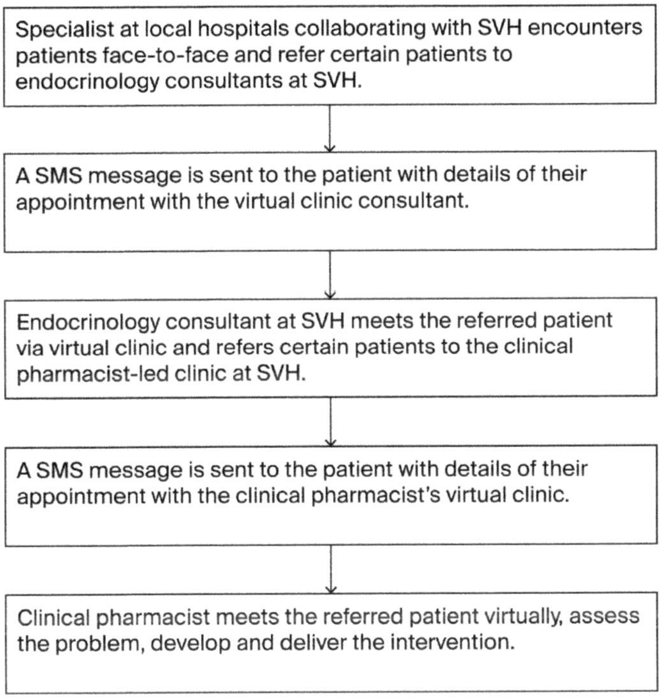

Figure 1. PLDC workflow.

Table 2. Pharmacist interventions.

Type of Intervention	**n (%)**
Provision of drug information or patient counselling including:	60 (34)
Medication name, doses, and time of administration (with or without food)	46
The importance of lifestyle modification (exercise, weight loss, diet advice)	35
The importance of adherence to prevent complications	24
Self-monitoring blood glucose and target level	23
The importance of screening for diabetic complications (e.g., eye check)	10
Managing acute complications (e.g., hypoglycemia symptoms and management)	7
Medication storage and stability/insulin storage and stability	5
Pregnancy complication	1
Drug monitoring (order laboratory test)	28 (16)
Update of patient's medication list	26 (15)
Referral to other healthcare professionals or clinics	21 (12)
Dose adjustment	19 (11)
Recommend discontinuation (suspend prescription)	6 (3)
Administration mode optimization	6 (3)
Monitoring results report	7 (4)
Recommend addition (new prescription)	3 (2)
Help with refill procedures	3 (2)

The impact of interventions was evaluated by two raters using the Clinical, Economic and Organization (CLEO) tool [28]. The raters had a high agreement rate (98%). Discussion was required to reach a consensus for 4 of the 179 interventions. The impact was evaluated as a potential minor clinical impact defined as the fact that the intervention can improve knowledge, satisfaction, and medication adherence or prevent harm. The majority of interventions did not change the cost of healthcare, but 49 interventions (27.5%) potentially increased costs due to the ordering of tests, referrals, or recommending a medication.

The mean consultation duration was 7.64 min (SD = 5.68, min = 1, max = 30). After each visit, the pharmacists entered free-text into the database containing a short summary about the patient's problem and any interventions or recommendations made to be shared with the physicians and other healthcare team members (five minutes per patient). This totaled 15.8 h (9.55 consultations and 6.25 documentations) across 23 clinics.

3.3. *Feasibility of Cost-Effectiveness Evaluation*

The rate of eligibility was 83.3%, as 16.6% of the 90 patients who attended the clinic were not diabetes patients and were consequently excluded. The average rate of recruitment was 21 patients per month (Table 3). Forty-one patients did not answer the phone call (missed appointment).

Table 3. Rate of eligibility and recruitment.

	Answered the Call (n = 90)		Did Not Answer the Call (n = 41)	Total
Month	**Eligible**	**Excluded**		
July	2	0	0	2
August	6	0	1	7
September	11	5	4	20
October	14	3	9	26
November	9	6	9	24
December	14	1	8	23
January	19	0	10	29
Total (%)	75 (57.3)	15 (11.4)	41 (31.3)	131

The collection of outcome measures was challenging. For many patients, no laboratory results for HbA1c were available through the telehealth platform. Among the follow-up patients (n = 26) who attended the first appointment before the data collection period, only two patients had HbA1c values before and after the intervention. Pharmacists asked patients about their HbA1c levels to assess their understanding of the test's meaning and their target goal. Forty-one patients (55%) reported knowing their last HbA1c reading. The mean self-reported HbA1c value was 9.91 (SD = 1.69).

The collection of resources used and volume was feasible. The main resource item was the pharmacists' time, which included the time required to read the referral, the virtual consultation time, and the time needed to document the clinic recommendations. The pharmacist's recommendations, such as ordering a lab test, recommending the addition of a medication, and referring patients to other clinics or healthcare practitioners, are another type of cost. To attach value to the resources used, we multiplied the hourly rate of employing a pharmacist by the visit time. The hourly rate of employing a pharmacist at the midpoint of the salary scale was calculated based on the monthly salary of SAR 20,500 (128 per hour) from published data. The cost of pharmacist consultation per patient was

SAR 269 (SD = 121, median 234, min 127, max 745). The total cost per patient, including recommendations such as ordering a test or referral, was SAR 370 (SD 177, median 333, min 127, max 865).

The clinic utilizes a digital platform for health practitioners to schedule patient appointments and provide counseling and a cloud-based digital health record for documenting patient progress notes. The costs of these telehealth platforms include setup, maintenance, software licensing, and internet connection. The clinic is equipped with a computer, headphones, microphones, and telephone. The clinic, including equipment, is not exclusive to the PLDC. These shared costs and fixed costs such as electricity are relevant from the perspective of the MoH; however, the costs attributed to PLDC patients are very small. Furthermore, these costs will be maintained even if PLDCs are terminated. Therefore, these costs were excluded from this study.

We originally planned to calculate ICER using the collected data. However, the incomplete data on pre- and post-HbA1c made this calculation unfeasible. As a result, we could not perform this analysis.

4. Discussion

In this descriptive feasibility study, we collected data prospectively from 75 patients who received pharmacist counseling virtually. Pharmacists were able to identify problems and make 179 interventions. The most common intervention was patient education and counseling about their disease and medications. Our secondary aim was to assess the feasibility of conducting a future cost-effectiveness study of PLDCs. It proved feasible to capture the details of pharmacist interventions using an observational study design. The data collection form was comprehensive and easy to fill out. Overall, while collection of relevant costs proved to be feasible, outcome measurement was not feasible and remained a challenge to be addressed.

Our findings concerning the reasons for referral and the content of patient education are consistent with those of Salhia et al. [31] who investigated the reasons for the referral of patients to Saudi MOH medication counseling clinics. During their study period, from May 2020 to December 2021, 28,998 patients were referred to pharmacists counseling either face-to-face (64.55%) or virtually (35.45%), with common reasons for referrals being patients with chronic diseases (50.84%), new medication addition (33.69%), or polypharmacy (22.71%). During the counseling session, the subjects discussed medication name, indication, dose and administration (85.62%), duration of therapy (68.42%), what to do if a dose was missed (44.51%), storage (39.69%), and lifestyle modifications (32.90%).

The types of interventions documented in our study are in concert with those of a previous systematic review [7,10] that reported that the most common pharmacist interventions for patients with diabetes were counseling and education on diabetes, medication, lifestyle modification, and self-monitoring; reinforcement of medication adherence or complication screening; adjustment of pharmacotherapy; and referrals to other healthcare professionals.

Forty-one patients (31%) did not answer the phone and consequently missed appointments. Missed appointments result in unused pharmacist time and decreased efficiency. Our rate of missed appointments was higher than that reported in the literature [32,33]. A UK study of outpatient services revealed that the rate of missed first appointments for remote consultations was higher than that of in-person appointments (12.5% vs. 9.2%), but follow-up appointments had similar rates [32]. The cited reasons for missed in-person appointments include competing work or family/childcare commitments and patients forgetting the appointment [34], and these reasons could be the same for virtual consultations. Future studies could identify individuals at risk of missing virtual PLDC appointments to help the development of interventions to mitigate this risk to help improve efficiency and avoid health inequalities.

Owing to incomplete data on pre- and post-HbA1c, it was not feasible to calculate the extra cost per extra 1% HbA1c reduction in order to decide whether investing in the virtual clinic was an efficient use of resources. A metanalysis [12] reported that telepharmacy is associated with a mean HbA1c reduction from baseline in observational studies (−1.55%; 95% CI, −2.07% to −1.02%) and in randomized controlled trials (−0.86%; 95% CI, −1.25% to −0.47%). However, the heterogeneity between included studies in the design of telepharmacy services make it inappropriate to extrapolate the findings to the SVH clinic.

Lack of access to patients' medical records and laboratory results was the main barrier to the provision of pharmaceutical services at the virtual PLDCs. Another challenge was the good proportion of patients who did not answer the scheduled phone call. These missed appointments lead to wasted time for pharmacists, the underutilization of resources, and potential delays in care for other patients.

4.1. Practice Implications

Our observations indicated that the current pharmacists' free-text note documentation missed many interventions identified by our data collection form. A study reported that electronic health record documentation of intensive care pharmacists' interventions increased the capture of interventions by 56% compared with progress notes entering [35]. We recommend replacing free-text documentation with a checklist that captures details of pharmacists' interventions to capture data fully and reflect the added value of pharmacists' interventions accurately.

The pharmacist at SVH does not have access to the patients' medical records at their local hospital. This lack of access compromises the ability of pharmacists to identify drug-related problems, make appropriate recommendations, and optimize medication therapy management [36]. The recent introduction of a shared clinic, where pharmacists and physicians from the local hospital attend the virtual clinic, could be part of the solution to this problem. The shared clinic offers the advantage of allowing pharmacists at SVH to obtain relevant clinical data and enables physicians to approve or disapprove their recommendations instantly. Access to patients' medical records, or integrating laboratory results and medication lists into the cloud-based digital health record platform, is recommended.

A high missed appointment rate reduces both access to care and provider productivity. The change in clinic time from morning to afternoon and sending a reminder message one day prior to the clinic may decrease the number of missed scheduled appointments. A Saudi study [37] reported that diabetic patients' attitudes, such as perceived privacy and usefulness of digital health services, significantly impact the perceived intention to use these services. Therefore, policy-makers, physicians, and pharmacists should develop strategies to increase patients' awareness of the benefits of pharmacists' consultations and address any concerns about privacy, trust, and ease of use.

The delivery of interventions can be improved if pharmacists engage patients in setting goals and actions for their planned behaviors, such as monitoring glucose blood levels, which have been shown to increase the likelihood of positive outcomes from pharmacist-led interventions [13,38,39]. Pharmacists have identified few cases of nonadherence and addressed the reasons behind it, such as the fear of side effects without the use of a standardized adherence tool. In the future, pharmacists may use tools to measure adherence levels, identify barriers and develop tailored interventions, although selecting a tool for clinical practice is not straightforward [40].

4.2. Future Research Recommendations

Future economic evaluations, whether performed alongside clinical trials or through model-based analyses, are warranted. Randomized controlled trials or observational studies conducted in a foreign country may not be able to inform policymaking in the Saudi context due to differences in clinical practices and healthcare financing systems. Therefore, we recommend local trials to assess the impact of virtual PLDCs on outcomes.

When planning a future cost-effectiveness study, access to and the use of patients' information in local hospitals need to be factored into the study design. For chronic conditions, a long-term time frame is crucial to accurately assess cost-effectiveness by capturing all relevant costs and benefits. For example, in a previous study, one event of non-severe hypoglycemia and one event of severe hypoglycemia were estimated to cost the Saudi MoH SAR 750 and SAR 1712, respectively [41]. Model-based economic evaluations integrate evidence from a variety of sources, including individual trials, meta-analyses, and expert opinion and account for long-term costs and benefits. Our feasibility study focused on assessing HbA1c reduction, as this is associated with lower overall and diabetes-related healthcare costs [42]. Further economic evaluations assessing long-term outcomes, such as mortality, complications, and quality-adjusted life years, are recommended.

Of the 131 patients scheduled for the clinic, 31% did not answer the phone call (missed appointments). Future research should investigate the reasons for missing virtual appointments. One reason could be that elderly patients often provide their caregivers' contact information, such as a son's or daughter's phone number, for scheduling and appointment reminders. As a result, all future communications, including reminders and virtual clinic calls, will be directed to the caregiver. If the caregiver is at work, they may not be available to assist the patient with their virtual appointment. Future work is needed to identify the support required to promote equitable access to care for all patients.

The majority of patients (97%) were from outside the capital city Riyadh, which suggests that the pharmacist was able to provide services to patients who might have otherwise missed them, thereby increasing access to services. However, an exploration of the virtual PLDC's impact on accessibility was beyond the scope of our investigation. Therefore, a future study specifically focused on accessibility is recommended to determine whether the virtual PLDC facilitates access to specialized pharmaceutical services for all regions of Saudi Arabia.

In our study, four patients were scheduled for the virtual PLDC via video conference, but two were switched to telephone due to technical issues. This suggests the need for further research to explore the impact of technological barriers on service delivery. The impact of technological disparities among different age groups, particularly older adults, on access to the service is a topic for future research.

Future surveys of the opinions and experiences of virtual PLDC users and their willingness to use the service again are needed. To develop a full picture of the pharmacists' intervention impact, additional studies will be needed that assess physicians' acceptance of pharmacists' recommendations.

4.3. Limitations

This study had several limitations. Our findings are constrained by data availability and quality. We did not assess the feasibility of assessing long-term outcomes, such as mortality, complications, or quality of life. As our study did not aim to investigate intervention effectiveness, a larger, adequately powered pragmatic study is needed to evaluate effectiveness. While pharmacists can directly make the majority of interventions (79%), actions such as ordering lab tests or starting/stopping medications require physician approval. Because our study did not measure physicians' acceptance of these interventions, this represents a major limitation.

5. Conclusions

Our detailed documentation of pharmacist–patient encounters revealed the ability of pharmacists to identify and manage the problems of diabetes patients at virtual PLDCs. While the collection of relevant costs proved to be feasible, measuring outcomes based on pre- and post-intervention data was not. Our feasibility study identified a few challenges that must be addressed when designing future cost-effectiveness studies.

Author Contributions: Conceptualization, S.A.-A. and A.M.; formal analysis, S.A.-A., A.M., N.A. and D.A.; investigation, A.M., N.A., D.A., R.A., W.A. and S.A.; methodology, S.A.-A. and A.M.; writing—original draft, S.A.-A.; writing—review and editing, S.A.-A., A.M., N.A., D.A., R.A., W.A. and S.A. All authors have read and agreed to the published version of the manuscript.

Funding: This research received no external funding.

Institutional Review Board Statement: The study was conducted according to the guidelines of the Declaration of Helsinki and approved by the Ministry of Health Research Ethics Committee (Reference: 24-67 E) on 21 July 2024.

Informed Consent Statement: Verbal informed consent was obtained from the participants. The rationale for utilizing verbal consent is that this observational research presents no more than minimal risk of harm to subjects and involves no intervention.

Data Availability Statement: The original contributions presented in this study are included in the article. For further inquiries, please contact the corresponding author.

Conflicts of Interest: The authors declare no conflicts of interest.

Abbreviations

The following abbreviations are used in this manuscript:

MoH	Saudi Ministry of Health
PLDC	pharmacist-led diabetes clinic
ICER	cost-effectiveness ratio

References

1. Ong, K.L.; Stafford, L.K.; McLaughlin, S.A.; Boyko, E.J.; Vollset, S.E.; Smith, A.E.; Dalton, B.E.; Duprey, J.; Cruz, J.A.; Hagins, H.; et al. Global, regional, and national burden of diabetes from 1990 to 2021, with projections of prevalence to 2050: A systematic analysis for the Global Burden of Disease Study 2021. *Lancet* **2023**, *402*, 203–234. [CrossRef]
2. Parker, E.D.; Lin, J.; Mahoney, T.; Ume, N.; Yang, G.; Gabbay, R.A.; ElSayed, N.A.; Bannuru, R.R. Economic costs of diabetes in the U.S. in 2022. *Diabetes Care* **2024**, *47*, 26–43. [CrossRef] [PubMed]
3. Abdulrhim, S.; Sankaralingam, S.; Ibrahim, M.I.M.; Awaisu, A. The impact of pharmacist care on diabetes outcomes in primary care settings: An umbrella review of published systematic reviews. *Prim. Care Diabetes* **2020**, *14*, 393–400. [CrossRef]
4. Al Assaf, S.; Zelko, R.; Hanko, B. The Effect of Interventions Led by Community Pharmacists in Primary Care for Adults with Type 2 Diabetes Mellitus on Therapeutic Adherence and HbA1c Levels: A Systematic Review. *Int. J. Environ. Res. Public Health* **2022**, *19*, 6188. [CrossRef]
5. Alabkal, R.M.; Medlinskiene, K.; Silcock, J.; Graham, A. Impact of Pharmacist-Led Interventions to Improve Clinical Outcomes for Adults with Type 2 Diabetes at Risk of Developing Cardiovascular Disease: A Systematic Review and Meta-analysis. *J. Pharm. Pract.* **2023**, *36*, 888–899. [CrossRef]
6. Coutureau, C.; Slimano, F.; Mongaret, C.; Kanagaratnam, L. Impact of Pharmacists-Led Interventions in Primary Care for Adults with Type 2 Diabetes on HbA1c Levels: A Systematic Review and Meta-Analysis. *Int. J. Environ. Res. Public Health* **2022**, *19*, 3156. [CrossRef] [PubMed]
7. Hassan, F.; Hatah, E.; Ali, A.M.; Wen, C.W. The intervention strategies and service model for pharmacist-led diabetes management: A scoping review. *BMC Health Serv. Res.* **2023**, *23*, 46. [CrossRef] [PubMed]

8. Jeong, S.; Lee, M.; Ji, E. Effect of pharmaceutical care interventions on glycemic control in patients with diabetes: A systematic review and meta-analysis. *Ther. Clin. Risk Manag.* **2018**, *14*, 1813–1829. [CrossRef] [PubMed]
9. Presley, B.; Groot, W.; Pavlova, M. Pharmacy-led interventions to improve medication adherence among adults with diabetes: A systematic review and meta-analysis. *Res. Soc. Adm. Pharm.* **2019**, *15*, 1057–1067. [CrossRef]
10. Pousinho, S.; Morgado, M.; Falcão, A.; Alves, G. Pharmacist Interventions in the Management of Type 2 Diabetes Mellitus: A Systematic Review of Randomized Controlled Trials. *J. Manag. Care Spec. Pharm.* **2016**, *22*, 493–515. [CrossRef]
11. Begnoche, B.R.; David Butler, C.; Carson, P.H.; Darr, A.; Jenkins, M.T.; Le, T.; McDaniel, R.B.; Mourad, H.; Shipman, C.J.; Stratton, T.P.; et al. ASHP Statement on Telehealth Pharmacy Practice. *Am. J. Health Syst. Pharm.* **2022**, *79*, 1728–1735. [CrossRef]
12. Cao, D.X.; Tran, R.J.C.; Yamzon, J.; Stewart, T.L.; Hernandez, E.A. Effectiveness of telepharmacy diabetes services: A systematic review and meta-analysis. *Am. J. Health Syst. Pharm.* **2022**, *79*, 860–872. [CrossRef]
13. Christy, A.; Fernanda, F.; Insani, W.N.; Abdulah, R. Pharmacist-Led Digital Health Interventions for Patients with Diabetes: A Systematic Review. *J. Multidiscip. Healthc.* **2025**, *18*, 101–112. [CrossRef]
14. Park, T.; Kim, H.; Song, S.; Griggs, S.K. Economic Evaluation of Pharmacist-Led Digital Health Interventions: A Systematic Review. *Int. J. Environ. Res. Public Health* **2022**, *19*, 11996. [CrossRef]
15. De Guzman, K.R.; Gavanescu, D.; Smith, A.C.; Snoswell, C.L. Economic evaluations of telepharmacy services in non-cancer settings: A systematic review. *Res. Soc. Adm. Pharm.* **2024**, *20*, 246–254. [CrossRef]
16. Ahmed, B.; Dannhauser, T.; Philip, N. A systematic review of reviews to identify key research opportunities within the field of eHealth implementation. *J. Telemed. Telecare* **2019**, *25*, 276–285. [CrossRef]
17. Scott Kruse, C.; Karem, P.; Shifflett, K.; Vegi, L.; Ravi, K.; Brooks, M. Evaluating barriers to adopting telemedicine worldwide: A systematic review. *J. Telemed. Telecare* **2018**, *24*, 4–12. [CrossRef]
18. Snoswell, C.L.; Chelberg, G.; De Guzman, K.R.; Haydon, H.M.; Thomas, E.E.; Caffery, L.J.; Smith, A.C. The clinical effectiveness of telehealth: A systematic review of meta-analyses from 2010 to 2019. *J. Telemed. Telecare* **2023**, *29*, 669–684. [CrossRef] [PubMed]
19. Baughman, D.J.; Jabbarpour, Y.; Westfall, J.M.; Jetty, A.; Zain, A.; Baughman, K.; Pollak, B.; Waheed, A. Comparison of Quality Performance Measures for Patients Receiving In-Person vs. Telemedicine Primary Care in a Large Integrated Health System. *JAMA Netw. Open* **2022**, *5*, e2233267. [CrossRef] [PubMed]
20. Seha Virtual Hospital. Available online: https://www.moh.gov.sa/en/Ministry/Projects/Pages/Seha-Virtual-Hospital.aspx (accessed on 16 March 2025).
21. Alsuwayni, B.; Alhossan, A. Impact of clinical pharmacist-led diabetes management clinic on health outcomes at an academic hospital in Riyadh, Saudi Arabia: A prospective cohort study. *Saudi Pharm. J.* **2020**, *28*, 1756–1759. [CrossRef] [PubMed]
22. Alqifari, S.F.; AlMharwal, B.; Aldawish, R.; Almokhlef, S.A. Impact of Pharmacist-Led Clinics on Health Outcomes of Patients with Diabetes at a Ministry of Health Diabetes & Endocrinology Center, Saudi Arabia: A Retrospective Study. *Cureus* **2022**, *14*, e25923. [CrossRef] [PubMed]
23. Alghadeer, S.M.; Alsuwayni, B.; Almuwayjid, A.K.; Almadi, M.S.; Mubarak, A.M.; Khunayn, R.M.B.; Al-Arifi, M.N. Glycemic Control and Management in Pharmacist-Led Diabetic Clinic vs. Physician-Led Diabetic Clinic. *Medicina* **2021**, *58*, 14. [CrossRef] [PubMed]
24. Faleh AlMutairi, M.; Tourkmani, A.M.; Alrasheedy, A.A.; Alharbi, T.J.; Bin Rsheed, A.M.; Aljehani, M.; AlRuthia, Y. Cost-effectiveness of telemedicine care for patients with uncontrolled type 2 diabetes mellitus during the COVID-19 pandemic in Saudi Arabia. *Ther. Adv. Chronic Dis.* **2021**, *12*, 20406223211042542. [CrossRef] [PubMed]
25. Bowen, D.J.; Kreuter, M.; Spring, B.; Cofta-Woerpel, L.; Linnan, L.; Weiner, D.; Bakken, S.; Kaplan, C.P.; Squiers, L.; Fabrizio, C.; et al. How We Design Feasibility Studies. *Am. J. Prev. Med.* **2009**, *36*, 452–457. [CrossRef]
26. Teresi, J.A.; Yu, X.; Stewart, A.L.; Hays, R.D. Guidelines for Designing and Evaluating Feasibility Pilot Studies. *Med. Care* **2022**, *60*, 95–103. [CrossRef]
27. Rotta, I.; Salgado, T.M.; Felix, D.C.; Souza, T.T.; Correr, C.J.; Fernandez-Llimos, F. Ensuring consistent reporting of clinical pharmacy services to enhance reproducibility in practice: An improved version of DEPICT. *J. Eval. Clin. Pract.* **2015**, *21*, 584–590. [CrossRef]
28. Vo, H.T.; Charpiat, B.; Chanoine, S.; Juste, M.; Roubille, R.; Rose, F.X.; Conort, O.; Allenet, B.; Bedouch, P. CLEO: A multidimensional tool to assess clinical, economic and organisational impacts of pharmacists' interventions. *Eur. J. Hosp. Pharm.* **2021**, *28*, 193–200. [CrossRef]
29. Allenet, B.; Bedouch, P.; Rose, F.-X.; Escofier, L.; Roubille, R.; Charpiat, B.; Juste, M.; Conort, O. Validation of an instrument for the documentation of clinical pharmacists' interventions. *Pharm. World Sci.* **2006**, *28*, 181–188. [CrossRef]
30. Pharmaceutical Care Network Europe. Classification for Drug Related Problems. Available online: https://www.pcne.org/upload/files/334_PCNE_classification_V9-0.pdf (accessed on 16 March 2025).
31. Salhia, H.; Mutlaq, A.; Alshaiban, A.; Alsaleh, A.; Alzahrani, R.; Alshennawi, M. Patterns in counselling services provided at Saudi Ministry of Health medication counselling clinics—Reasons for referrals and subjects discussed: A cross-sectional study. *Saudi Pharm. J.* **2023**, *31*, 1157–1166. [CrossRef]

32. Kerr, G.; Greenfield, G.; Hayhoe, B.; Gaughran, F.; Halvorsrud, K.; Pinto da Costa, M.; Rehill, N.; Raine, R.; Majeed, A.; Costelloe, C.; et al. Attendance at remote versus in-person outpatient appointments in an NHS Trust. *J. Telemed. Telecare* **2025**, *31*, 721–731. [CrossRef]
33. Adepoju, O.E.; Chae, M.; Liaw, W.; Angelocci, T.; Millard, P.; Matuk-Villazon, O. Transition to telemedicine and its impact on missed appointments in community-based clinics. *Ann. Med.* **2022**, *54*, 98–107. [CrossRef] [PubMed]
34. Parsons, J.; Bryce, C.; Atherton, H. Which patients miss appointments with general practice and the reasons why: A systematic review. *Br. J. Gen. Pract.* **2021**, *71*, e406–e412. [CrossRef]
35. Vlashyn, O.O.; Murphy, C.V.; Cape, K.; Phelps, M.K.; Nunez, S.M.; Hafford, A.; Jordan, T.A.; Smetana, K.S. Evaluation of an electronic health record documentation tool use to improve pharmacist intervention tracking in the intensive care unit. *J. Am. Coll. Clin. Pharm.* **2024**, *7*, 358–366. [CrossRef]
36. Kestin, R.; Howe, A.; Moose, J.; Marciniak, M.W.; Rhodes, L.A. Impact of health information exchange access on medication management recommendations in a community-based pharmacy setting. *J. Am. Pharm. Assoc.* **2024**, *64*, 102104. [CrossRef] [PubMed]
37. Al-Sulimani, T.S.; Bouaguel, W. Understanding Factors Influencing Diabetic Patients' Intention to Use Digital Health Services in Saudi Arabia Using the Technology Acceptance Model. *Int. J. Environ. Res. Public Health* **2024**, *21*, 889. [CrossRef]
38. Craske, M.E.; Hardeman, W.; Steel, N.; Twigg, M.J. Components of pharmacist-led medication reviews and their relationship to outcomes: A systematic review and narrative synthesis. *BMJ Qual. Saf.* **2024**, *33*, 808–822. [CrossRef]
39. Deters, M.A.; Laven, A.; Castejon, A.; Doucette, W.R.; Ev, L.S.; Krass, I.; Mehuys, E.; Obarcanin, E.; Schwender, H.; Laeer, S. Effective Interventions for Diabetes Patients by Community Pharmacists: A Meta-analysis of Pharmaceutical Care Components. *Ann. Pharmacother.* **2018**, *52*, 198–211. [CrossRef]
40. Rickles, N.M.; Mulrooney, M.; Sobieraj, D.; Hernandez, A.V.; Manzey, L.L.; Gouveia-Pisano, J.A.; Townsend, K.A.; Luder, H.; Cappelleri, J.C.; Possidente, C.J. A systematic review of primary care-focused, self-reported medication adherence tools. *J. Am. Pharm. Assoc.* **2023**, *63*, 477–490.e1. [CrossRef]
41. AlHarbi, M.; Othman, A.; Nahari, A.A.; Al-Jedai, A.H.; Cuadras, D.; Almalky, F.; AlAzmi, F.; Almudaiheem, H.Y.; AlShubrumi, H.; AlSwat, H.; et al. Burden of Illness of Type 2 Diabetes Mellitus in the Kingdom of Saudi Arabia: A Five-Year Longitudinal Study. *Adv. Ther.* **2024**, *41*, 1120–1150. [CrossRef]
42. Lage, M.J.; Boye, K.S. The relationship between HbA1c reduction and healthcare costs among patients with type 2 diabetes: Evidence from a U.S. claims database. *Curr. Med. Res. Opin.* **2020**, *36*, 1441–1447. [CrossRef]

healthcare

MDPI

Article

Telemedicine-Supported Intervention Versus Standard Care for Managing Cardiovascular Risk Factors in a Socially Deprived Urban Population: A Prospective Study

Angelica Gherman [1,2,†], Codrina Mihaela Levai [2,3,†], Ovidiu Alin Haţegan [4,*], Călin Marius Popoiu [5,*], Emil Robert Stoicescu [6,7,8] and Anca Laura Maghiari [9]

1 Ph.D. School Department, "Victor Babeş" University of Medicine and Pharmacy of Timisoara, 300041 Timisoara, Romania; angelica.gherman@umft.ro
2 Research Center for Medical Communication, "Victor Babeş" University of Medicine and Pharmacy of Timisoara, Eftimie Murgu Square No. 2, 300041 Timisoara, Romania; codrinalevai@umft.ro
3 Discipline of Medical Communications, Department 2—Microscopic Morphology, "Victor Babeş" University of Medicine and Pharmacy of Timisoara, 300041 Timisoara, Romania
4 Discipline of Anatomy and Embriology, Medicine Faculty, Vasile Goldis Western University of Arad, Revolution Boulevard 94, 310025 Arad, Romania
5 Department of Pediatric Surgery, "Victor Babeş" University of Medicine and Pharmacy of Timisoara, 300041 Timisoara, Romania
6 Radiology and Medical Imaging University Clinic, "Victor Babeş" University of Medicine and Pharmacy of Timisoara, Eftimie Murgu Square No. 2, 300041 Timisoara, Romania; stoicescu.emil@umft.ro
7 Research Center for Pharmaco-Toxicological Evaluations, "Victor Babeş" University of Medicine and Pharmacy of Timisoara, Eftimie Murgu Square No. 2, 300041 Timisoara, Romania
8 Field of Applied Engineering Sciences, Specialization Statistical Methods and Techniques in Health and Clinical Research, Faculty of Mechanics, "Politehnica" University Timisoara, Mihai Viteazul Boulevard No. 1, 300222 Timisoara, Romania
9 Department of Anatomy and Embriology, "Victor Babeş" University of Medicine and Pharmacy of Timisoara, 300041 Timișoara, Romania; boscu.anca@umft.ro
* Correspondence: hategan.ovidiu@uvvg.ro (O.A.H.); mcpopoiu@umft.ro (C.M.P.)
† These authors contributed equally to this work.

Abstract: Background: Cardiovascular disease (CVD) remains a leading cause of morbidity and mortality, particularly in socioeconomically disadvantaged populations. Telemedicine offers a potential strategy to support risk factor management in such groups with limited access to care. Our aim was to assess the effectiveness of a telemedicine-supported intervention compared to usual care in improving cardiovascular risk parameters among adults from a socially deprived urban population. **Materials and Methods:** In this controlled intervention study, adult patients with one or more cardiovascular risk factors were recruited from a primary care center in a low-income urban neighborhood in Timişoara, Romania. Participants were allocated to either usual care or a six-month telemedicine-supported intervention group. The intervention consisted of regular phone calls by trained staff focusing on medication adherence, self-monitoring of blood pressure and glucose, smoking cessation, and lifestyle advice. No physical visits were delivered. Primary outcomes included changes in systolic and diastolic blood pressure, fasting glucose, and lipid profile. Data were collected at baseline and at six months. **Results:** A total of 144 patients were allocated to the telemedicine group and 142 to the usual care group. After 6 months, diastolic blood pressure decreased by 3.9 mmHg in the telemedicine group compared to 0.3 mmHg in the standard care group ($p < 0.001$). LDL-cholesterol was reduced by 18.0 mg/dL with telemedicine versus 5.7 mg/dL with usual care ($p < 0.001$). In contrast, fasting glucose improved more in the standard care group (−10.9 mg/dL vs. −2.0 mg/dL, $p < 0.001$). Patient satisfaction in the telemedicine group was high, with 84% rating the program as very useful. **Conclusions:** Basic telemedicine-supported interventions may represent a feasible and effective strategy for improving cardiovascular risk factors such as diastolic

 https://doi.org/10.3390/healthcare13172202

blood pressure and LDL-cholesterol in socially deprived populations. High satisfaction suggests strong acceptability; however, given the small sample size, short follow-up, and single-center design, these findings should be interpreted cautiously and confirmed in larger studies.

Keywords: cardiovascular risk factors; telemedicine; health disparities; blood pressure; cholesterol; fasting glucose; urban population; patient satisfaction

1. Introduction

Cardiovascular diseases (CVDs) are the leading cause of death globally, accounting for an estimated 17.7 million deaths in 2015, according to the World Health Organization, with a disproportionate burden falling on socially deprived populations [1–3]. Beyond mortality, CVD represents the most expensive health burden worldwide, with annual indirect costs projected to rise from USD 237 billion to USD 368 billion by 2035 [1]. Individuals living in underserved urban communities often face significant barriers to healthcare access, including transportation difficulties, limited health literacy, and strained healthcare infrastructure [4,5]. These challenges contribute to suboptimal management of cardiovascular risk factors, ultimately worsening health outcomes [6,7].

Cardiovascular risk factors comprise modifiable and non-modifiable variables, such as age, sex, elevated blood pressure, abnormal lipid profiles, and impaired glucose metabolism, that can collectively contribute to the development and clinical manifestation of CVD [8]. A sedentary lifestyle and the frequent intake of energy-dense, nutrient-poor foods high in saturated fats and sugars are also closely linked to the onset of atherosclerosis and metabolic disorders such as metabolic syndrome, diabetes mellitus, and hypertension, conditions that are highly prevalent in individuals with cardiovascular disease [9,10]. According to a recent investigation, behavioral factors have a greater impact on the management of cardiovascular diseases than preventative medicine [11,12]. Additionally, new research indicates that lowering certain risk factors, such as total cholesterol, arterial hypertension, and body mass index (BMI), may lower the death rate from cardiovascular disease [12,13]. Despite the fact that exercise and a balanced diet reduce the risk of CVD, heavy smokers who also followed these recommendations still had a 3.8-fold higher risk of CVD, which is consistent with previous research [12,14,15].

Telemedicine encompasses various modalities, including synchronous video consultations, asynchronous data exchange, remote patient monitoring, and mobile health applications, each tailored to enhance healthcare delivery and accessibility [16]. This field has emerged as a promising strategy to bridge gaps in care delivery, offering remote monitoring, counseling, and follow-up without the need for frequent in-person visits. While telemedicine interventions have shown efficacy in various clinical settings, evidence remains limited regarding their effectiveness in low-resource, high-risk urban populations [17–19]. It will be more important to assess the quality of care being provided and provide evidence that it is being maintained as telemedicine develops into a standard service in environments with limited resources [19]. In particular, the impact of basic, low-cost telemedicine solutions, as opposed to app-based or technologically advanced systems, requires further investigation to determine their feasibility and clinical utility in real-world primary care settings.

This study aimed to evaluate the effectiveness of a basic telemedicine intervention compared to usual care in improving cardiovascular risk profiles over a six-month period in a socially deprived urban population. The outcomes of interest included changes in blood pressure, lipid and glucose levels, BMI, and patient satisfaction, with the goal of informing scalable solutions to reduce health disparities.

2. Materials and Methods

2.1. Study Design

This was a prospective, quasi-experimental controlled study conducted in a primary care setting. Participants were consecutively enrolled during routine visits and allocated to either a telemedicine-supported intervention group or a standard care group. No randomization was performed; instead, allocation was structured to achieve comparable group sizes.

2.2. Population

This study targeted adults aged 40–80 years living in a socioeconomically deprived urban area of Timișoara, Romania. Eligible participants were those with at least one cardiovascular risk factor, defined as hypertension, dyslipidemia, impaired fasting glucose, or elevated BMI. Individuals with a known history of cardiovascular disease, severe psychiatric or cognitive disorders, or inability to provide informed consent were excluded.

Eligible participants were identified consecutively during routine visits at the primary care center. All eligible patients were informed about the study procedures and purpose, and those who agreed provided written informed consent. Enrollment continued until the planned sample size of 300 participants was reached.

Participants were allocated in equal numbers to the two study arms: 150 to the telemedicine-supported intervention group and 150 to the standard care group. Over the 6-month follow-up period, 286 participants (95.3%) completed the study, including 144 in the telemedicine arm and 142 in the standard care arm. Fourteen patients did not complete follow-up: in the telemedicine group, three moved away from the study area and three could not be contacted despite repeated attempts; in the standard care group, four moved away, three were lost to contact, and one withdrew consent. No adverse events related to the intervention were reported.

In the intervention group, telemedical care was delivered by trained general practitioners and nurses affiliated with the primary care center. Patients received monthly structured telephone consultations lasting approximately 15–20 min for six months. Each call followed a standardized checklist and included review of blood pressure and glucose self-monitoring logs, reinforcement of medication adherence, lifestyle counseling (dietary habits, physical activity, and smoking cessation), and reminders to complete laboratory evaluations. Nurses conducted most consultations under physician supervision, with cases requiring medical decision-making escalated to the supervising general practitioner.

The control group received standard care through local health services, consisting of usual clinic referrals and routine follow-up if patients chose to attend, without additional structured telephone support.

2.3. Data Collection

Data were collected at baseline and after six months for both groups. These assessments included measurements of systolic and diastolic blood pressure and BMI, laboratory analysis of fasting glucose and lipid profiles (total cholesterol, low-density lipoprotein (LDL) cholesterol, high-density lipoprotein (HDL) cholesterol, triglycerides), and a questionnaire capturing lifestyle behaviors and access to healthcare. Systolic and diastolic blood pressure were measured with validated automated sphygmomanometers (Omron M6, Omron Healthcare, Kyoto, Japan). Measurements were performed in a seated position, after 5 min of rest, on the right arm supported at heart level. Three readings were taken at one-minute intervals, and the average of the last two was recorded. Body weight and height were measured with participants wearing light clothing and no shoes, using calibrated scales and stadiometers. BMI was calculated as weight (kg)/height (m^2). All laboratory tests were performed in accredited clinical laboratories. Venous blood samples were obtained after an overnight fast of at least 8 h. Standardized enzymatic methods were used for glucose and lipid profile (total cholesterol, LDL-c, HDL-c, triglycerides). In the intervention group, follow-up interviews were conducted at six months to assess patient satisfaction with telemedicine and perceived level of engagement, using a 5-point Likert scale questionnaire.

2.4. Outcomes

The primary outcomes were the changes from baseline to six months in systolic blood pressure (SBP), diastolic blood pressure (DBP), fasting glucose, and lipid levels. Secondary outcomes included changes in BMI, the proportion of patients who completed laboratory or primary care follow-up, self-reported lifestyle changes (improved diet or physical activity), and patient satisfaction within both groups.

2.5. Statistical Analysis

All analyses were conducted using IBM SPSS Statistics, version 29.0 (IBM Corp, Armonk, NY, USA) and Microsoft Excel for Microsoft 365 (Microsoft Corp., Redmont, WA, USA). Continuous variables were reported as means and standard deviations, and categorical variables were summarized using frequencies and percentages. Between-group comparisons at baseline and at six months were assessed using independent-sample t-tests for continuous variables and chi-square tests for categorical variables. Paired t-tests were used for within-group comparisons over time. To assess whether the change from baseline to 6 months differed significantly between the two groups, we calculated a p-value for interaction ('p-value (difference in Δ from baseline)'), reflecting the difference in trajectories of the parameters across the 6-month period. To evaluate the magnitude of differences in changes between groups from baseline to six months, Cohen's d effect sizes were calculated. Effect sizes were interpreted as small (0.2), moderate (0.5), or large (0.8). Achievement of therapeutic goals was assessed by comparing the proportion of patients in each group who met predefined metabolic targets at the 3-month follow-up. A two-sided p-value < 0.05 was considered statistically significant for all tests.

3. Results

3.1. Study Population

Out of 300 initially enrolled participants, 150 were allocated to the telemedicine group and 150 to the standard care group. Of these, 286 completed the study: 144 in the telemedicine arm and 142 in the standard care arm. The baseline characteristics of the two groups were generally comparable (Table 1). The mean age in the telemedicine group was 60.35 ± 7.47 years, while in the standard care group it was slightly higher at 62.38 ± 9.26 years, a difference that reached statistical significance (p = 0.03). The gender distribution was similar between groups, with women representing 53.5% in the telemedicine group and 45.8% in the standard care group (p = 0.55). No statistically significant differences were noted at baseline for the main cardiovascular and behavioral risk parameters (all p-values > 0.05), except for DBP (p = 0.02). The prevalence of hypertension (71.52% vs. 70.42%), diabetes mellitus (38.20% vs. 40.84%), and dyslipidemia (64.58% vs. 66.19%) was comparable across groups, with no statistically significant differences (all p > 0.60). Likewise, the proportions of patients receiving antihypertensive therapy (68.75%

vs. 70.42%), lipid-lowering therapy (54.16% vs. 55.63%), and antidiabetic treatment (33.33% vs. 35.21%) were balanced between the telemedicine and standard care arms (all $p > 0.70$).

Table 1. Baseline clinical parameter comparison between telemedicine and standard care groups.

Parameter	Telemedicine (Baseline)	Standard Care (Baseline)	p-Value (Baseline)	Telemedicine (6 Months)	Standard Care (6 Months)	p-Value (6 Months)	p-Value (Difference in Δ from Baseline)
Age (years)	60.35 ± 7.47	62.38 ± 9.26	0.03	–	–	–	–
Gender (male/female, %)	46.5/53.5	54.2/45.8	0.55	–	–	–	–
Smoking	21.5%	23.2%	0.83	22.2%	23.2%	0.94	1
Physically active (%)	48.6%	50.7%	0.81	52.08%	54.92%	0.71	0.98
Healthy diet reported (%)	61.8%	58.4%	0.64	79.83%	63.38%	0.003	0.001
BMI (kg/m^2)	28.34 ± 3.66	27.57 ± 3.98	0.21	27.52 ± 4.35	27.15 ± 4.60	0.65	0.57
Systolic BP (mmHg)	141.23 ± 12.49	142.24 ± 13.75	0.27	136.02 ± 11.09	138.05 ± 12.72	0.16	0.08
Diastolic BP (mmHg)	88.99 ± 7.48	88.63 ± 6.48	0.02	85.06 ± 6.73	88.95 ± 6.59	<0.001	<0.001
Fasting glucose (mg/dL)	126.09 ± 20.59	125.31 ± 20.11	0.74	124.10 ± 19.01	114.38 ± 17.91	<0.001	<0.001
Total cholesterol (mg/dL)	161.76 ± 37.85	167.26 ± 41.99	0.24	149.71 ± 39.57	152.99 ± 45.01	0.27	0.20
HDL-c (mg/dL)	46.86 ± 7.71	46.18 ± 8.39	0.66	46.50 ± 7.80	48.48 ± 7.34	0.03	0.13
LDL-c (mg/dL)	136.03 ± 20.03	136.24 ± 20.96	0.21	118.02 ± 18.05	130.54 ± 19.66	<0.001	<0.001
Triglycerides (mg/dL)	166.41 ± 41.34	165.83 ± 38.12	0.90	162.46 ± 33.74	167.21 ± 41.27	0.28	0.07

Abbreviations: BMI—body mass index; BP—blood pressure; HDL—high-density lipoprotein; LDL—low-density lipoprotein. The last column indicates whether the change from baseline to 6 months differed significantly between telemedicine and standard care.

3.2. Six-Month Parameter Comparisons

At 6 months, improvements were noted across most parameters in both groups, but were significantly greater in the telemedicine group for DBP and LDL-cholesterol. However, improvements in BMI, SBP, triglycerides, and total cholesterol did not significantly differ between groups. Moreover, HDL-cholesterol and fasting glucose have shown important changes only in the standard care group. BMI decreased modestly in both groups, from 28.34 ± 3.66 to 27.52 ± 4.35 in the telemedicine group and from 27.57 ± 3.98 to 27.15 ± 4.60 in the standard care group. Although the reduction was slightly larger in the telemedicine group (mean change of −0.82 vs. −0.42), this difference was not statistically significant ($p = 0.57$). SBP declined by an average of 5.21 mmHg in the telemedicine group and 4.19 mmHg in the standard care group, with the between-group difference at 6 months approaching statistical significance ($p = 0.08$). DBP showed a statistically significant change in favor of the telemedicine group. The telemedicine group experienced a mean reduction of 3.93 mmHg, compared to a negligible change in the standard care group, where values slightly increased (88.63 ± 6.48 to 88.95 ± 6.59; $p < 0.001$). Fasting glucose improved more substantially in the standard care group, dropping from 125.31 ± 20.11 to 114.38 ± 17.91 mg/dL, with a mean reduction of 11.71 mg/dL. In contrast, the telemedicine group saw a smaller decrease from 126.09 ± 20.59 to 124.10 ± 19.01 mg/dL (−1.99 mg/dL), with a between-group p-value < 0.001. Total cholesterol decreased in both groups but to a slightly greater extent in the standard care arm (−14.27 mg/dL vs. −12.05 mg/dL in telemedicine). However, the *p*-value for between-group comparison at 6 months was not statistically significant ($p = 0.20$). HDL-cholesterol increased slightly in both groups (+3.01 mg/dL in telemedicine vs. +2.3 mg/dL in standard care), but the between-group difference did not reach statistical significance ($p = 0.13$). LDL-cholesterol saw a substantial reduction in the telemedicine group, from 136.03 ± 20.03 to 118.02 ± 18.05 mg/dL (−18.01 mg/dL), whereas in the standard care group, LDL dropped more modestly from 136.24 ± 20.96 to 130.54 ± 19.66 mg/dL (−5.70 mg/dL), with a *p*-value < 0.001. Triglycerides decreased by 3.95 mg/dL in the telemedicine group and slightly increased by 1.38 mg/dL in the standard care group ($p = 0.07$). Smoking status, dietary habits, and physical activity were obtained via self-reported questionnaires. These variables were not included among the primary clinical parameters due to potential reporting bias and subjectivity, in contrast to the objectively measured laboratory and anthropometric outcomes.

3.3. *Achievement of Therapeutic Goals*

Comparative analysis of cardiovascular and metabolic parameters revealed that patients in the telemedicine group were more likely to achieve therapeutic targets within the 3-month follow-up period than those receiving usual care.

For fasting glucose, however, the pattern was reversed: 66% of participants in the standard care group reached levels below 110 mg/dL by three months, compared to 43% in the telemedicine group ($p < 0.01$). In contrast, 71% of patients in the telemedicine group achieved systolic blood pressure values below 140 mmHg within the same timeframe, versus 66% in the standard care group. For diastolic blood pressure both groups showed almost the same achievement by the 3-month follow-up.

Lipid parameters followed a comparable pattern. In the telemedicine group, a greater proportion of patients reached total cholesterol levels below 200 mg/dL and LDL-cholesterol levels below 130 mg/dL by three months, compared to those in the usual care group. Triglyceride targets (<150 mg/dL) were also achieved more frequently among telemedicine patients during this period. These thresholds were used as pragmatic indicators of metabolic improvement, rather than guideline-based therapeutic targets that depend on individual cardiovascular risk categories.

3.4. *Effect Sizes*

The analysis of effect sizes for the change from baseline to six months between the telemedicine and standard care groups showed variable magnitudes across parameters, generally favoring the telemedicine group (Table 2, Figure 1).

Table 2. Cohen's d effect sizes for cardiometabolic measures.

Parameter	Cohen's *d* (95% CI)
BMI	0.08 (−0.14 to 0.31)
Systolic BP	−0.17 (−0.40 to 0.06)
Diastolic BP	−0.58 (−0.82 to −0.34)
Fasting Glucose	0.52 (0.29 to 0.76)
Total Cholesterol	−0.07 (−0.30 to 0.15)
HDL-c	−0.26 (−0.49 to −0.02)
LDL-c	−0.66 (−0.90 to −0.42)
Triglycerides	−0.12 (−0.35 to 0.10)

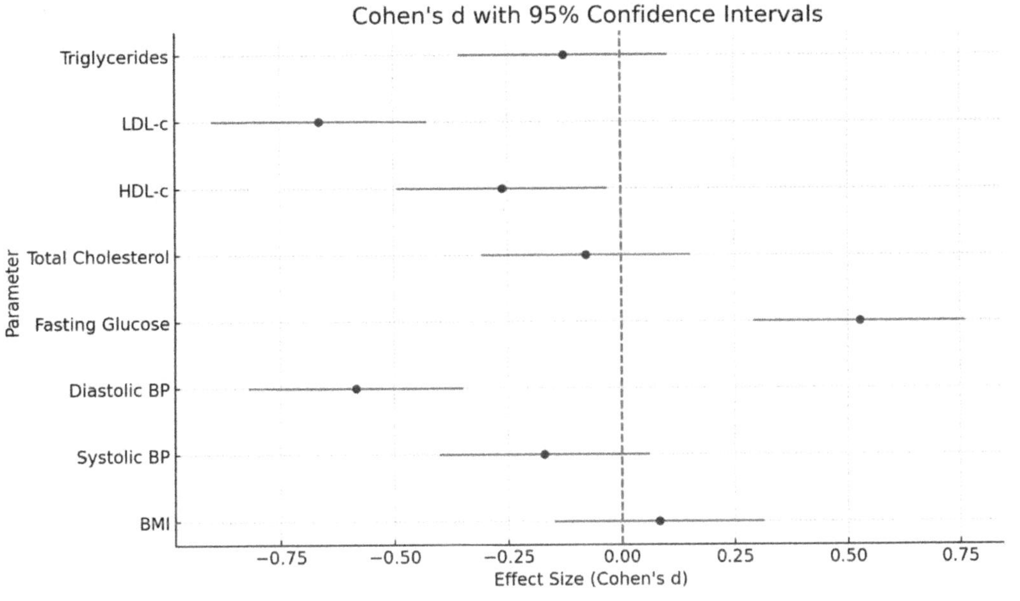

Figure 1. Forest plot of Cohen's d effect sizes for cardiometabolic parameters.

LDL-cholesterol exhibited the largest effect (Cohen's d = 0.68, 95% CI: 0.40 to 0.97), with a moderate-to-large benefit of telemedicine in reducing LDL levels compared to standard care. Fasting glucose also showed a moderate effect size (d = 0.53, 95% CI: 0.26 to 0.81). DBP demonstrated a similar moderate effect (d = 0.60, 95% CI: 0.32 to 0.88). In contrast, other parameters such as SBP, BMI, HDL-cholesterol, triglycerides, and total cholesterol had small or negligible effect sizes (d ranging from 0.01 to 0.27), and most of their confidence intervals crossed zero.

3.5. Satisfaction Results

Patient satisfaction was assessed at 6 months across several domains using a structured questionnaire with a 5-point Likert scale (1 = very unsatisfied, 5 = very satisfied) (Table 3). Results indicate a significantly higher satisfaction in the telemedicine group (mean = 4.2, SD = 0.6) compared to the usual care group (mean = 3.4, SD = 0.7). The difference was statistically significant ($p < 0.001$).

Table 3. Patient satisfaction ratings across groups.

Domain	Telemedicine (Mean ± SD)	Standard Care (Mean ± SD)	p-Value
Accessibility of care	4.6 ± 0.5	3.9 ± 0.7	<0.001
Time efficiency	4.5 ± 0.6	3.8 ± 0.8	<0.001
Communication with medical team	4.2 ± 0.7	4.4 ± 0.6	0.03
Comfort and convenience	4.7 ± 0.5	4.0 ± 0.8	<0.001
Understanding of treatment plan	4.4 ± 0.6	4.3 ± 0.6	0.21
Perceived effectiveness	4.5 ± 0.6	4.2 ± 0.7	0.006
Trust in care provider	4.3 ± 0.6	4.5 ± 0.5	0.03
Technical ease of use	4.5 ± 0.5	—	—

Patients reported greater accessibility (mean 4.6 ± 0.5 vs. 3.9 ± 0.7, $p < 0.001$), while time efficiency also favored telemedicine (4.5 ± 0.6 vs. 3.8 ± 0.8, $p < 0.001$). Similarly, comfort and convenience scored markedly higher in the telemedicine group (4.7 ± 0.5 vs. 4.0 ± 0.8, $p < 0.001$) However, some domains revealed a slight preference for in-person care. Usual care was rated higher in communication with the medical team (4.4 ± 0.6 vs. 4.2 ± 0.7, $p = 0.034$), and trust in the care provider (4.5 ± 0.5 vs. 4.3 ± 0.6, $p = 0.031$).

No statistically significant difference was observed in patients' understanding of their treatment plans (4.4 ± 0.6 vs. 4.3 ± 0.6, $p = 0.217$), indicating that both care models communicated therapeutic goals effectively. Additionally, technical ease of use received a high average score of 4.5 ± 0.5 in the telemedicine group. Overall, the results support the feasibility and acceptability of telemedicine in delivering patient-centered care, while also highlighting areas where in-person care may retain an advantage.

3.6. Dropout Rate and Adherence

The study completion rate was high in both arms, with only minor dropout due to relocation or loss of contact (14 patients in total, 6 patients from the telemedicine group and 8 patients from the standard care group). No adverse events related to the telemedicine intervention were reported.

Adherence to lifestyle recommendations was self-reported to be higher in the telemedicine group during interim follow-up calls. At 6 months, a greater proportion of participants in the telemedicine group reported adopting healthier behaviors, with some differences reaching statistical significance. Improved dietary habits were reported by 79.8% of individuals in the telemedicine group, compared to 63.4% in the usual care group ($p = 0.001$). Increased physical activity, defined as engaging in at least 150 min of moderate activity per week, was reported by 52.1% of telemedicine participants and 54.9% of those in the control group ($p = 0.71$), showing no significant difference. Smoking prevalence remained relatively stable in both groups, with 22.2% of participants in the telemedicine group and 23.2% in the usual care group reporting current smoking at 6 months ($p = 0.94$). However, only the change in reported dietary habits showed a statistically significant difference over time between groups (p for interaction = 0.001), while changes in smoking and physical activity did not (p for interaction = 1.0 and 0.98, respectively).

4. Discussion

This study was carried out in a socially disadvantaged urban community with little access to digital technology. We addressed the often-overlooked digital divide by deliberately avoiding reliance on smartphone apps and instead using simple telephone-based telemedicine. Through familiar and easily available communication techniques, participants who could have been excluded from traditional mHealth initiatives were actively engaged. Low-tech telemedicine models have the potential to overcome healthcare gaps in underprivileged communities, as seen by the better clinical outcomes and increased satisfaction seen in the telemedicine group. This strategy could be modified for wider application in comparable high-risk, resource-constrained contexts due to its simplicity and scalability.

The study demonstrates that a structured, low-tech telemedicine intervention significantly improved multiple cardiovascular risk factors in a socially vulnerable adult population over a six-month period. Compared with standard care, the telemedicine group achieved more pronounced reductions in systolic and diastolic blood pressure, LDL-cholesterol, and triglycerides, with moderate-to-large effect sizes.

Our results align with findings from previous randomized trials and meta-analyses evaluating digital health interventions in chronic disease management. Other telemedicine-based interventions demonstrated overall beneficial effects on key cardiovascular risk factors, yielding small but statistically significant reductions in HbA1c among patients with diabetes (g = −0.432, $p < 0.001$), moderate reductions in systolic blood pressure (g = −0.775, $p < 0.001$), small reductions in diastolic blood pressure (g = −0.447, $p < 0.001$), and moderate reductions in body weight among overweight individuals (g = −0.628, $p < 0.001$) [20]. Pogosova et al. showed that the intervention group showed significantly greater reductions in weight, waist circumference, BMI, diastolic blood pressure, total and LDL-cholesterol, and body fat mass compared to controls. Lean mass was higher, and both anxiety and depression scores were significantly lower in the intervention group [21]. A meta-analysis by Omboni et al. reported that telemonitoring and teleconsultations significantly reduced both systolic and diastolic blood pressure, with average reductions of 4.7 mmHg and 2.5 mmHg, respectively, changes comparable to our observed improvements in SBP and DBP [22]. Another study exhibited no significant changes in BMI, blood pressure (both systolic and diastolic), or lipid profiles, including total cholesterol, HDL-c, LDL-c, and triglycerides, in either hospital-based or home-based cardiac rehabilitation programs. These parameters remained largely stable from baseline to post-intervention, with p-values > 0.05 for both within-group and between-group comparisons [23]. A follow-up study of an mHealth intervention involving motivational calls and SMS found no significant impact on blood pressure after 5 years, though a trend toward reduced hypertension risk was noted. However, meaningful reductions in body weight (−5.42 kg) and BMI (−2.56 kg/m^2) were observed, especially among those who received at least half of the scheduled calls. Unlike our study, these changes in BMI and weight became evident due to the longer follow-up period of 5 years [24]. Our observed reductions in fasting glucose levels are different from the findings of the TELESAGE study, where patients receiving remote diabetes management achieved better glycemic control and treatment adherence than those in usual care [25]. Similarly, a telemedicine-supported lifestyle intervention led to a modest but statistically significant reduction in HbA1c at 6 months compared to usual care (−0.13%, 95% CI −0.25 to −0.01; $p = 0.04$). However, this effect was not maintained at 12 months once individualized feedback and health literacy support were discontinued [26].

Compared to high-tech platforms relying on apps or wearables, our study used only monthly phone calls conducted by nurses or general practitioners. This approach not only achieved measurable health improvements, but did so among patients in a socially deprived urban area, a population often overlooked in digital health research. Similar low-tech interventions have shown efficacy in India, sub-Saharan Africa, and Latin America, where phone-based follow-up improved blood pressure and glycemic outcomes in hypertensive or diabetic patients [27–29]. However, few of these studies have included a broad set of cardiometabolic outcomes or stratified by socioeconomic vulnerability.

Notably, the improvements in LDL-cholesterol in our telemedicine group, although modest in magnitude, suggest favorable lipid modulation through lifestyle and medication adherence. In contrast to our findings, some previous studies have reported minimal effects of telemedicine on lipid profiles. For example, a trial by Margolis et al. observed no significant differences in LDL-c at 6 months, suggesting that results may vary depending on patient engagement, baseline risk, and the intensity of the intervention. A meta-analysis of 54 studies found that telemedicine interventions modestly reduced blood pressure and HbA1c levels, while effects on lipid profiles and BMI were inconsistent and clinically insignificant [30]. Our more pronounced improvement in triglycerides (−3.95 mg/dL) and total cholesterol (−12.05 mg/dL) may reflect the combined effect of dietary counseling, physical activity encouragement, and regular feedback via phone.

In a trial by Garcia et al., lipid levels improved significantly after the one-year follow-up. LDL-c decreased from 108.4 ± 40.6 to 48.7 ± 14.4 mg/dL. The proportions of patients achieving LDL-c <100, <70, and <55 mg/dL increased from 44.5%, 17.6%, and 7.2% at baseline to 100%, 95.4%, and 81.5% at study end [31].

The speed of achieving clinical targets was also superior in the telemedicine group. These findings suggest that structured support may facilitate attainment of blood pressure and lipid targets through improved adherence and monitoring. However, this effect did not extend to glycemic control, where patients in the standard care group achieved fasting glucose targets more frequently. Possible explanations include differences in medication use, variability in self-monitoring, and the relatively short follow-up period. A study from the United States evaluated changes in HbA1c among patients with poorly controlled type 2 diabetes (HbA1c > 8%) enrolled in a pharmacy-driven telehealth program. The analysis compared glycemic outcomes between two time periods: pre-COVID-19 and during COVID-19. After 3 months, the COVID-19 group showed a mean HbA1c reduction of 2.0%, compared to 1.3% in the pre-COVID group ($p = 0.305$); at 6 months, the reductions were 2.2% vs. 1.2%, respectively ($p = 0.249$) [32]. Another study reported after just three months of intervention that patients using the cellular phone-based telemedicine system showed a significantly greater reduction in HbA1c levels compared to those using standard self-monitoring. While the control group experienced a modest and non-significant decrease of 0.20%, the telemedicine group achieved a meaningful drop of 0.61% ($p < 0.001$), with even greater improvement (0.81%) among those starting with HbA1c $\geq$ 8% [33].

Patient satisfaction was another key strength of the telemedicine arm. Higher scores in accessibility, convenience, and perceived effectiveness are consistent with large-scale surveys conducted during the COVID-19 pandemic, where telemedicine was broadly endorsed for chronic disease follow-up [34]. Importantly, trust and provider communication were slightly favored in the usual care group, echoing the concern that some aspects of rapport may be diluted in remote settings—a limitation that should be addressed in future hybrid models of care. However, another study showed that among 1026 respondents, 71% preferred in-person visits and 29% preferred telemedicine, exposing a significant difference ($p < 0.0001$). Overall, telemedicine was seen as convenient and accessible, especially for chronic or mobility-limited patients, but in-person care remained the preferred choice for most [35]. In another research work involving large-sized sample groups, patient satisfaction with telemedicine was similar to in-person visits, with early lower scores for clinical communication improving over time. Telemedicine was rated higher for appointment access early in the pandemic, but in-person visits were slightly preferred for doctor interaction and care explanations [36].

Despite these promising outcomes, several limitations merit consideration. First, although random allocation was used, full blinding was not possible due to the nature of the intervention, which could introduce bias in patient-reported outcomes. Second, self-reported lifestyle improvements may overestimate behavioral change. Third, the duration of follow-up (6 months) is relatively short, and long-term sustainability of benefits remains uncertain.

In summary, this study provides compelling evidence that structured, low-tech telemedicine can effectively reduce cardiovascular risk factors in disadvantaged populations. The observed improvements, comparable to or exceeding those seen in more technologically complex interventions, show the importance of inclusivity and simplicity in digital health strategies. Our findings support broader implementation of basic telemedicine tools, not as replacements for in-person care, but as scalable complements that can help bridge health equity gaps in cardiovascular prevention.

5. Conclusions

This study suggests that a simple, low-cost telemedicine intervention may help improve selected cardiovascular and metabolic outcomes in a socially deprived urban population. Patients receiving structured phone-based support achieved better control of diastolic blood pressure and LDL-cholesterol and were more likely to reach treatment targets within three months. However, patients from the standard care group reached better fasting glucose levels. The intervention was well accepted, with high satisfaction and good adherence. Taken together, these findings support the feasibility and acceptability of low-tech telemedicine as a potentially scalable strategy to improve care in underserved settings. Nonetheless, the results should be interpreted with caution due to the relatively small sample size, short follow-up period, and single-center design, and confirmation in larger, multicenter trials is warranted.

Author Contributions: Conceptualization, C.M.L.; methodology, A.G.; validation, E.R.S.; formal analysis, E.R.S.; investigation, A.G., O.A.H.; data curation, E.R.S.; writing—original draft preparation A.G., C.M.L., O.A.H.; writing—review and editing, C.M.P., A.L.M.; visualization, A.G.; supervision, A.L.M., C.M.P. All authors have read and agreed to the published version of the manuscript.

Funding: We would like to acknowledge "Victor Babes" University of Medicine and Pharmacy Timisoara for their support in covering the costs of publication for this research paper.

Institutional Review Board Statement: This study was conducted in accordance with the Declaration of Helsinki, and approved by the Research Ethics Committee of Victor Babes University of Medicine and Pharmacy Timisoara (approval no 77/08.01.2024).

Informed Consent Statement: Informed consent was obtained from all subjects involved in the study. Written informed consent has been obtained from the patients to publish this paper.

Data Availability Statement: The data presented in this study are available on request from the corresponding author due to privacy and ethical restrictions.

Conflicts of Interest: The authors declare no conflicts of interest.

Abbreviations

The following abbreviations are used in this manuscript:

BMI	body mass index
COVID-19	coronavirus disease 2019
CVD	cardiovascular disease
DBP	diastolic blood pressure
HDL	high-density lipoprotein
LDL	low-density lipoprotein
SBP	systolic blood pressure

References

1. Dunbar, S.B.; Khavjou, O.A.; Bakas, T.; Hunt, G.; Kirch, R.A.; Leib, A.R.; Morrison, R.S.; Poehler, D.C.; Roger, V.L.; Whitsel, L.P. Projected Costs of Informal Caregiving for Cardiovascular Disease: 2015 to 2035: A Policy Statement from the American Heart Association. *Circulation* **2018**, *137*, E558–E577. [CrossRef]
2. Olvera Lopez, E.; Ballard, B.D.; Jan, A. Cardiovascular Disease. In *StatPearls*; StatPearls Publishing: Treasure Island, FL, USA, 2025.
3. Schultz, W.M.; Kelli, H.M.; Lisko, J.C.; Varghese, T.; Shen, J.; Sandesara, P.; Quyyumi, A.A.; Taylor, H.A.; Gulati, M.; Harold, J.G.; et al. Socioeconomic Status and Cardiovascular Outcomes: Challenges and Interventions. *Circulation* **2018**, *137*, 2166–2178. [CrossRef]
4. Cacciatore, S.; Mao, S.; Nuñez, M.V.; Massaro, C.; Spadafora, L.; Bernardi, M.; Perone, F.; Sabouret, P.; Biondi-Zoccai, G.; Banach, M.; et al. Urban Health Inequities and Healthy Longevity: Traditional and Emerging Risk Factors across the Cities and Policy Implications. *Aging Clin. Exp. Res.* **2025**, *37*, 143. [CrossRef]
5. Wolfe, M.K.; McDonald, N.C.; Holmes, G.M. Transportation Barriers to Health Care in the United States: Findings from the National Health Interview Survey, 1997–2017. *Am. J. Public Health* **2020**, *110*, 815–822. [CrossRef]
6. Acquah, I.; Hagan, K.; Javed, Z.; Taha, M.B.; Valero-Elizondo, J.; Nwana, N.; Yahya, T.; Sharma, G.; Gulati, M.; Hammoud, A.; et al. Social Determinants of Cardiovascular Risk, Subclinical Cardiovascular Disease, and Cardiovascular Events. *J. Am. Heart Assoc.* **2023**, *12*, e025581. [CrossRef]

7. Bazoukis, G.; Loscalzo, J.; Hall, J.L.; Bollepalli, S.C.; Singh, J.P.; Armoundas, A.A. Impact of Social Determinants of Health on Cardiovascular Disease. *J. Am. Heart Assoc.* **2025**, *14*, e039031. [CrossRef]
8. Bays, H.E.; Taub, P.R.; Epstein, E.; Michos, E.D.; Ferraro, R.A.; Bailey, A.L.; Kelli, H.M.; Ferdinand, K.C.; Echols, M.R.; Weintraub, H.; et al. Ten Things to Know about Ten Cardiovascular Disease Risk Factors. *Am. J. Prev. Cardiol.* **2021**, *5*, 100149. [CrossRef] [PubMed]
9. US Preventive Services Task Force; Curry, S.J.; Krist, A.H.; Owens, D.K.; Barry, M.J.; Caughey, A.B.; Davidson, K.W.; Doubeni, C.A.; Epling, J.W.; Kemper, A.R.; et al. Risk Assessment for Cardiovascular Disease with Nontraditional Risk Factors: US Preventive Services Task Force Recommendation Statement. *JAMA* **2018**, *320*, 272. [CrossRef]
10. Benjamin, E.J.; Virani, S.S.; Callaway, C.W.; Chamberlain, A.M.; Chang, A.R.; Cheng, S.; Chiuve, S.E.; Cushman, M.; Delling, F.N.; Deo, R.; et al. Heart Disease and Stroke Statistics—2018 Update: A Report From the American Heart Association. *Circulation* **2018**, *137*, e67–e492. [CrossRef] [PubMed]
11. Lavie, C.J.; Ozemek, C.; Carbone, S.; Katzmarzyk, P.T.; Blair, S.N. Sedentary Behavior, Exercise, and Cardiovascular Health. *Circ. Res.* **2019**, *124*, 799–815. [CrossRef] [PubMed]
12. Adhikary, D.; Barman, S.; Ranjan, R.; Stone, H. A Systematic Review of Major Cardiovascular Risk Factors: A Growing Global Health Concern. *Cureus* **2022**, *14*, e30119. [CrossRef]
13. Capewell, S.; Ford, E.S.; Croft, J.B.; Critchley, J.A.; Greenlund, K.J.; Labarthe, D.R. Cardiovascular Risk Factor Trends and Options for Reducing Future Coronary Heart Disease Mortality in the United States of America. *Bull. World Health Organ.* **2010**, *88*, 120–130. [CrossRef]
14. Chow, C.K.; Jolly, S.; Rao-Melacini, P.; Fox, K.A.A.; Anand, S.S.; Yusuf, S. Association of Diet, Exercise, and Smoking Modification with Risk of Early Cardiovascular Events After Acute Coronary Syndromes. *Circulation* **2010**, *121*, 750–758. [CrossRef] [PubMed]
15. Roth, G.A.; Huffman, M.D.; Moran, A.E.; Feigin, V.; Mensah, G.A.; Naghavi, M.; Murray, C.J.L. Global and Regional Patterns in Cardiovascular Mortality From 1990 to 2013. *Circulation* **2015**, *132*, 1667–1678. [CrossRef] [PubMed]
16. Mechanic, O.J.; Persaud, Y.; Kimball, A.B. Telehealth Systems. In *StatPearls*; StatPearls Publishing: Treasure Island, FL, USA, 2025.
17. Chandwani, R.; De, R.; Dwivedi, Y.K. Telemedicine for Low Resource Settings: Exploring the Generative Mechanisms. *Technol. Forecast. Soc. Change* **2018**, *127*, 177–187. [CrossRef]
18. Haleem, A.; Javaid, M.; Singh, R.P.; Suman, R. Telemedicine for Healthcare: Capabilities, Features, Barriers, and Applications. *Sens. Int.* **2021**, *2*, 100117. [CrossRef]
19. Wootton, R.; Bonnardot, L. Telemedicine in Low-Resource Settings. *Front. Public Health* **2015**, *3*, 3. [CrossRef]
20. Jaén-Extremera, J.; Afanador-Restrepo, D.F.; Rivas-Campo, Y.; Gómez-Rodas, A.; Aibar-Almazán, A.; Hita-Contreras, F.; Carcelén-Fraile, M.D.C.; Castellote-Caballero, Y.; Ortiz-Quesada, R. Effectiveness of Telemedicine for Reducing Cardiovascular Risk: A Systematic Review and Meta-Analysis. *J. Clin. Med.* **2023**, *12*, 841. [CrossRef]
21. Pogosova, N.; Yufereva, Y.; Sokolova, O.; Yusubova, A.; Suvorov, A.; Saner, H. Telemedicine Intervention to Improve Long-Term Risk Factor Control and Body Composition in Persons with High Cardiovascular Risk: Results from a Randomized Trial: Telehealth Strategies May Offer an Advantage over Standard Institutional Based Interventions for Improvement of Cardiovascular Risk in High-Risk Patients Long-Term. *Glob. Heart* **2021**, *16*, 21. [CrossRef] [PubMed]
22. Omboni, S.; Gazzola, T.; Carabelli, G.; Parati, G. Clinical Usefulness and Cost Effectiveness of Home Blood Pressure Telemonitoring: Meta-Analysis of Randomized Controlled Studies. *J. Hypertens.* **2013**, *31*, 455–468. [CrossRef]
23. Bravo-Escobar, R.; González-Represas, A.; Gómez-González, A.M.; Montiel-Trujillo, A.; Aguilar-Jimenez, R.; Carrasco-Ruíz, R.; Salinas-Sánchez, P. Effectiveness and Safety of a Home-Based Cardiac Rehabilitation Programme of Mixed Surveillance in Patients with Ischemic Heart Disease at Moderate Cardiovascular Risk: A Randomised, Controlled Clinical Trial. *BMC Cardiovasc. Disord.* **2017**, *17*, 66. [CrossRef]
24. Bernabe-Ortiz, A.; Pauschardt, J.; Diez-Canseco, F.; Miranda, J.J. Sustainability of mHealth Effects on Cardiometabolic Risk Factors: Five-Year Results of a Randomized Clinical Trial. *J. Med. Internet Res.* **2020**, *22*, e14595. [CrossRef]
25. Zhao, Y.; Sun, H.; Zhang, W.; Xi, Y.; Shi, X.; Yang, Y.; Lu, J.; Zhang, M.; Sun, L.; Hu, D. Elevated Triglyceride–Glucose Index Predicts Risk of Incident Ischaemic Stroke: The Rural Chinese Cohort Study. *Diabetes Metab.* **2021**, *47*, 101246. [CrossRef]
26. Mueller, S.; Dinges, S.M.T.; Gass, F.; Fegers-Wustrow, I.; Treitschke, J.; von Korn, P.; Boscheri, A.; Krotz, J.; Freigang, F.; Dubois, C.; et al. Telemedicine-Supported Lifestyle Intervention for Glycemic Control in Patients with CHD and T2DM: Multicenter, Randomized Controlled Trial. *Nat. Med.* **2025**, *31*, 1203–1213. [CrossRef]
27. Varghese, C.; Nongkynrih, B.; Onakpoya, I.; McCall, M.; Barkley, S.; Collins, T.E. Better Health and Wellbeing for Billion More People: Integrating Non-Communicable Diseases in Primary Care. *BMJ* **2019**, *364*, l327. [CrossRef]
28. Shetty, A.S.; Chamukuttan, S.; Nanditha, A.; Raj, R.K.C.; Ramachandran, A. Reinforcement of Adherence to Prescription Recommendations in Asian Indian Diabetes Patients Using Short Message Service (SMS)—A Pilot Study. *J. Assoc. Physicians India* **2011**, *59*, 711–714.

29. Casas, L.A.; Alarcón, J.; Urbano, A.; Peña-Zárate, E.E.; Sangiovanni, S.; Libreros-Peña, L.; Escobar, M.F. Telemedicine for the Management of Diabetic Patients in a High-Complexity Latin American Hospital. *BMC Health Serv. Res.* **2023**, *23*, 314. [CrossRef] [PubMed]
30. Mihevc, M.; Virtič Potočnik, T.; Zavrnik, Č.; Klemenc-Ketiš, Z.; Poplas Susič, A.; Petek Šter, M. Managing Cardiovascular Risk Factors with Telemedicine in Primary Care: A Systematic Review and Meta-Analysis of Patients with Arterial Hypertension and Type 2 Diabetes. *Chronic Illn.* **2025**, *21*, 3–24. [CrossRef] [PubMed]
31. García, R.V.; García, J.E.P.; Navas, W.D.; Salmerón, D.M.; Mateos, D.B. Impact of a Virtual Lipid Clinic on Lipid-Lowering Therapy, LDL Cholesterol Levels, and Outcomes in Patients with Acute Coronary Syndrome. *J. Clin. Lipidol.* **2022**, *16*, 635–642. [CrossRef]
32. Woodhouse, A.G.; Orvin, C.; Rich, C.; Crosby, J.; Keedy, C.A. Diabetes outcomes before and during telehealth advancements surrounding COVID-19. *J. Am. Pharm. Assoc.* **2022**, *62*, 214–217. [CrossRef]
33. Lee, Y.J.; Jeong, M.H.; Kim, J.H.; Park, J.; Kim, H.Y.; A Seo, J.; Kim, S.G.; Kim, N.H.; Choi, K.M.; Baik, S.H.; et al. Cellular phone-based telemedicine system improves blood glucose control in type 2 diabetes patients with inadequate glycemic control. *Korean Diabetes J.* **2009**, *33*, 232–240. [CrossRef]
34. Fisk, M.; Livingstone, A.; Pit, S.W. Telehealth in the Context of COVID-19: Changing Perspectives in Australia, the United Kingdom, and the United States. *J. Med. Internet Res.* **2020**, *22*, e19264. [CrossRef]
35. Moulaei, K.; Sheikhtaheri, A.; Fatehi, F.; Shanbehzadeh, M.; Bahaadinbeigy, K. Patients' Perspectives and Preferences toward Telemedicine versus in-Person Visits: A Mixed-Methods Study on 1226 Patients. *BMC Med. Inform. Decis. Mak.* **2023**, *23*, 261. [CrossRef] [PubMed]
36. Kee, D.; Verma, H.; Tepper, D.L.; Hasegawa, D.; Burger, A.P.; Weissman, M.A. Patient Satisfaction with Telemedicine Among Vulnerable Populations in an Urban Ambulatory Setting. *Mayo Clin. Proc. Digit. Health* **2024**, *2*, 8–17. [CrossRef] [PubMed]

healthcare

MDPI

Review

Implementation of Telehealth Among Older People: A Challenge and Opportunity for Latin America and the Caribbean—A Literature Review

Rafael Pizarro-Mena [1,2,*,†], Elena S. Rotarou [2,3,†], Hendrik Adrián Baracaldo-Campo [4,†], Samuel Duran-Aguero [1,†], Solange Parra-Soto [5], Felipe Retamal-Walter [6], Patrick Alexander Wachholz [7,†], Silvia Maranzano [8,†], Victoria Tirro [9,†], Sara Aguilar-Navarro [10], Isabel Barrientos-Calvo [11,†], Valeria Carpio-Arias [12,†], Clarissa Botello [13,†], María Fernanda López [14,†], Roni Mukamal [15], Alessandra Tieppo [16], Igor Cigarroa [17,18,†], Fausto Medola [19,†] and Gloria Riveros-Basoalto [20]

[1] Facultad de Ciencias de la Rehabilitación y Calidad de Vida, Universidad San Sebastián, Sede Los Leones, Santiago 7500000, Chile; samuel.duran@uss.cl
[2] Núcleo Milenio Estudios en Discapacidad y Ciudadanía—DISCA (NCS2022_039), Santiago 7500000, Chile; elena.rotarou@uss.cl
[3] Facultad de Medicina, Universidad San Sebastián, Sede Los Leones, Santiago 7500000, Chile
[4] Facultad de Ciencias de la Salud, Universidad Autónoma de Bucaramanga—UNAB, Floridablanca 680003, Colombia; hbaracaldo@unab.edu.co
[5] Departamento de Nutrición y Salud Pública, Facultad Ciencias de la Salud y de los Alimentos, Universidad del Bio-Bio, Chillán 3780000, Chile; sparra@ubiobio.cl
[6] School of Health and Rehabilitation Sciences, The University of Queensland, Brisbane QLD 4072, Australia; f.retamalwalter@uq.edu.au
[7] Faculdade de Medicina de Botucatu, Universidade Estadual Paulista—UNESP, São Paulo 18618-687, CEP, Brazil; patrick.wachholz@unesp.br
[8] Departamento de Educación Física, Universidad Nacional de Luján, Delegación San Fernando, Buenos Aires 164, Argentina; sprivada@unlu.edu.ar
[9] Departamento de Ciencias del Comportamiento, Escuela de Psicología, Facultad de Ciencias, Universidad Metropolitana, Estado Miranda 76819, Venezuela; vtirro@unimet.edu.ve
[10] Instituto Nacional de Ciencias Médicas y Nutrición Salvador Zubirán, Ciudad de Mexico 14000, Mexico; sgan30@hotmail.com
[11] Unidad de Investigación Hospital Nacional de Geriatría y Gerontología, Universidad de Costa Rica, San José 11501-2060, Costa Rica; isacrisba80@gmail.com
[12] Grupo de Investigación en Alimentación y Nutrición (GIANH), Escuela Superior Politécnica del Chimborazo, Riobamba 060104, Ecuador; tannia.carpio@espoch.edu.ec
[13] Departamento de Medicina, Facultad de Medicina, Universidad Nacional de Panama, Ciudad de Panama 0816-01552, Panama; clarissabotello24@gmail.com
[14] Facultad de Psicología y Ciencias Sociales, Universidad Flores, Buenos Aires C1406EEE, Argentina; licmflopez@gmail.com
[15] Servicio de Geriatria e Gerontologia, Departamento de Clínica Médica da Faculdade de Medicina, Universidade Federal do Espírito Santo, Vitória 29055-420, ES, Brazil; ronimukamal@yahoo.com.br
[16] Universidade Anhembi Morumbi, São Paulo 03164-000, CEP, Brazil; atieppo@uol.com.br
[17] Escuela de Kinesiología, Facultad de Ciencias de la Salud, Universidad Católica Silva Henriquez, Santiago 7500000, Chile; icigarroac@ucsh.cl
[18] Facultad de Ciencias de la Salud, Universidad Arturo Prat, Victoria 4720000, Chile
[19] Departamento de Design, Faculdade de Arquitetura, Artes, Comunicação e Design (FAAC), Universidade Estadual Paulista "Júlio de Mesquita Filho"—UNESP, Bauru 17033-360, CEP, Brazil; fausto.medola@unesp.br
[20] Bibliotecóloga Referencista, Vicerrectoría Académica, Universidad San Sebastián, Santiago 7500000, Chile; gloria.riveros@uss.cl
* Correspondence: rafael.pizarro@uss.cl; Tel.: +56-992331171
† The authors also belong to Red Interuniversitaria de Envejecimiento Saludable de Latinoamérica y Caribe (RIES-LAC).

Abstract: Although the COVID-19 pandemic negatively affected the health and quality of life of older people (OP), it provided an opportunity for the implementation of telehealth in the areas of Gerontology and Geriatrics, globally and in the countries of Latin America and the Caribbean, which enabled the continuity of healthcare interventions. Therefore, this literature review aimed to (a) conceptualize telehealth in OP through the lens of Gerontology and Geriatrics; (b) analyze the implementation, facilitators, and barriers of telehealth for OP during the COVID-19 pandemic at both global and Latin American and Caribbean regional levels; (c) identify lessons learned and considerations for improving implementation and reducing barriers to telehealth for OP; and (d) discuss challenges related to the integration of telehealth for OP in the region. The databases consulted were PubMed, Scopus, and Scielo; scientific articles in both English and Spanish were considered, including research conducted globally and in Latin American and Caribbean countries that contributed to the objectives of the literature review; the search was conducted from the year 2020 onwards. In addition, government documents and non-governmental technical guidelines from countries in the region were included, whether they focused specifically on older populations or the general population; the search was not limited to a specific time period. Initially, in our search strategy, 1631 scientific articles and 20 governmental and non-governmental documents were identified for the literature review. After eliminating duplicate and applying the inclusion and exclusion criteria, 84 documents were selected for the literature review (46 analyzed the implementation, barriers, and facilitators of telehealth during the COVID-19 pandemic). This literature review presents a conceptual analysis of the implementation and facilitators of, as well as barriers to, telehealth among OP during the COVID-19 pandemic from the perspective of healthcare providers and OP themselves. The paper synthesizes a number of international and Latin American experiences and proposes several recommendations for the implementation of telehealth for OP in the Latin American and Caribbean region. Despite the ongoing challenges regarding telehealth research and training, this review describes telehealth for OP as an intervention approach that improves the provision of holistic care, favoring OP autonomy, functionality, and overall quality of life. This review also proposes telehealth as a regular intervention approach to clinical practice in Gerontology and Geriatrics in the region. Collaborative endeavors are needed to further regulate and promote public policy on telehealth, telemedicine and telerehabilitation for OP.

Keywords: older people; telehealth; telegerontology; telegeriatrics; Latin America; COVID-19

1. Introduction

Worldwide, the population aged 60 and over will increase from 900 million to more than 1.4 billion people between 2015 and 2030. This represents a 64% increase in just 15 years, making it the fastest-growing age group [1]. Although the situation varies significantly across regions, the Latin America and the Caribbean region is on the verge of an unprecedented shift in its history, with projections indicating an increase from 76 million older persons (OP) today to 147 million by 2037 [1]. Although the region as a whole has entered a stage of accelerated aging, in half of the countries (some of which are among the least developed), the process is still incipient and moderate, with the most significant changes expected to occur between now and 2030 [1].

Although the Coronavirus SARS-CoV-2 (COVID-19) pandemic was a global public health emergency between 2020 and 2023, its health consequences remain a priority for the region [2]. Quarantines, isolation measures, and mobility restrictions were public health strategies implemented during the pandemic. Among OP, longer quarantine periods were observed, overlooking their heterogeneity, health and illness history, life trajectories, and the diverse ways in which people age. This approach disregarded their role as agents of change and full-rights citizens [3], shifting from physical distancing to a form of social exclusion. This distancing had a negative impact on the overall health of OP, defined as a geriatric emergency [3] associated with physical inactivity [4,5], increased susceptibility to chronic diseases and geriatric syndromes [3], and related mental health issues [6,7].

Specifically, various bio-psycho-social challenges were identified among OP during the COVID-19 pandemic. For example, low levels of physical activity (PA) were associated with immunosenescence, increased risk of chronic diseases, frailty, cognitive decline, and mortality [8]; a decrease in muscle mass, muscle strength, and the number of steps per day [4]; sleep problems, insomnia, and daytime sleepiness [3,9]; worsening of pre-existing conditions, such as diabetes, hypertension, angina pectoris, cardiac events, and psychiatric conditions [10]. Poor appetite control was also described (including possible excessive consumption of ultra-processed foods, risk of malnutrition, weight gain or loss), along with reduced exposure to sunlight and vitamin D [9]. The loss of daily routines and the reduction in physical and social contact led to a sense of isolation from the rest of the world, boredom, frustration, uncertainty about the future, and fear of infection [11,12], resulting in stress, distress, and agitation. The situation was further aggravated by the inability to carry out Activities of Daily Living (ADLs) [11,12]. This was accompanied by limited participation in community activities, formal physical activity, and adherence to medical regimens, and public health recommendations [13]. Additionally, the discontinuation of participation in cognitive stimulation activities, workshops, social gatherings, group therapies, and/or volunteer work contributed to increased cognitive decline and depressive symptoms, resulting in reduced social contact and heightened feelings of loneliness [3]. A complex and bidirectional relationship was even described between mental health problems and social disconnection [10], leading to the emergence of social frailty among OP [13]. All these bio-psycho-social challenges affected the resilience that OP had developed throughout their aging process prior to the pandemic.

This global health situation also affected the implementation and continuity of government-led programs for OP, due to lack of access [14]. Likewise, it disrupted in-person research with OP, forcing projects to either suspend operations or implement remote, contactless methods [15,16]. In this context, and as alternatives to help OP maintain their ADLs, the World Health Organization (WHO) encouraged continued social engagement through virtual means and regular physical activity at home [17]. In doing so, the pandemic accelerated innovation in telecommunications and normalized the use of previously underutilized services and products, such as telehealth [15,18], understood as, a modality that utilizes Information and Communication Technologies (ICTs) to pro-vide health services, medical care, and information regardless of distance [19]. This led to an earlier-than-expected implementation of telehealth globally, across various contexts, programs, and services, and for different health conditions, chronic diseases, and geriatric syndromes [20–32]. In turn, telehealth maintained and/or improved health outcomes by increasing access to care for OP with limited resources, those living in remote geographic areas, individuals with cognitive and/or physical disabilities, or with limited access to transportation; it also enhanced follow-up and quality of care, reduced costs, and facilitated the collection of collateral information during the pandemic [20,33–38]. Additionally, it led to the establishment of new models of care [39]. In this context, at the beginning of the pandemic, a scoping review describing the implementation of telehealth for OP, showed a greater experience of telehealth in high-income countries in the Northern Hemisphere. It also indicated a lack of consistency in the concepts associated with telehealth for OP [40], that is, for the field of action of Gerontology and Geriatrics.

Despite a growing body of literature describing the implementation of telehealth in the health systems of some Latin American countries, some countries stand out as having pushed more than others to adopt telemedicine in their health systems, as Argentina, Brazil,

Chile, Colombia and Mexico [41], as well as some of the main facilitators and barriers to telehealth in the region [42], these studies have not focused specifically on OP. Therefore, this literature review aimed to (a) conceptualize telehealth in OP through the lens of Gerontology and Geriatrics; (b) analyze the implementation, facilitators, and barriers of telehealth for OP during the COVID-19 pandemic at both global and Latin American and Caribbean regional levels; (c) identify lessons learned and considerations for improving implementation and reducing barriers to telehealth for OP; and (d) discuss challenges related to the integration of telehealth for OP in the region.

2. Materials and Methods

Search Strategy

A literature review was chosen as the methodological approach, as it allows for a broader and more diverse identification of the available literature, as well as a more flexible and context-sensitive exploration [43]. To achieve the objectives of this literature review [43], a bibliographic search was conducted to answer the question: How was telehealth implemented for older people during the COVID-19 pandemic at the global level and in Latin America and the Caribbean region? The keywords and search terms (MeSH/DeCS), in both English and Spanish, were as follows: older adult, older person, older people, old age, aging, aged, elderly, telehealth, telemedicine, telerehabilitation, Covid, Pandemic, SARS-CoV-2, Coronavirus, implement, facilitator, and barrier. The search strategy is described in Appendix A, Table A1.

The databases consulted were PubMed, Scopus, and Scielo. Scientific articles in both English and Spanish were considered, including research conducted globally and in Latin American and Caribbean countries that contributed to the objectives of the literature review. The search was conducted from the year 2020 onwards.

In addition, government documents and non-governmental technical guidelines from countries in the region were included, whether they focused specifically on older populations or the general population. To do this, the research team, made up of members from different countries (Mexico, Costa Rica, Panama, Venezuela, Colombia, Brazil, Ecuador, Argentina, and Chile), reviewed the websites of the health ministries, professional associations, and other non-governmental organizations from countries in the region. The documents included addressed the implementation of telehealth in the countries of the region. The search was not limited to a specific time period.

Conference abstracts, scientific conference reports, dissertations, research reports, theses, case studies, protocols, letters to the editor, and editorials were excluded. The inclusion and exclusion criteria are described in Appendix A, Table A2.

The literature review process followed the steps outlined in references [44,45], depending on the type of document. In the case of scientific articles, the steps included were: search strategy, article identification, removal of duplicates, title and abstract screening, full-text review, selection, data compilation into tables, analysis, interpretation of results and discussion, and referencing. For governmental and non-governmental documents, the steps were: search, identification, full-text review focused on the implementation of telehealth for both OP and the general population in countries of the region, selection, data compilation into tables, analysis, interpretation of results and discussion, and referencing. A reference librarian, part of the research team, contributed to the various stages of the literature review process. This professional contributed to the process by helping with defining keywords, formulating the search strategy, identifying articles, removing duplicates, retrieving the full text of articles for review (from the university's institutional databases), proposing tables for organizing the results, and compiling the bibliography.

Initially, 1631 scientific articles and 20 governmental and non-governmental documents were identified for the literature review. A total of 254 duplicates were found and removed. After applying the inclusion and exclusion criteria, 84 documents were selected for the literature review (76 scientific articles, 4 governmental documents, and 4 non-governmental documents). Figure 1 presents a flowchart of the article selection process for the literature review.

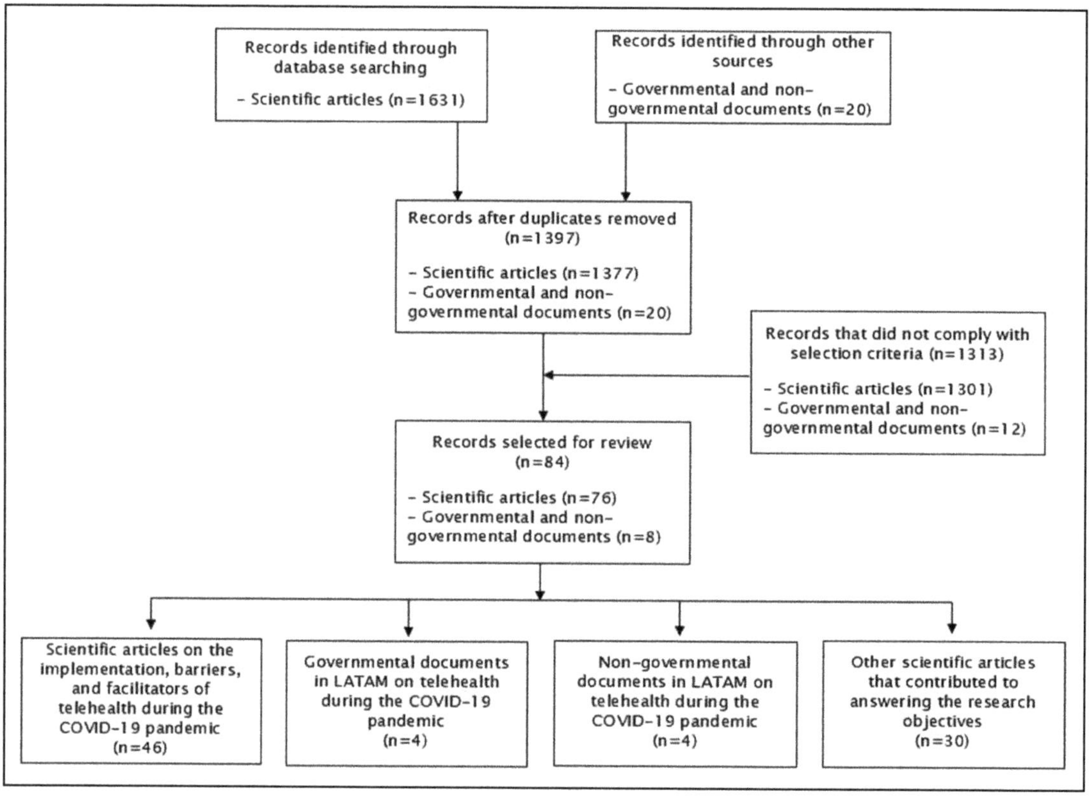

Figure 1. Flowchart of the article selection process for the literature review, classified by type of document. Abbreviation: LATAM: Latin America.

3. Results

3.1. Conceptualization of Telehealth in Gerontology and Geriatrics

Guidelines from various international, governmental, and non-governmental organizations, both prior to and during the COVID-19 pandemic, they were identified, and thus, established conceptual frameworks related to telehealth [19,46–50]. Consequently, telehealth is understood as a modality that utilizes Information and Communication Technologies (ICTs) to provide health services, medical care, and information regardless of distance [19]. Telehealth is also a tool for disseminating information on the care and prevention of chronic diseases, as well as epidemics [19]. Telehealth is also part of AgeTech, understood as the use of advanced technologies for OP, including both existing devices (such as eyeglasses, walkers, and prosthetics) and emerging technologies (digital media, ICTs, mobile technologies, wearables, and smart home systems) [51], which experienced significant growth during the COVID-19 pandemic [51].

Three key components of telehealth are described: tele-education, telemedicine, and tele-assistance [19,47]. Specifically, telemedicine focuses on the provision of remote health services in the areas of health promotion, prevention, diagnosis, treatment, and rehabilitation. These services are delivered by healthcare professionals who use ICTs to exchange data, with the aim of facilitating access and timely delivery of services for populations facing limited healthcare availability, access barriers, or both, in their geographic area [19,46]. Telerehabilitation, in turn, focuses on the provision of rehabilitation services remotely through the application of telecommunication, remote sensing, operational, and information technologies. Its purpose is to serve individuals, professionals, and systems by minimizing barriers of distance, time, and cost [19,46,50]—a concept that was further reinforced during the COVID-19 pandemic [50]. In summary, telerehabilitation is a branch of telemedicine [50], and telemedicine is a branch of telehealth [19]. Regarding its modality, there are three ways to implement telehealth, telemedicine, and telerehabilitation: synchronous (in real time between the professional and the user); asynchronous (at different times and/or for later review); or hybrid (a combination of both) [19,46].

Telehealth has been incorporated into public health systems in some countries of the region [41]. For example, in the case of Chile, telehealth is understood as a strategy based on the Comprehensive Family and Community Health Care Model, within the context of Integrated Health Service Networks. It facilitates the provision of remote services in the areas of health promotion, prevention, diagnosis, treatment, rehabilitation, and palliative care [19], with a person-centered approach that considers the sociocultural context and life course. The aim is to maintain optimal health status and continuity of care for the population, thereby improving equity in access, rights, timeliness, and quality of care [19]. This intervention was implemented during the pandemic to ensure continuity of care for OP in primary healthcare (PHC) programs [52].

Integrating the conceptualization of telehealth (its components and branches) previously described [19] within the fields of Gerontology (the science of aging) [45,53] and Geriatrics (a branch of this science that focuses on addressing the needs, problems, and geriatric syndromes of OP across different levels of healthcare) [45,54], we propose the concept of Telegerontology, expanding on previous definitions [55]. Additionally, we expand the concept of Telegeriatrics as proposed by the Brazilian Society of Gerontology and Geriatrics [56] for broader application in the region, as summarized in Table 1 and Figure 2.

Table 1. Concepts of TeleGerontology and TeleGeriatrics for use in the Latin America and Caribbean region.

Concept	Definition
TeleGerontology	Provision of gerontology services at a distance, through the application of telecommunication, information technology, and computerized data transmission, to support aging and old age across biological, functional, psycho-affective, social, and environmental dimensions of older people and their surroundings; while also understanding what technologies older persons use and how they use information and communication technologies.
TeleGeriatrics	Use of telemedicine to provide older people with access to specialists who can deliver medical services and specialized care to this population [56], with emphasis on health promotion, prevention, assessment, diagnosis, treatment, rehabilitation, palliative care, and management of health problems, chronic conditions, and geriatric syndromes affecting them and their families.

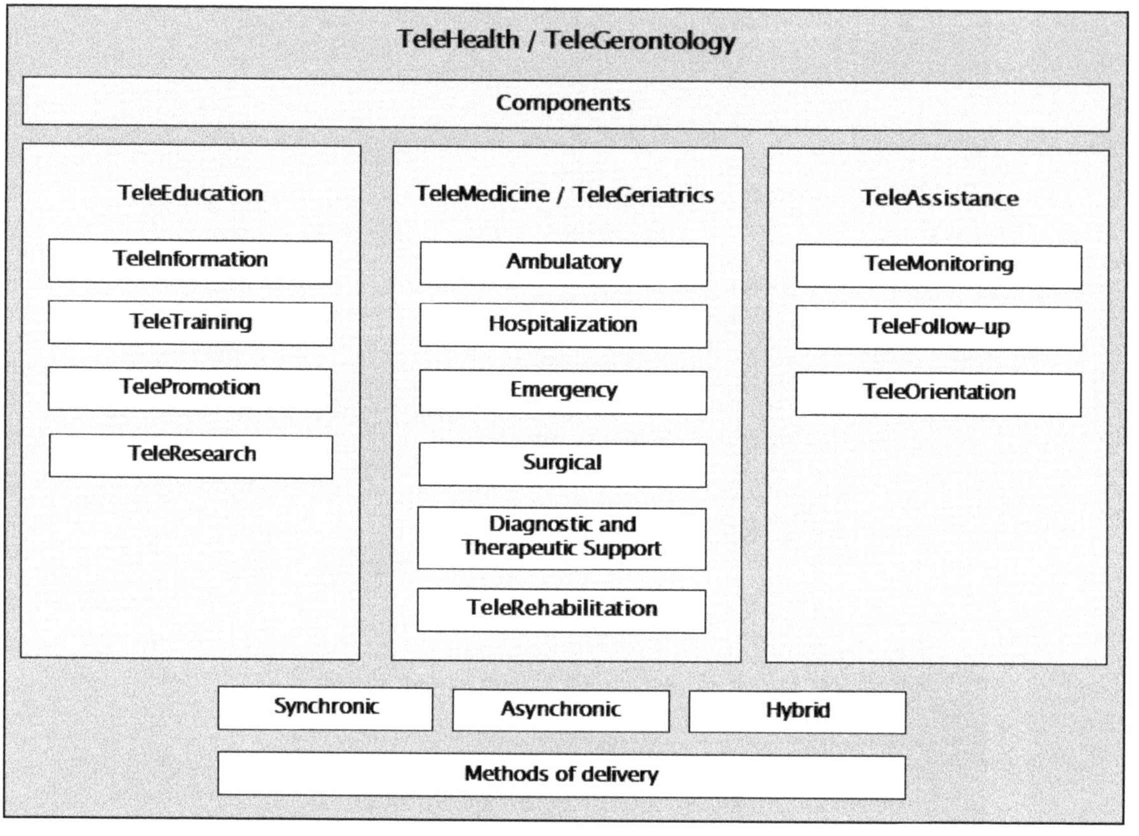

Figure 2. Components of telehealth, their relationship with the branches of telemedicine and telerehabilitation, and their modalities of delivery; with emphasis on the care of older persons, incorporating the concepts of TeleGerontology and TeleGeriatrics. Own elaboration based on the document "National Telehealth Program in the context of Integrated Health Services Networks" [19].

These updated concepts, which reflect the regional experience of Latin America and the Caribbean, allow for a more precise understanding of the scope of Telehealth (as a care modality) in the fields of Gerontology and Geriatrics, as well as in the daily approach to OP in different contexts, programs, and services; concepts that can also be used in other regions globally (Table 1). Update and integrate these new concepts "Telegerontology" and "Telegeriatrics" into previously published concepts in the field of Telehealth [19], provides a more appropriate representation for the fields of Gerontology and Geriatrics (Figure 2).

3.2. *Overview of the Implementation, Barriers, and Facilitators of Telehealth for Older People*

This literature review has compiled a total of 46 scientific articles that address the implementation, barriers, and facilitators of telehealth for OP (Appendix A, Table A3). Among these, an integrative review article, published prior to the COVID-19 pandemic, has been included to provide an initial comparative perspective on the barriers and facilitators of telehealth for OP.

Several types of research have been identified: Quantitative (20), Qualitative (12) and Mixed Methods (6). Within quantitative research, primarily through cross-sectional studies. Within qualitative research, primarily through semi-structured interviews. A similar trend can be observed in research using mixed methods. This reflects the need and the resources that researchers had available at the beginning of the pandemic to address this research topic, as well as the diversity of information collected. Furthermore, there are studies that have included some type of intervention (10), primarily analyzed at the end of the intervention.

Most studies focused exclusively on OP, healthy individuals and/or those with various chronic diseases (23), followed by groups of physicians and/or healthcare professionals (7), and then both groups combined (6). In the case of studies using exclusively quantitative methods (excluding mixed methods), the sample sizes ranged from 8 to 3257 OP. For studies using exclusively qualitative methods (excluding mixed methods), the sample sizes ranged from 7 to 98 OP. This reflects the diversity of stakeholders who have reported the information. Two studies presented data on the number of consultations with the Telehealth service.

Globally, the United States is the main country of origin for these studies (15), followed by Canada (5). Specifically in Latin America and the Caribbean, eleven articles on this topic have been identified, published in Chile (5), Mexico (2), Brazil (2), and Peru (2).

Eight review articles were included, providing a broader perspective to support the objectives of this literature review. Three of these review articles specifically included information from countries in Latin America and the Caribbean.

Next, and in the following three sections, we present a narrative and detailed analysis of the research findings, with regard to implementation, barriers, and facilitators of telehealth for OP.

3.3. Implementation of Telehealth for Older People During COVID-19

Older people are the fastest-growing group of ICT users [15]. A study in 1067 OP in Italy conducted during the pandemic identified that smartphones were the most commonly used devices for internet access (59%), WhatsApp was the most frequently used app (57%), internet users were younger than non-users (63 vs. 78 years old), and they had higher educational levels [57]. Furthermore, a study conducted in Chile among 680 OP who used technology during the pandemic showed that 91% of participants considered having internet access useful in their daily lives, and 86% stated that the internet enabled them to access knowledge they would not have obtained otherwise. In addition, participants reported using social media in their everyday lives, including WhatsApp (95%), Facebook (82%), and YouTube (60%) [58].

Regarding the use of telehealth among OP, it increased from 4.6% before the COVID-19 pandemic to 21.1%, with 1 in 3 OP having used telemedicine during the pandemic [32]. Since the onset of the pandemic, there has been growing interest and acceptance of telehealth among OP, with studies indicating that active collaboration between OP and their healthcare providers has been linked to increased acceptance of remote services [40]. It was also reported that OP were more motivated and able to quickly learn new technologies in the context of the pandemic [59], enabling them to continue with their ADLs, exchange informal support with family and neighbors, rely on formal support from community organizations, and remain physically active as part of their resilience [60].

A scoping review investigating the use of telehealth in geriatrics revealed that telehealth interventions targeting OP at the onset of the pandemic focused predominantly on curative services, rather than on promotional—preventive care and rehabilitation [40]. However, these services were predominantly available in high-income countries of the Northern Hemisphere, compared to those in the Global South and middle- to low-income countries [40], such as those in the Latin American region. In addition, there was a greater focus on research about telehealth for OP based on information provided by healthcare providers, both during the beginning of the pandemic [61–63], and prior to it [64].

Several international experiences [13,65–71] demonstrated that telehealth made it possible to ensure continuity of care for OP and reduce the risk of infection during the pandemic [23,72,73]. However, at the global level, there is still a lack of studies that explore in depth issues such as the safety, usefulness, usability, scalability, cost-effectiveness, facilitators and barriers, and demand for the use of telehealth in gerontology and geriatrics. Therefore, there is a clear need for research in these areas now that the COVID-19 pandemic has ended [40], so that the lessons learned can help identify the specific needs of OP when designing and managing future telehealth interventions [65].

Potential uses of telehealth for OP include: remote monitoring of chronic diseases (e.g., vital signs, weight, blood glucose), receiving laboratory results and medical reports, access to personal medical records, and medical/professional consultations via videoconference [9]. Potential uses of telerehabilitation for OP have also been proposed, including: facilitating transitions of care between different healthcare settings (e.g., acute care hospitals, rehabilitation centers, long-term care facilities, home care), preventing falls and reducing functional decline, cognitive rehabilitation, targeted therapy for specific conditions (e.g., heart disease, osteoarthritis), addressing loneliness and social isolation, and monitoring safety in the home environment [9].

A systematic review exploring the application and implementation of telehealth services for OP during the pandemic identified the following services: triage and monitoring, remote monitoring and treatment, online follow-up for residents in healthcare facilities, and the use of online services involving various types of telehealth applications. These applications included phone calls, live videoconferencing, online programs, smartphone apps, Internet of Things (IoT), cloud computing, and social media—mostly reported in countries in the Northern Hemisphere [66]. To ensure the security and privacy of telehealth services, the U.S. Department of Health and Human Services provided a list of video communication providers that comply with the Health Insurance Portability and Accountability Act (HIPAA) [47].

Regarding the specific analysis of the implementation of telehealth with OP during the pandemic, a qualitative study conducted in 2020 through interviews with geriatricians, primary care physicians, and emergency doctors in both rural and urban settings in the United States described telehealth as a more flexible, value-based, and user-centered mode of care [61]. The authors identified several benefits of using telehealth with OP, including the reduction in delayed care and the increase in timely attention, improved efficiency of physicians, enhanced communication with caregivers and OP, reduced travel burdens for the elderly, and greater facilitation of health education and outreach [61]. The same study described several challenges, including unequal access in rural areas and the care of OP with cognitive impairments [61]. Other reported benefits have included greater time efficiency and the delivery of visual information through videoconferencing, as well as increased convenience and safety [34,74,75].

Moreover, in the context of PHC in the United States, a qualitative study conducted in 2021—including interviews with 29 OP and three focus groups with professionals—found that telemedicine contributed to continuity of care. Also, in this same country, another research mixed-method carried out in 80 OPs identified socio-emotional connection and comfort as benefits, and technological barriers and loss of the face-to-face experience as challenges [76]. It was particularly convenient when there was a pre-existing or established doctor–patient relationship or when addressing minor health concerns. It was also beneficial for individuals with reduced mobility, as it reduced their exposure to potentially high-risk environments [23].

From a telehealth management perspective, a series of strengths, weaknesses, threats, and opportunities related to telehealth for OP were synthesized at the beginning of the COVID-19 pandemic [40]. Identifying them would allow for the design and implementation of more optimal telehealth strategies for OP (in both intervention and/or research contexts), whether during a pandemic or under normal circumstances. This also highlights the need to further explore this analysis both during and after the pandemic.

Implementation of Telehealth for Older People, Before and During COVID-19 in Latin America and the Caribbean

In the Americas, in the 20 years prior to the COVID-19 pandemic, there has been an increase in resources and technical capacity, an improvement in digital education, patient empowerment in their treatment, and greater public interest in telemedicine; he formation of interdisciplinary teams, academic and professional networks, and virtual medical consultations, have been considered particularly successful [42]. During the pandemic, Chile, Brazil, Colombia, Mexico, Argentina and Peru were the countries that made the most progress in the field of telehealth in Latin America, both within their health systems and/or through legislation, increasing its use in recent years [41].

Specifically regarding OP, during the pandemic, the Chilean Ministry of Health urged the teams of the primary healthcare program "Más Adultos Mayores Autovalentes (+AMA)" to implement the intervention through telehealth modalities (synchronous, asynchronous, and/or supported by manuals), depending on local resources and training [52]. This approach incorporated local experiences and was seen as an adaptation to alternative forms of contact. Other countries in the region have also developed recommendations for implementing telehealth for OP. For instance, at the end of 2023, the Brazilian Society of Gerontology and Geriatrics published the Telegeriatrics Guide [56]. However, there are still few guidelines or recommendations on telehealth with an emphasis on gerontology and geriatrics in the region.

Additional benefits have been reported regarding the implementation of telehealth with OP from the perspective of healthcare personnel and patients. A user satisfaction survey conducted during the COVID-19 pandemic in Peru reported that, out of a total of 129 healthcare workers, more than 55% of professionals expressed satisfaction with telehealth [77]. On the other hand, approximately 77% of 377 patients (including 44 OP) reported being satisfied with telehealth services. [77].

Specifically, published experiences have been identified on the implementation of telehealth interventions focused on OP in countries of the region, such as the psychosocial teleassistance program of Peru's Social Security, which provided 154,280 follow-ups and 36,492 teleassistance services to OP—mainly involving emotional support and social counseling [78]; the TeleCOVID-MG program in two municipalities in Brazil, which offered support to OP [79]; a multidisciplinary intervention conducted in Mexico involving 44 OP with colorectal or gastric cancer from a geriatric oncology clinic, where geriatric assessments, treatment toxicity evaluations, physical exams, and treatment prescriptions were performed using platforms such as WhatsApp or Zoom [80]; a semi-presential technological platform (mobile dental clinic combined with a digital platform) designed to support urgent and priority dental care for OP in five regions of Chile [81]; and telehealth-based evaluations, such as the use of the Phototest to identify mild cognitive impairment in OP with memory complaints from rural areas in southern Chile [82]. Additionally, there are reported experiences that have included OP (average age of 68 years), such as a multidisciplinary supportive care program for individuals with advanced cancer in Mexico. In this program, the most common interventions were psychological care (33%), pain and symptom management (25%), and nutritional counseling (13%). Half of the interventions were delivered via videoconference [83]. Also, in Chile, an online course on healthy aging was implemented for the community and health professionals, which included 20% of OP [84].

Additionally, some interventions initially delivered in person were later continued via telehealth. One example is Brazil's Playful Living Program, aimed at delivering clown-based performances to OP with aphasia [85]. This telehealth-based intervention included not only clowning but also dance, storytelling, and cooking (safe complementary therapies), delivered through individual and group video calls. It involved the participation of professionals and undergraduate and graduate students from the fields of Speech and Language Therapy, Theater, Psychology, Dance, Culinary Arts, Psychiatry, and Public Health [85]. In addition, to facilitate access for OPs, they received donated technological devices; to improve affordability, they were provided with internet credit donations necessary to stay connected; and to support digital capacity, assistance was offered to help them use the technology [85]. Also in Chile, +AMA—the government program that began in 2015, [52], transitioned from an in-person format to an asynchronous telehealth modality, as a pilot in one of the cities where it is implemented. In its in-person format, it is a health promotion and prevention intervention within PHC, which provides physical activity, cognitive stimulation, and education to OP in the community. During the pandemic, the local team transitioned to an asynchronous telehealth modality through videos uploaded to YouTube and infographics stored on Facebook, which were shared weekly via WhatsApp with OP groups so they could carry out the activities [71]. Monthly telephone follow-ups were conducted. Additionally, during the final month of the intervention, a manual containing the same exercises/activities (including a weekly check-up schedule) was delivered in person to the OP, along with other materials. This intervention has been described in detail previously [71].

3.4. Telehealth Facilitators for Older People, Before and During COVID-19

Before the COVID-19 pandemic, an integrative review identified several facilitators that contributed to the acceptance of telehealth by OP with chronic physical conditions. These included: devices with fewer buttons, automatic information transmission, use of low-tech platforms (such as telephones or televisions), devices that provided reminders or alerts (either visual or audio-guided), and user-friendly images [64]. In addition, a systematic mixed-methods review analyzing telemedicine in OP in primary healthcare settings (mostly from studies published before the pandemic) identified the most frequently cited facilitator as location and travel time savings [86].

During the pandemic, qualitative studies involving healthcare providers described additional facilitators of telehealth use in OP [34,63,69]. The first study, conducted in 2020, interviewed 13 healthcare providers in the United States (including medical/clinical directors, program managers, clinical nurses/managers, and clinical social work managers) who provided synchronous telehealth via videoconference to medically complex OP. It identified the following facilitators: assessment of patient needs, collection of information from OP, and increased scheduling capacity [63]. The second study, conducted in the same year, interviewed 33 geriatricians and primary care physicians in the United States to explore their experiences with telemedicine and to identify strategies used to maintain continuity of care for OP [69]. This study reported that many physicians successfully bridged the digital divide by assessing OP's technological readiness in advance, educating them about telehealth privacy and utility, being flexible with telehealth modalities, using the home or available facilities, making accommodations for disabilities, and involving caregivers [69]. The third study, conducted between 2020 and 2021, interviewed 29 geriatric care physicians in Canada and identified the presence of a caregiver and administrative support as key facilitators of telemedicine use with OP [34]. Additionally, a mixed-methods study conducted in 2020 interviewed 30 professionals—geriatricians, geriatric psychiatrists, and geriatric nurses in Canada—regarding the use of telemedicine technologies with frail OP, their families, and caregivers. The study identified several facilitators, including relative advantage, adaptability, tension for change, available resources, access to knowledge, networks and communication, compatibility, knowledge and beliefs, self-efficacy, champions, external agents, execution, and reflection and evaluation [87].

Other features of synchronous telehealth visits via videoconference have been highlighted as additional opportunities for intervention, as they allow professionals to observe the OP's home environment [75]—something that in-clinic visits rarely offer. For example, gait assessments revealed mobility obstacles in the home that increased the risk of falls and injuries [65]. Additionally, medication reviews allowed providers to observe how medications were stored and administered [65]. Inviting professionals into the OPs home environment also enabled more direct conversations. Those OPs and caregivers who had previously participated in a video visit reported being more likely to accept a video call visit in the future [65]. At the same time, the use of audio and video equipment of adequate quality (including adaptive devices such as pocket speakers) facilitated these virtual assessments [88]. For its part, regarding asynchronous telehealth, it has been shown that the volume of follow-up, response time, and the quality-related variables involved in service delivery are critically important to ensure patient/user satisfaction, programmatic success, and the sustainability of the intervention [20]. Among the methodologies used, the use of WhatsApp has been described as reducing loneliness among OP [89], and more generally, the use of technology (in various forms) is considered a strategy to address loneliness in OP living alone [90].

A mixed-methods study conducted in the United States in 2020, involving 3 patients, 4 caregivers, 19 physicians, 5 medical assistants, and 2 programers, identified customer service support and the existence of protocols to guide patients in the use of telemedicine as key facilitators of video consultations [91]. Specifically regarding OP, a qualitative study conducted in New Zealand in 2021 aimed at identifying facilitators for the use of telehealth in underserved rural populations—through seven focus groups and thirteen individual interviews across four diverse communities—found that the term *telehealth* was not initially understood by many participants and required clarification [92]. Those who had used telehealth reported positive experiences—such as saving time and costs—and were likely to use it again [92]. Facilitators also included trust in telehealth technology (reliable and accessible internet access, and access to digital devices); trust in the user experience through the relationship between the consumer and healthcare provider (such as the availability of user support); and trust in the healthcare system (regarding wait times, communication and coordination, and cost) [92]. Additionally, facilitators included access to culturally appropriate healthcare services, the type of consultation (enabling access to specialized services), and the implementation of telehealth (through a fixed community center or a mobile bus unit, with support available—especially when combined with non-health services such as online banking) [92].

Telehealth Facilitators for Older People During COVID-19 in Latin America and the Caribbean

From the perspective of healthcare providers in the Latin American region, evidence on facilitators of telehealth for OP during the pandemic is limited. However, insights can be drawn from the perspective of OP telehealth users, as demonstrated in a qualitative study conducted in Chile in 2020. This study used in-depth semi-structured interviews with 26 community-dwelling self-sufficient OP (14 participated in the telehealth intervention, and 12 served as non-intervention controls) [71]. These OP participated in the government intervention program +AMA [52]. This is a multicomponent intervention (Physical Activity, Cognitive Stimulation, and Education) that, during the pandemic, was delivered through an asynchronous telehealth modality (videos, infographics, and a manual) to ensure continuity of care [52]. The OP had previously participated in the same intervention in its in-person format in earlier years. Following thematic analysis, the OP identified the following as facilitators: participating in the intervention alongside others, prior experience with the in-person modality, good digital literacy, self-motivation, commitment to the program, and the emergence of natural leaders [71]. In addition, the OP identified several positive aspects of this modality, such as the sustainability of the effects between the in-person and telehealth formats, the bio-psycho-social benefits achieved through telehealth, the fact that telehealth helped establish a routine, the guidance and instructions provided by professionals, and the flexibility to carry out the intervention at any time and place, which fostered a sense of autonomy and flexibility [71].

3.5. Telehealth Barriers for Older People, Before and During COVID-19

Prior to the pandemic, the aforementioned review [64], also described intrinsic barriers to the use of technology. These included font size, the use of unusual characters (which are difficult to read), soft graphics and poor color contrast, devices with widgets (which pose challenges for fine eye-hand motor coordination), the use of a computer mouse (difficult for individuals with hand arthritis), lack of experience using a smartphone or computer, multiple screen transitions required to complete tasks, multi-layered menu bars, inappropriate smartphone size (either too large or too small), and difficulties handling devices among many OP with reduced grip strength [64]. Delays in responses, lack of feedback, and technical problems can lead to frustration and decrease motivation for OP to continue engaging in self-care activities. Likewise, for OP who are not accustomed to using technology, telehealth can represent a significant cultural shift [64]. Moreover, in the previously mentioned mixed-methods systematic review [86], the most frequently cited barrier was user habits or preferences.

During the COVID-19 pandemic, additional barriers were described. A quantitative study involving surveys with 16 primary care physicians from a U.S.-based program serving 873 community-dwelling OP aimed to identify barriers to synchronous (video-based) telehealth. The study found that over one-third of these OP participated in video-based telehealth visits for the first time between April and June 2020. It also reported that most required assistance from a family member and/or paid caregiver to complete the visit. Among OP who had not used telehealth, 27% were unable to engage via video due to factors such as cognitive or sensory impairments, while 14% lacked access to a caregiver who could assist them with the technology [62]. Similarly, physicians were unaware of their OP patients' internet connectivity, ability to afford mobile phone plans, or access to video-capable devices [62]. In another qualitative study conducted in 2020, involving interviews with 13 synchronous (video-based) telehealth providers in the United States who worked with medically complex OP, the reported barriers included cognitive and sensory abilities, access to technology, reliance on caregivers and aides, addressing sensitive topics, and incomplete examinations [63]. A mixed-methods study conducted in 2020 in Canada, which interviewed 30 professionals (geriatricians, geriatric psychiatrists, and geriatric nurses), identified several barriers to telemedicine for frail OP, their families, and caregivers. These included complexity, quality of design and presentation, patient needs and resources, readiness for implementation, and cultural factors [87]. More recently, a qualitative study conducted between 2020 and 2021 with 29 geriatric care physicians in Canada identified several barriers to telemedicine, including difficulties using technology, patients' sensory impairments, lack of hospital support, and a high volume of pre-existing patients [34].

In the previously mentioned 2020 study conducted in the United States with 33 participants (including 3 patients, caregivers, physicians, medical assistants, and programers), the identified barriers to video consultations included difficulties navigating technology, concerns about privacy, and lack of technical support [91]. Additionally, a quantitative study conducted in 2021 in Canada, involving surveys with 39 healthcare providers, 40 patients with multiple comorbidities, and 22 caregivers from outpatient clinics at a tertiary hospital—who had received phone visits—expressed interest in future telehealth visits. They identified similar barriers: lack of access to technology and skills, the perception that telehealth may be inferior to in-person visits, lack of administrative support, limited technological skills among both healthcare professionals and patients, and limited access to infrastructure and internet [93].

Also, in a qualitative study conducted in 2021 in the United States involving 29 OP from primary care, participants expressed concerns about the lack of eye contact, which they felt led healthcare professionals to overlook essential details. They also identified issues related to poor communication due to language or hearing barriers [23]. Similarly, in a qualitative study conducted in 2021 with 20 OP in Canada, identified barriers to telehealth included the need for physical examination and touch, lack of nonverbal communication, difficulties using technology, and systemic barriers to access [74]. Furthermore, in a qualitative study conducted with 14 OP in Israel, they expressed concern about the potential for poorer quality of telemedicine sessions compared to in-person sessions, and they also expressed a lack of trust in telemedicine services and frustration with the lack of face-to-face interaction and communication [94]. Additionally, in a mixed-methods study conducted in 2021 in the United States with 249 OP residing in independent living facilities in the community, the main barriers to video visits included not knowing how to connect to the platform, lack of familiarity with technology and the internet, difficulty hearing, limited English proficiency, and lack of interest in seeing providers outside the clinic setting [95]. In addition to the above, in a qualitative study of 78 OP in Singapore, they preferred in-person consultations due to a perceived lack of human interaction and diagnostic accuracy, low digital literacy, and a lack of access to telehealth-compatible devices [96].

Telehealth Barriers for Older People During COVID-19 in Latin America and the Caribbean

In the Latin American region, while there is limited evidence on telehealth barriers for OP during the pandemic from the perspective of providers, there is information from the perspective of OP users. A quantitative study, which surveyed 237 OP in Brazil participating in the TeleCOVID-MG program, identified certain personal barriers such as being over 80 years old, having lower educational levels, and experiencing hearing and visual impairments—all of which were associated with the need for support during teleconsultations. This need for support was also associated with hospitalization and mortality [79]. Also, in a quantitative study conducted in 2020 in Chile surveying 34 OP, participants received physical exercise and pain education videos over a 4-week period to be performed independently at home (asynchronous telehealth) [97]. The average adherence was 2 days per week over 2.5 weeks, with the main barrier identified as a lack of willingness to perform the activities. This reluctance was more common among individuals who had engaged in group physical exercise before the pandemic [97]. Additionally, in the previously described 2020 study [71], OP who participated in the asynchronous telehealth intervention reported pain during physical activity and the complexity of the cognitive exercises as barriers [71]. Additionally, those who did not participate in the intervention (controls) reported low digital literacy and lack of support from others as barriers. They also cited lack of motivation, lack of time, low digital literacy, limited knowledge of how to use social media, and poor internet connection, as reasons for not engaging in telehealth [71].

Recognizing the various benefits, facilitators, and barriers that telehealth presented for OP during the COVID-19 pandemic—summarized in Table 2—will be essential when designing and implementing future interventions.

Table 2. Summary of telehealth benefits, facilitators, and barriers among older people during the COVID-19 pandemic: Global and Latin America and Caribbean perspectives.

Context	Benefits	Facilitators	Barriers
Technological/ Telehealth	- Provided visual information through video conferences. - Offered a more flexible, value-based, and user-centered mode of care.	- Adaptability of telehealth. - Flexibility with the types of telehealth modalities used. - Using the home or available facilities. - Existence of protocols to guide OP in using telehealth. - Promotion of self-efficacy and self-management among OP. - OP's trust in telehealth technology (access to reliable and affordable internet, and to digital devices). - Education of OP about the privacy and usefulness of telehealth.	- Telehealth complexity. - Quality of design and presentation. - Limited knowledge of how to use social media. - OP's difficulty navigating technology. - Limited access to infrastructure and internet. - Poor internet connection. - Lack of eye contact, which can lead professionals to overlook essential details. - Need for physical examination and touch.
Organizational/ Governance	- Contribution to continuity of care. - Provision of greater convenience and safety. - Reduction in delayed care. - Increase timely access to care. - Improvement of time efficiency of interventions. - Improvement of efficiency of physicians/professionals.	- OP's trust in healthcare system (including wait times, communication and coordination, and cost). - Scheduling capacity for care. - Making adaptations for disabilities. - Presence of a caregiver and/or family member. - Type of consultation (allowing access to specialized services). - Videoconferencing facilitating home assessments for OP (environment, medication management). - Follow-up volume, response time, and quality-related variables involved in service delivery. - Provision of customer service. - Having previously participated in the same intervention in person. - Administrative support. - Access to culturally appropriate healthcare services.	- Concerns about privacy and lack of technical support. - Physicians'/professionals' lack of awareness regarding their OP patients' internet connectivity, ability to afford mobile phone plans, or access to video-capable devices. - Professionals' difficulties navigating technology. - High volume of pre-existing patients. - Lack of support in the hospital setting.
Human/ Psychosocial	- For OP with reduced mobility, reduction in exposure to potentially high-risk environments. - Improvement in communication with caregivers and OP. - Facilitation of health education.	- OP's trust based on consumer–health provider relationship (ease of access to user support). - OP's needs assessment. - Gathering information from OP. - Assessment of technological readiness in advance. - More direct conversations through videoconferencing. - Good digital literacy among OP. - OP's motivation to use telehealth. - Natural and/or community leaders who support other OP in using telehealth.	- Being over 80 years old. - Lower educational level among OP. - OP's needs and resources. - Dependence on a family member to complete the videoconference. - Presence of cognitive or sensory impairments in OP. - Lack of communication due to language or hearing barriers. - Addressing sensitive topics and incomplete examinations. - Lack of motivation, willingness, and/or time among OP to engage in telehealth. - No or low digital literacy among OP. - Pain during physical activity and the complexity of cognitive stimulation exercises. - Perception that telehealth may be inferior to in-person visits. - Lack of interest among OP in seeing providers outside the clinic. - Not speaking the native language. - Cultural factors.
Financial	- Reduced the travel burden for OP.	- Time and cost savings. - Flexibility to carry out the intervention anytime and anywhere (asynchronous telehealth).	- Requiring a paid caregiver to complete the videoconference.

4. Discussion

4.1. Lessons Learned and Considerations to Improve the Implementation of Telehealth and Reduce Barriers for Older People

Recent studies have identified a trend and preference among OP and professionals for using telehealth in combination with in-person interventions, rather than relying solely on telehealth [23,71,74,76,94,96]. This includes starting with initial in-person appointments, followed by telehealth and/or additional in-person visits [75].

In general, the three principles for delivering telehealth to OP proposed by The Collaborative for Telehealth and Aging (C4TA) from the United States—a group composed of providers, geriatric experts, telehealth specialists, and advocates—can be followed [98]. First, care must be person-centered; therefore, telehealth programs should be designed to meet the needs and preferences of OP by considering their goals, family and caregivers, language characteristics, and their readiness and ability to use technology [98]. Second, care must be equitable and accessible; thus, telehealth programs should address both individual and systemic barriers to care for OP by taking into account issues of equity and access [98]. Third, care must be integrated and coordinated across systems and individuals [98]. In addition, we present more specific considerations below to reduce telehealth barriers for OP. These recommendations are presented for application in various countries worldwide, including those in Latin America and the Caribbean, based on the findings identified in this literature review.

4.1.1. Intrinsic and Extrinsic Factors

A review of OP's perceptions of technology showed that a one-size-fits-all approach does not work, and that technologies must be adapted to individual needs [99]. It should also not be assumed that all OP face difficulties accessing virtual care. [88]. Therefore, it is important to identify OP's perceptions of ICTs in order to encourage their use, considering intrinsic factors, such as control-oriented attitudes, independence, and the need or requirement for safety; and extrinsic factors, such as usability, feedback, and costs [99].

Active listening should be encouraged, as well as discussing both the advantages and disadvantages of telehealth, considering existing recommendations in these areas [23]. It is important to emphasize the positive benefits that promote autonomy [99], adapt to OP's lifestyles and expectations, and offer personalized interventions that take into account individual preferences and capabilities [5]. Also, the option to choose between a phone or videoconference assessment should be offered [88], all with the aim of preventing rejection or dropout. Therefore, technologies must be perceived as reliable and effective, if long-term use is to be achieved [99].

4.1.2. Digital Health Literacy

It has been reported that older age, low educational level, low income, depressive symptoms, low cognitive functioning, disability, limited support networks, complex application interfaces, and lack of digital health literacy are negatively associated with the use of telehealth [32,57,100–104]. It is important to note that when introducing new ICTs, the steep learning curve that OP may experience should be acknowledged, and support should be provided to help them become familiar with these technologies [5]. In addition, they may feel less comfortable, lack access to the necessary technology, and/or have sensory difficulties (such as impaired hearing or vision), which can hinder their use of telehealth [65]. Likewise, the "digital divide" resulting from socioeconomic status, age, geographic location, and cultural factors should also be taken into account [5].

In terms of Assessment, this could be achieved through the use of in-person or online surveys, as previously reported [73], to identify OP's readiness for telehealth. This includes internet use, access to internet-connected devices, experiences and concerns related to this mode of intervention, and perceived barriers—ultimately enabling the development of training programs [73].

In terms of Training, a commonly expressed need among OP has been for professionals to provide educational sessions, workshops, and tutorials on how to use remote care [94]. In this regard, a meta-analysis—where the majority of studies included were from the United States—which aimed at evaluating the effectiveness of digital health literacy interventions for OP, found that these interventions led to significant improvements in OP's knowledge and self-efficacy [105]. Additionally, it has been reported that in-person teaching, guided by a conceptual framework and delivered over a minimum of four weeks, had a more significant effect [105]. This approach also helps to strengthen relationships and bonds, which later foster trust when using telehealth [88].

In addition, programs aimed at increasing digital health literacy and competencies should include physicians, professionals, and OP, as this is essential to ensure that all parties have the knowledge, confidence, and ability to equitably benefit from emerging innovations, such as telehealth [33]. To this end, experiences such as the one implemented in Chile—where an online course on healthy aging was offered to both the community and healthcare professionals [84]—can be followed, as well as other international initiatives, such as volunteer programs involving university students that increased access to telehealth services for OP during the pandemic [106]. Likewise, training and capacity building for the personnel who will deliver telehealth should be encouraged, provided by clinical professionals with experience in telehealth, along with updates on new digital assessment tools [75].

In terms of Intervention, it is recommended that professionals use a coaching model for OP, which increases OP's sense of responsibility in each session and enhances relationship-centered communication skills [9]. At the same time, review techniques should be used to ensure that OP adequately understand instructions and training. It is also important to listen to both the content and the emotions expressed by OP [9].

In addition, a series of actions should be considered with the OP, their family member and/or caregiver before a telehealth appointment, that include: explaining the format and purpose of the visit, practicing with providers beforehand, reminding the OP and their support network when and how the call will take place, explaining the need for future in-person consultations, obtaining photo documentation and/or encouraging family participation—all with the aim of ensuring better preparation for subsequent telehealth sessions [75]. This presents a challenge for OP, as it increases their responsibility to report on their health status and to engage in self-examination [9]. During the telehealth appointment, it is recommended to ask the OP to repeat the information and review it again at the end of the session or to write it down, provide opportunities to ask questions during the visit, look at the camera and be more expressive to ensure the message is understood—including careful placement of the microphone to avoid blocking the mouth. If multiple people are present, it is helpful to practice participation and decide in advance who will lead the conversation. All of this aims to improve communication [75].

4.1.3. Support, Adaptations, and Complements

OP should be supported in navigating the telehealth platform as needed, and assistance should be provided to promote self-efficacy and self-management. [23]. Social support and the involvement of a caregiver or family member during telehealth increase the likelihood of use [107] and facilitate the use of technology (e.g., Zoom). During the assessment, their participation can also be helpful for obtaining collateral information and may aid in remembering appointments [88], which becomes even more relevant for OP with disabilities [103].

A commonly expressed need among OP has been to simplify telehealth infrastructure [94]. It has also been reported that when enablers are present (having a cellphone/PC/tablet, knowing how to use them, and having internet access), these factors cease to be barriers [32]. Therefore, regarding telehealth and data use, it is recommended to use lower bandwidth if the platform allows it, provide a tablet and data loan service, use high-quality headsets/microphones that do not cover the mouth [75], use adequately functioning audio and video equipment (including adaptive devices such as pocket speakers) [88], and include a chat feature during the video call [23], all of which can facilitate telehealth.

Specifically for OP in rural areas or with disabilities, telehealth interventions can be adapted with a health promotion focus, drawing on international experiences in which context was adjusted (shorter, smaller, and longer-duration activities) and equity was addressed (e.g., phone formats, automatically generated subtitles) without altering the content [108]. Specifically, and based on the authors' experience, we present a series of recommendations to consider when implementing telehealth with OP with disabilities, in order to reduce barriers and, as a result, improve access, use, and satisfaction with telehealth in this population group (Table 3). These recommendations can help make telehealth equitable and accessible, as well as integrated and coordinated across systems and individuals [98].

Table 3. Recommendations and strategies for implementing telehealth for older people with disabilities, aimed at reducing telehealth barriers.

Type of Disability of Older People	Strategies to Reduce Telehealth Barriers
Visual disability	- Use of screen readers compatible with telehealth platforms. - Adaptation of platforms with voice commands and audio navigation. - High contrast and enlarged font in interfaces. - Usage instructions in audio format. - Training for caregivers on providing remote assistance to OP with low vision or blindness. - Preliminary ophthalmologic evaluation to personalize accessibility. - Implementation of virtual assistants with spoken responses. - Availability of educational materials in braille or audio. - Training in the use of accessible mobile technologies. - Periodic usability assessments of accessible platforms.
Hearing disability	- Inclusion of sign language interpreters in sessions. - High-quality real-time automatic subtitles. - Use of platforms with live chat as an alternative to videoconferencing. - Training for professionals in clear written communication. - Availability of informational materials in sign language. - Visual alerts for notifications and reminders. - Promotion of asynchronous telehealth (email, secure messaging). - Hearing evaluation prior to determining the modality of remote care. - Technological adaptation guides for OP with hearing loss. - Incorporation of sound amplification technologies.
Motor disability	- Interfaces compatible with adaptive devices (trackballs, switches). - Design of simplified navigation platforms (few clicks). - Automation of voice command functions. - Keyboard/mouse configuration adjustments to facilitate use. - In-home training on the use of adapted tablets. - Remote support for personalized equipment setup. - In-home technical assistance when necessary. - Inclusion of caregivers or family members in the telehealth experience. - Assessment of home's physical environment to ensure accessibility. - Use of ergonomic physical supports to hold devices.

Table 3. *Cont.*

Type of Disability of Older People	Strategies to Reduce Telehealth Barriers
Intellectual disability	- Simple interface design with icons and guided steps. - Use of visual and auditory reminders to schedule sessions. - Digital skills training with the support of a family member and/or caregiver. - Structured repetition of key instructions during the session. - Educational materials adapted in plain language. - Inclusion of caregivers and/or family members in telehealth sessions. - Neuropsychological assessment to tailor technology use. - Shortening session duration based on attention span. - Promotion of digital routines with step-by-step tasks. - Support through digital mentoring (telecompanionship).
Psychosocial disability	- Inclusion of emotional and psychological support before and after sessions. - Use of platforms that ensure confidentiality and privacy. - Reduction in the number of different professionals involved in remote telehealth care. - Flexible scheduling to avoid stressful situations. - Empathetic language adapted to the emotional state of the person. - Inclusion of support networks (family members, caregivers, peers). - Assessment of emotional readiness to use technology. - Digital skills training programs with psychosocial support. - Feedback spaces to express fears and barriers. - Access to mental health resources through integrated platforms.

It has even been suggested that in cases where telehealth cannot be implemented at all, support for OP should be provided via telephone or social media. Periodic home visits may also be carried out, delivering infographics, guidelines, and/or manuals for use and later feedback [52], following the example of rural schools where due to geographic inaccessibility, this is a common practice to facilitate interventions. In this context, it was found that using a manual as the sole intervention tool is less effective compared to videos or a combination of both (video plus manual) [71], due to a social presence effect.

A strategy that could improve manual delivery and follow-up/support was drawn from a telehealth study during the pandemic, where the manual included a calendar with scheduled dates that OP were instructed to mark [13]. In this way, the number of sessions completed was self-reported during biweekly phone calls, incorporating motivational, psychological, and practical elements, along with goal-setting and an emphasis on independence—allowing OP to choose the physical activity of their preference. This approach enhanced adherence and empowerment [13], enabling positive relationships between users and professionals, addressing questions, monitoring health and intervention progress, and fostering self-efficacy in OP.

4.1.4. Conceptual Framework for the Implementation and Presentation of Research Related to Telehealth for Older People

Implementation science encompasses a broad range of applicable methodologies to improve the dissemination, implementation, and scalability of effective interventions in behavioral, clinical, healthcare, public health, global health, and educational settings, with the aim of improving the quality of care and health outcomes, while taking into account local realities, and ensuring sustainable implementation at scale [109]. This could be an interesting conceptual framework for the implementation of telehealth in different population groups, and specifically among OP. Unlike most publication guidelines, which apply to a specific research methodology, the Standard for Reporting Implementation Studies (StaRI) and its accompanying checklist cover the wide range of study designs used in implementation research [110]; therefore, this checklist can guide and facilitate the reporting of interventions and research related to the implementation of telehealth for OP. Furthermore, when designing and implementing these interventions, researchers should consider the barriers and facilitators identified in this literature review. The need for a comprehensive description of the context, implementation strategies, and interventions, as well as the presentation of various effectiveness, process, and cost-effectiveness outcomes, poses a challenge for journals with strict word limits for research articles and may require innovative solutions and the use of online Supplementary Materials [110], as well as for researchers themselves.

4.2. Challenges for Telehealth for Older People in Latin America and the Caribbean

4.2.1. Considerations from a Perspective of Future Pandemics

It is essential that responses to this past crisis (and to similar ones in the future) identify and prioritize OP, who may be at particular risk of being left behind or excluded during the pandemic response and subsequent recovery phases [14]. This is especially important in less developed countries, which are less likely to have access to ICTs and where needs are even greater [14], as may be the case in countries in the region.

As a result, it is necessary to ensure that community-based services and support for OP are maintained despite future physical distancing measures [14]. This presents a challenge for professional teams in social and health programs—at the institutional level (hospitals, long-term care facilities), in primary healthcare, and in the community—who have traditionally worked in face-to-face modalities, and who faced both the need and the opportunity to shift to telehealth in order to ensure continuity of care during the pandemic. In this sense, telehealth for OP should become a regular component of clinical practice for professionals in Gerontology and Geriatrics. Therefore, professional teams should always design and implement their in-person interventions with the awareness that, in situations like a pandemic, they may need to rapidly transition—within days—to a telehealth model to continue providing care.

It has been reported that, during quarantine periods, preventive telehealth strategies focused on cognitive, behavioral, social, positive, and brief interventions—delivered either online or in person—can improve mental well-being, social affiliation, and support, and reduce perceived loneliness [6]. On the other hand, cognitive skills and social support networks can help OP foster meaningful connection and a sense of belonging, improving social connection and promoting healthy relationships with oneself and others [6]. The minimum components that an intervention should include to protect the psychological and mental health of OP during a pandemic are: developing problem- and emotion-focused coping strategies; strengthening social skills and family relationships; and engaging in regular physical activity [111]. In addition, religion and spirituality have been strongly associated with positive psychological well-being, as they provide support, a sense of belonging, life purpose, and helping alleviate distress in the face of adversity [13]; this will be interesting to investigate and include as part of Telesalud's interventions with OP of the Latin American and Caribbean region, where there is a high Christian and Catholic proportion.

4.2.2. Considerations from a Management Perspective: Design, Implementation, and Evaluation

In addition, investment is needed in care and support services to ensure that they are adapted to the individual needs of OP, advancing in the design, implementation, and management of cost-effective telehealth interventions that prioritize low cost and take into account the diversity and specific needs of OP [15]. These services should be designed to be accessible and aligned with the changes associated with normal aging, considering and differentiating by sex, age, educational level, functional status, cognitive status, digital literacy, context, among other factors. This approach promotes well-being, helps maintain autonomy and independence [14], and improves quality of life. Furthermore, interventions should include OP and their families in the design, user testing, and standardization of telehealth services.

At the same time, it is necessary to support OP and their caregivers so they can access digital communication or alternative ways to stay in contact with their families and social networks, when physical movement is restricted [14]. For this reason, it is also recommended to include OP and their caregivers in learning programs, as well as to regularly improve their access to ICTs [14]. It is both a challenge and a responsibility for professionals to conduct digital health literacy workshops, thereby fostering better performance of the telehealth strategies implemented.

It would also be essential to design, translate, adapt, and/or validate tools that assess motivation, competence, usability, and/or user satisfaction with mobile devices and telehealth, given that very few tools currently exist [112] and there are still challenges and opportunities in identifying valid tools for the OP population [113], —especially in Spanish or Portuguese in the region—following some early-stage experiences in certain countries [77,97]. These tools could complement those used in the Comprehensive Gerontological Assessment (CGA) [45,114], which is the cornerstone of evaluation in this field, thereby facilitating professional training. Furthermore, there is an opportunity to digitize many scales, questionnaires, or clinical tests routinely used in CGA—either through apps or video consultations—as has already been done with cognitive assessment tools in Chile and other countries [38,82,115,116]. Questionnaires or written materials may even be provided to OP before virtual visits to improve the quality of the evaluation [88]. This entire set of tools could be used to assess telehealth in OP and their caregivers, as part of the CGA, as previously recommended [45].

4.2.3. Considerations from a Research Perspective

In parallel, it is necessary to advance qualitative, quantitative, and mixed-methods research with an interdisciplinary focus involving OP, recognizing the specificities and strengths of the region. This will help explore in greater depth how telehealth was implemented during the COVID-19 pandemic from the perspectives of physicians, professionals (in their diversity), and OP themselves, using methodological strategies already employed—such as online surveys, due to their feasibility and reach [117]. It will also be highly relevant to investigate the benefits, facilitators, and barriers—such as those documented in this article (Table 2)—as experienced by both OP and healthcare providers, as well as the effects of different telehealth modalities (synchronous, asynchronous, or hybrid) on the biopsychosocial health and quality of life of OP, considering previous research, which showed that older people were more likely to recover from negative emotions, improve their well-being, and enhance their quality of life during the COVID-19 pandemic through telehealth services [118].

4.2.4. Considerations from an Academic Training Perspective

The fact that healthcare providers themselves may possess greater knowledge about managing telehealth with OP—following a gerontological and geriatric care model, alongside other intervention modalities—will enable them to develop more appropriate interventions with OP, their families, and caregivers, from a more ethical perspective and with a focus on promoting their rights. Likewise, this new knowledge needs to be incorporated into the training and curriculum of undergraduate and postgraduate students/professionals, as well as into continuing education programs for professionals who work or will work in the health and psychosocial fields with OP.

4.2.5. Considerations from a Healthcare System and Public Policy Perspective

Finally, some countries of the region already incorporate the telehealth as part of the strategies from their health ministries, such as Argentina, Brazil, Chile and Colombia [41]. Also telehealth guidelines in OP emanating from non-governmental organizations such as the Brazilian Society of Gerontology and Geriatrics [56], which can be replicated in other geriatric societies or professional associations in the region, with a focus on OP. These and other countries in the region must demonstrate the viability, scalability, profitability, availability and sustainability throughout the health system, of the telehealth with emphasis on gerontology and geriatrics. Therefore, having greater knowledge of telehealth in gerontology and geriatrics in Latin America and the Caribbean region will generate lessons learned and experiences that can be used to improve public policies, regulations, and health systems in countries where implementation barriers still persist [41], in light of other international experiences [119].

One of the limitations of our literature review is that the methodological quality of the scientific articles was not assessed, given the diversity of designs included in this literature review. However, its strengths include an updated concept of TeleGerontology and TeleGeriatrics; a broad and exhaustive review of the global and regional literature on the implementation, barriers, and facilitators of telehealth for OP during the COVID-19 pandemic; lessons learned and considerations for improving telehealth implementation and reducing barriers for OP, both globally and regionally; and the challenges for telehealth for OP in Latin America and the Caribbean (as a present and future opportunity) in aspects related to future pandemics, management (design, implementation, and evaluation), research, academic training, and the healthcare system and public policies.

5. Conclusions

During the COVID-19 pandemic, the effectiveness of telehealth was demonstrated, as it provided continuity and access to gerontological and geriatric care services, while reducing the risk of infection among OP by minimizing the need to visit healthcare facilities. Telehealth, thus, became a new modality of intervention with OP and their support networks, accelerating its adoption by several decades.

As a result, the pandemic was an opportunity to evaluate the current systems for delivering social and healthcare services, both for the general population and for OP. This highlights the importance of assessing, designing, and implementing strategies in a telehealth modality, considering all levels of healthcare, in order to ensure the continuity of regular interventions.

The increase in population aging is one of the major challenges in the coming decades, and one in which the needs and requirements among demographic cohorts will vary considerably, in light of individuals' life course. In this context, the documented benefits of telehealth support its role as a fundamental and routine component of gerontological and geriatric care, particularly for reaching OP who face barriers to accessing healthcare services, including those in rural and remote areas. Similarly, telehealth is an excellent alternative for ensuring continuity of specialized care in situations involving physical isolation (e.g., pandemics, natural disasters, disability, and critical care), which restrict the social and healthcare participation of those affected. In fact, during the early months of the pandemic, telehealth served as a care alternative for OP with various health conditions. A proactive approach to identifying and addressing telehealth barriers can help maximize virtual interactions for the older population and mitigate healthcare inequities.

In the future, it will be necessary to gather local experiences accumulated during the pandemic, as well as to advance research, university education, professional training, and the development of guidelines, regulations, and public policies on telehealth in the fields of gerontology and geriatrics, reflecting the specific needs and context of the region.

Finally, the recommendations emerging from this review are highly relevant for healthcare professionals who work directly with older people, as well as for decision-makers, in guiding effective intervention strategies for the implementation of healthcare services for individuals with limited access to specialized care. Telehealth should help reduce fragmentation, improve data sharing, enhance communication among stakeholders, and address the sustainability of interventions.

Author Contributions: Conceptualization, R.P.-M. and E.S.R.; methodology, R.P.-M., E.S.R. and G.R.-B.; resources, R.P.-M.; writing—original draft preparation, R.P.-M., E.S.R., H.A.B.-C., S.D.-A., S.P.-S., F.R.-W., P.A.W., S.M., V.T., S.A.-N., I.B.-C., V.C.-A., C.B., M.F.L., R.M., A.T., I.C., F.M. and G.R.-B.; writing—review and editing, R.P.-M., E.S.R., H.A.B.-C., S.D.-A., S.P.-S., F.R.-W., P.A.W., S.M., V.T., S.A.-N., I.B.-C., V.C.-A., C.B., M.F.L., R.M., A.T., I.C., F.M. and G.R.-B.; supervision, E.S.R.; project administration, R.P.-M.; funding acquisition, R.P.-M. All authors have read and agreed to the published version of the manuscript.

Funding: This work was supported by the ANID Millennium Science Initiative Program (NCS2022_039).

Institutional Review Board Statement: Not applicable.

Informed Consent Statement: Not applicable.

Data Availability Statement: No new data were created or analyzed in this study. Data sharing is not applicable to this article.

Conflicts of Interest: The authors declare no conflicts of interest.

Appendix A

Table A1. Search strategy.

Databases	Syntax Descriptors	Results
Pubmed	(("older adult"[Title/Abstract] OR "older person"[Title/Abstract] OR "older people"[Title/Abstract] OR "old age"[Title/Abstract] OR aging[Title/Abstract] OR aged[Title/Abstract] OR elderly[Title/Abstract]) AND (telehealth[Title/Abstract] OR telemedicine[Title/Abstract] OR telerehabilitation[Title/Abstract]) AND (Covid*[Title/Abstract] OR Pandemic*[Title/Abstract] OR SARS-CoV-2[Title/Abstract] OR Coronavirus[Title/Abstract]) AND (implement*[Title/Abstract] OR facilitator*[Title/Abstract] OR barrier*[Title/Abstract])) Filters: English, Spanish	313
Scopus	((("older adult" OR "older person" OR "older people" OR "old age" OR aging OR aged OR elderly) AND (telehealth OR telemedicine OR telerehabilitation) AND (covid* OR pandemic* OR sars-cov-2 OR coronavirus) AND (implement* OR facilitator* OR barrier*))) AND (LIMIT-TO (DOCTYPE, "ar")) AND (LIMIT-TO (LANGUAGE, "English") OR LIMIT-TO (LANGUAGE, "Spanish"))	1299
Scielo	(ab:((older adult OR older person OR older people OR old age OR aging OR aged OR elderly) AND (telehealth OR telemedicine OR telerehabilitation))) Filtros aplicados: (Tipo de literatura: Artículo)	19
	Total export	**1631**
	Total duplicates	254
	Total articles	**1377**

Date of the Exporting records 23 January 2025.

Table A2. Inclusion and Exclusion Criteria.

Inclusion Criteria	Exclusion Criteria
(a) Scientific articles: • Databases: PubMed, Scopus, and Scielo. • Language: English and Spanish • Aims: Research conducted globally and in Latin American and Caribbean countries that contributed to the objectives of the literature review. • Date: from the year 2020 onwards. (b) Government documents and non-governmental documents: • Databases: Websites of the health ministries, professional associations, and other non-governmental organizations from countries in the region • Language: English and Spanish • Aims: documents conducted in Latin American and Caribbean countries that contributed to the objectives of the literature review. The documents included addressed the implementation of telehealth in the countries of the region. • Date: The search was not limited to a specific time period.	• Conference abstracts • Scientific conference reports • Dissertations • Research reports • Theses • Case studies • Protocols • Letters to the editor • Editorials

Table A3. Description of the 46 scientific articles on the implementation, barriers, and facilitators of telehealth during the COVID-19 pandemic, included in the literature Review.

N°	Title	Country	Year	Aim	Type of Research	Sample Size (n=)	Results
1	Perceived Facilitators and Barriers, From the Perspective of Users, of a Multicomponent Intervention in Older People Using an Asynchronous Telehealth Modality During the COVID-19 Pandemic: A Qualitative Research [71]	Chile	2025	Examine the facilitators and barriers, from the users' perspective, of a promotional-preventive multicomponent intervention in older people using an asynchronous telehealth modality during the COVID-19 pandemic, as a continuation of the face-to-face intervention.	Qualitative. Intervention. In-depth semi-structured interviews	26 OP	Six themes were identified: positive aspects of telehealth, telehealth facilitators, preference for face-to-face modality over telehealth modality, telehealth barriers, reasons for not performing telehealth, and coping strategies in the pandemic: specifically, as facilitators, participating in the company of others, having participated in the same intervention previously (face-to-face modality), good knowledge of digital literacy, self-motivation, commitment to the program, and the emergence of innate leaders, and as barriers, pain during physical activity, complexity of cognitive exercises included in cognitive stimulation, poor digital literacy, and not having support from others.
2	Satisfaction of healthcare workers and patients regarding telehealth service in a hospital in Peru [77]	Peru	2022	Evaluate the level of satisfaction of healthcare workers and patients with the telehealth service of the Hospital III Regional Honorio Delgado (HRHD), as well as the maturity level of the telehealth service implementation.	Quantitative. Cross-sectional survey	129 (physicians and nonphysician professionals) 377 patients (44 OP)	Non-physician professionals' satisfaction with the telehealth service was higher than that of physicians (72.5% vs. 18.3%). Of patients, 77.6% stated they were satisfied with the service. Regarding the maturity level, the HRHD telemedicine service had 32% of items in null status, 40.8% in started, 25.2% in advanced, and 2% in ready conditions.
3	Psychosocial telemonitoring and teleorientation for older adults in the Social Security (EsSalud) during the first six months of the COVID-19 pandemic in Peru [78]	Peru	2022	Describe the experience of implemented Psychosocial telemonitoring and teleorientation for elderly patients during COVID-19 pandemic.	Quantitative. Cross-sectional	154,280 follow-ups and 36,492 remote care services were provided to OP	The main interventions provided were emotional support (75.5%) and social counseling (53.8%). The most recorded moods were calmness and worry. Feelings of worry, stress, sadness, and fear are higher in the reports with COVID-19 compared to those without COVID-19.
4	Understanding the Personal Barriers of Elderly Patients for Carrying out Teleconsultations During COVID-19 Pandemic: An Observational Study [79]	Brazil	2024	Describe the socioeconomic, clinical, and functional characteristics of elderly patients who were supported by a COVID-19 telehealth program.	Quantitative. Cross-sectional	237 OP	Age greater than 80 years, lower educational level, hearing, and visual impairments were characteristics associated with the need for support for teleconsultations. The need for support was associated with hospitalization and mortality.
5	Providing geriatric oncology care using telemedicine for older patients with cancer during the COVID-19 pandemic in Mexico [80]	Mexico	2023	Describe experience using readily available telemedicine tools to deliver specialist multidisciplinary care to older adults with cancer at a Mexican medical center during the COVID-19 pandemic.	Quantitative. Intervention. Cross-sectional	44 OP with cancer	Only 20% of patients had webcam-equipped computers, and 50% of visits were performed using a caregiver's device. Seventy-five percent of visits took place using WhatsApp, and 23% using Zoom. The average visit lasted 23 min, with only 2% not completed due to technical issues. A geriatric assessment was successfully conducted in 81% of telemedicine visits, and chemotherapy was prescribed remotely in 32%.

Table A3. *Cont.*

N°	Title	Country	Year	Aim	Type of Research	Sample Size (n=)	Results
6	Implementation of a Teledentistry Platform for Dental Emergencies for the Elderly in the Context of the COVID-19 Pandemic in Chile [81]	Chile	2022	Develop and implement a "semi-presential" technology platform to support urgent and priority dental care for the elderly in the context of the COVID-19 pandemic among the Chilean population.	Quantitative. Intervention. Cross-sectional	135 OP	53.3% required immediate or urgent treatment, and 24.4% were derived to specialists from whom 60.6% needed immediate or urgent treatment. 74.3% of teleconsultations were derived to an oral pathology specialist.
7	Clinical utility of Phototest via teleneuropsychology in Chilean rural older adults [82]	Chile	2022	Analyze the clinical utility of the Phototest, through telemedicine, to identify mild cognitive impairment in rural older adults with memory complaints, during the COVID-19 pandemic.	Quantitative. Cross-sectional Case–control	111 (rural OP with mild cognitive impairment) 130 (healthy controls)	To identify mild cognitive impairment, using a cutoff score of 27–28 points, the Phototest showed a sensitivity of 96.6% and a specificity of 81.8%; indicators superior to those of the MMSEm.
8	Providing Supportive and Palliative Care Using Telemedicine for Patients with Advanced Cancer During the COVID-19 Pandemic in Mexico [83]	Mexico	2021	Describe how transformed a multidisciplinary supportive and palliative care program into a telemedicine intervention for patients with advanced cancer during the COVID-19 pandemic.	Quantitative. Intervention. Cross-sectional	45 patients with Advanced Cancer (Median age was 68 years)	The most common interventions were psychological care (33%), pain and symptom control (25%), and nutritional counseling (13%). Half of the interventions were provided by video conferencing. The most common patient-reported barrier was limited experience using communication technology.
9	Implementation of a virtual telehealth course for Chilean older adults and health students [84]	Chile	2023	Assess the perception and impact of an online course about healthy aging aimed at the community and healthcare professionals.	Quantitative. Intervention. Cross-sectional survey	386 attendants (20,46% OP)	All respondents acquired new knowledge and were willing to participate again. The frequency of interest about self-care is three times greater than about caring for another person, In an older person, the interest is 101 more times about self-care than caring for another person. Ninety five percent of respondents felt more active and 84% felt more accompanied.
10	Playing remotely in times of crisis: A program to overcome social isolation [85]	Brazil	2022	Examine the feasibility of an intergenerational remote intervention program designed to promote the well-being and social connection of vulnerable older adults, mainly people with aphasia and dementia during the COVID-19 pandemic in the south of Brazil.	Mixed-method. Quantitative (Cross-sectional) Qualitative (participative observation)	34 OP with stroke-induced cognitive impairments, dementia and individuals without any neurological conditions	The initial period of the program achieved 83.7% of adherence and sustainability for additional 3 months. Preliminary results suggest feasibility and acceptability, considering formal and informal support in digital inclusion. Participatory observations describe that the structure of sessions and activities were well received. The analysis of participants' perceptions detects the thematic saliency of feelings of social connection and a sense of having learned with the group.
11	Experience in the use of videos for the promotion of physical exercise at home in online mode in older adults in Chile during the COVID-19 pandemic [97]	Chile	2022	Describe the usability, actionability and understanding of videos to promote exercise at home online during the COVID-19 pandemic, analyzing the characteristics of the population, their satisfaction, adherence and barriers to physical exercise.	Quantitative. Intervention. Cross-sectional survey	34 OP	The videos as understandable and actionable. Usability was lower in people who perceived a lower level of technological management. Average adherence was 2 days a week for 2.5 weeks. The main perceived barrier was the lack of will, which showed a greater tendency in people who performed physical exercise in a group way before the restrictions due to the COVID-19 pandemic.

Table A3. *Cont.*

N°	Title	Country	Year	Aim	Type of Research	Sample Size (n=)	Results
12	Telemedicine in primary care of older adults: a qualitative study [23]	Canada	2024	Identify potential facilitators and barriers to telemedicine use in primary care for older adults and develop recommendations accordingly.	Qualitative. Semi-structured interviews and focus groups	29 OP 15 Healthcare professionals (family physicians, nurses, social workers, and physiotherapists)	Telemedicine contributed to maintaining the continuity of care and was particularly convenient when there was an existing or established patient-physician relationship or for addressing minor health issues. Telemedicine was found to be beneficial for people with limited mobility, reducing their exposure to potentially high-risk environments. However, participants expressed concerns about the lack of visual contact, causing essential details to be overlooked. Additionally, issues related to miscommunication due to language or hearing barriers were identified. Healthcare professionals perceived that most older adults did not consider phone consultations a medical act. Participants were open to a hybrid approach, combining in-person consultations and telemedicine, based on their specific health conditions.
13	The Effect of a Tele-Health Intervention Program on Home-Dwelling Persons with Dementia or MCI and on Their Primary Caregivers during the Stay-at-Home-Order Period in the COVID-19 Pandemic Outbreak: Evidence from Taiwan [26]	Taiwan	2022	The results could serve as an important reference for policymakers to evaluate whether the Tele-Health intervention program is an appropriate policy instrument for delivering various supportive care services to persons with dementia or mild cognitive impairment and their primary caregivers.	Quantitative. Intervention Case–control	8 OP dementia and mild cognitive impairment (Case) 8 OP dementia and mild cognitive impairment (control group)	The Telehealth intervention program significantly increased the well-being of the participants and their primary caregivers, but the negative correlations between the Tele-Health intervention program and family functioning were also found to be significant.
14	Telehealth Use Among Older Adults During COVID-19: Associations With Sociodemographic and Health Characteristics, Technology Device Ownership, and Technology Learning [32]	USA	2022	Examine rates and correlates of telehealth (video call) use among those aged 70+, and tested the significance of access to information and communication technology device ownership and knowledge of how to use the internet and devices as telehealth-enabling factors.	Quantitative. Cross-sectional survey	3257 OP	Telehealth use increased to 21.1% from 4.6% pre-pandemic. In logistic regression models without technology-enabling factors, older age and lower income were negatively associated with telehealth use; however, when technology-enabling factors were included, they were significant while age and income were no longer significant. Insuring that older adults have ICT devices and internet access may reduce health disparities and improve telehealth care delivery.
15	Geriatric care physicians' perspectives on providing virtual care: a reflexive thematic synthesis of their online survey responses from Ontario, Canada [34]	Canada	2024	Understand the perspectives of geriatric care providers on using telemedicine with older adults through telephone, videoconferencing and eConsults.	Qualitative. Cross-sectional survey (thematic analysis)	29 Geriatric care physicians	Identified difficulty using technology, patient sensory impairment, lack of hospital support and pre-existing high patient volumes as barriers against using telemedicine, whereas the presence of a caregiver and administrative support were facilitators. Perceived benefits of telemedicine included improved time efficiency, reduced travel, and provision of visual information through videoconferencing. Ultimately, participants felt telemedicine served various purposes in geriatric care, including improving accessibility of care, providing follow-up and obtaining collateral history. Main limitations are the absence of, or incomplete physical exams and cognitive testing.

Table A3. *Cont.*

N°	Title	Country	Year	Aim	Type of Research	Sample Size (n=)	Results
16	Digital literacy as a potential barrier to implementation of cardiology tele-visits after COVID-19 pandemic: the INFO-COVID survey [57]	Italy	2023	Evaluate digital literacy among cardiology outpatients.	Quantitative. Cross-sectional survey	1067 OP	For internet access, there was a splitting between "never" (42.1%) and "every day" (41.0%). In the total population, the most used devices for internet access were smartphones (59.0%), and WhatsApp represented the most used app (57.3%). Internet users were younger compared to non-internet users (63 vs. 78 years old, respectively) and with a higher educational level. Age and educational level were associated with non-use of internet.
17	Technology Learning and the Adoption of Telehealth Among Community-Dwelling Older Adults During the COVID-19 Outbreak [59]	USA	2022	Examine changes in the prevalence of telehealth utilization in older adults before and during the COVID-19 outbreak, and to investigate the relationship between learning a new technology and the adoption of telehealth during the outbreak.	Quantitative. Cross-sectional survey	1769 OP	The older adults substantially increased the utilization of telehealth during the outbreak. Additionally, learning a new technology is related to the adoption of both emails and video calls to access telehealth. The findings suggest that older adults may be motivated and able to quickly learn a new technology that is required to access telehealth during the COVID-19 outbreak.
18	Exploring Factors Enhancing Resilience Among Marginalized Older Adults During the COVID-19 Pandemic [60]	USA	2022	Explore daily activities of marginalized older adults and how they coped with various challenges during the COVID-19 pandemic when there was state-wide quarantine enforcement.	Qualitative. In-depth semi-structured interviews	18 OP	COVID-19 influenced not only the physical health but also the mental health of older adults. However, they overcame adversity by using technology to continue daily activities, exchanging informal support with family and neighbors, relying on formal support from community organizations, and keeping themselves physically active in their neighborhoods.
19	Perspectives on Telehealth for older adults during the COVID-19 pandemic using the quadruple aim: interviews with 48 physicians [61]	USA	2022	Understand experiences of frontline physicians caring for older adults via telehealth during the COVID-19 pandemic.	Qualitative. Semi-structured interviews	18 Geriatricians 15 Primary care physicians 15 Emergency physicians	Frontline physicians described telehealth as a more flexible, value-based, and patient-centered mode of healthcare delivery. Benefits of using telehealth to treat older adults included reducing deferred care and increasing timely care, improving efficiency for physicians, enhancing communication with caregivers and patients, reducing patient travel burdens, and facilitating health outreach and education. Challenges included unequal access for rural, older, or cognitively impaired patients. Physicians noted that payment parity with in-person visits, between video and telephone visits, and relaxation of restrictive regulations would enhance their ability to continue to offer telehealth.

Table A3. *Cont.*

N°	Title	Country	Year	Aim	Type of Research	Sample Size (n=)	Results
20	Barriers to telehealth access among homebound older adults [62]	USA	2021	Identify major barriers to video-based telehealth use among homebound older adults.	Quantitative. Cross-sectional survey	16 physicians	More than one-third (35%) of homebound patients (mean age of 82.7; 46.6% with dementia; mean of 4 comorbidities/patient) engaged in first-time video-based telehealth encounters between April and June 2020 during the first COVID-19. The majority (82%) required assistance from a family member and/or paid caregiver to complete the visit. Among patients who had not used telehealth, providers deemed 27% "unable to interact over video" for reasons including cognitive or sensory impairment and 14% lacked access to a caregiver to assist them with technology. Physicians were not knowledgeable of their patients' internet connectivity, ability to pay for cellular plans, or video-capable device access.
21	"There Is Something Very Personal About Seeing Someone's Face": Provider Perceptions of Video Visits in Home-Based Primary Care During COVID-19 [63]	USA	2021	Examine provider perceptions of video visits during the first wave of the COVID-19 crisis in New York City.	Qualitative. Semi-structured interviews	6 Medical/clinical director 3 Nurse/nursing coordinator 3 Social worker/social work coordinator 1 Program manager	Providers reported a combination of commercial (health system-supported) and consumer (e.g., FaceTime) technological platforms was essential. Video visit benefits included triaging patient needs, collecting patient information, and increasing scheduling capacity. Barriers included cognitive and sensory abilities, technology access, reliance on caregivers and aides, addressing sensitive topics, and incomplete exams.
22	Telehealth for the cognitively impaired older adult and their caregivers: lessons from a coordinated approach [65]	USA	2022	Describe the 'Coordinated Care At Risk/Remote Elderly' program (CCARRE) to demonstrate a unique approach to reaching culturally diverse and vulnerable population using telehealth, and share some of the lessons learned as a result of early difficulties faced.	Quantitative. Intervention. Cross-sectional	85 OP with cognitive complaints	Recognized unique factors that could improve patient care, lessen burden and optimize access to community resources. Lessons learned from the experience are shared: the televisit approach; start on the phone & move to video; use the video visit to conduct a 'real-time' safety evaluation; the 'virus' approach; address advance care planning & goals of care; address caregiver stress & caregiver needs, including providing behavioral management techniques; address daily activities—cognitively, socially & physically. appropriate things patients can/should be doing; the multidisciplinary approach; address social determinants of health; consider cultural/racial factors & language barriers; and link with local community-based organizations to establish seamless connections.
23	Telemedicine Care of Dementia Patients During the COVID-19 Pandemic [67]	Germany	2023	Evaluate the potential use of telemedicine in older people with incipient cognitive deficits in the context of dementia.	Quantitative. Intervention. Cross-sectional survey	90 OP at risk of developing dementia or with dementia disease	More than 80% of the physicians and neuropsychologists rated the technical process of video consultations as good/very good. A general assessment of the cognitive deficits by physicians and neuropsychologists correlated extremely highly with the results of the subsequent specific testing (MMST and ACE) in F2F and video consultations. Overall, could not find any significant differences in patients' satisfaction between video consultations and classical face-to-face contact presentation.

Table A3. *Cont.*

N°	Title	Country	Year	Aim	Type of Research	Sample Size (n=)	Results
24	Strategies to Ensure Continuity of Care Using Telemedicine with Older Adults during COVID-19: A Qualitative Study of Physicians in Primary Care and Geriatrics [69]	USA	2022	Understand the experiences using telemedicine during the COVID-19 pandemic to examine strategies used to maintain continuity of care with their patients, ages 65 and older.	Qualitative. Semi-structured interviews	18 geriatricians 15 Primary care physicians	Many physicians successfully bridged the digital divide by: assessing patients' technological readiness in advance, being flexible with telehealth modes, using available home or facility-based staff, educating patients on telehealth privacy and usefulness, making accommodations for disabilities, and involving caregivers.
25	Development and implementation of an interdisciplinary telemedicine clinic for older patients with cancer-Preliminary data [70]	USA	2023	Develop the Cancer and Aging Interdisciplinary Team (CAIT) clinic model to provide timely GA and treatment recommendations independent of patient's physical location.	Quantitative. Intervention. Cross-sectional	50 OP with cancer	68% were 80 years of age or older (range 67–99). All the evaluations were hybrid. The median days between receiving a referral and having the appointment was 8. GA detected multiple unidentified impairments. About half of the patients (52%) went on to receive chemotherapy (24% standard dose, 28% with dose modifications). The rest received radiation (20%), immune (12%) or hormonal (4%) therapies, 2% underwent surgery, 2% chose alternative medicine, 8% were placed under observation, and 6% enrolled in hospice care. Feedback was extremely positive.
26	COVID-19 transforms health care through telemedicine: Evidence from the field [72]	USA	2020	Provide data on the feasibility and impact of video-enabled telemedicine use among patients and providers and its impact on urgent and nonurgent healthcare delivery from one large health system (NYU Langone Health) at the epicenter of the COVID-19 outbreak in the United States.	Quantitative. Cross-sectional	1336 telemedicine visits	Between March 2nd and April 14th 2020, telemedicine visits increased from 102.4 daily to 801.6 daily (683% increase) in urgent care after the system-wide expansion of virtual urgent care staff in response to COVID-19. Of all virtual visits post expansion, 56.2% and 17.6% urgent and nonurgent visits, respectively, were COVID-19-related. Telemedicine usage in urgent care (21.7%, in 55 and over) and non-urgent care (40.9%, in 55 and over).
27	Telemedicine Preparedness Among Older Adults With Chronic Illness: Survey of Primary Care Patients [73]	USA	2022	About their telemedicine preparedness, including internet usage, internet-capable devices, telemedicine experiences and concerns, and perceived barriers.	Quantitative. Cross-sectional survey	30 OP with chronic illness	Most participants (70%) reported having a device that could be used for telemedicine and using the internet. However, about half had only a single connected device, and messaging and video calling were the most commonly used applications. Few used email and none used online shopping or banking. Nearly all respondents recognized avoiding travel and COVID-19 exposure as telemedicine benefits. The most common concerns were loss of the doctor-patient connection and inability to be examined.

Table A3. *Cont.*

N°	Title	Country	Year	Aim	Type of Research	Sample Size (n=)	Results
28	The Impact of COVID-19 on Older Adults' Perceptions of Virtual Care: Qualitative Study [74]	Canada	2022	Understand older adults' perspectives and experiences of virtual care during the pandemic.	Qualitative. Semi-structured interviews	20 OP	Participants were generally satisfied with the virtual care they received during the pandemic. Participants described the benefits of virtual care (e.g., increased convenience, efficiency, and safety), the limitations of virtual care (e.g., need for physical examination and touch, lack of nonverbal communication, difficulties using technology, and systemic barriers in access), and their perspectives on the future of virtual care. Half of our participants preferred a return to in-person care after the COVID-19 pandemic, while the other half preferred a combination of in-person and virtual services. Many participants who preferred to access in-person services were not opposed to virtual care options, as needed; however, they wanted virtual care as an option alongside in-person care. Participants emphasized a need for training and support to be meaningfully implemented to support both older adults and providers in using virtual care.
29	Rapid implementation of telehealth in geriatric outpatient clinics due to COVID-19 [75]	Australia	2021	Evaluate the rapid implementation of telehealth in outpatient geriatric clinics at a tertiary public hospital in Victoria, in response to COVID-19.	Mixed-method. Quantitative (Cross-sectional survey) Qualitative (Semi-structured interviews)	24 Geriatricians	Half of the appointments needed to be re-scheduled due to language barrier, poor connection, hard of hearing and inability to perform assessments. Advantages included time efficiency and ability to visualize the home. Preference for the future was initial appointments as face–face, but reviews as either telehealth or face–face.
30	Telehealth access and experiences of older adults with HIV during the COVID-19 pandemic: Lessons for the future [76]	USA	2024	Assess the telehealth capability and experiences of older people with HIV at an urban HIV clinic.	Mixed-method. Quantitative (Cross-sectional survey) Qualitative (Focus group)	80 OP	One-third did not have internet access or an email address. A total of 65% had at least one telehealth-capable device but 12.5% of respondents with a device did not know how to use it. Themes were grouped into benefits (social/emotional connection and convenience) and challenges (technological barriers and missed in-person experience).
31	Understanding the Experience of Geriatric Care Professionals in Using Telemedicine to Care for Older Patients in Response to the COVID-19 Pandemic: Mixed Methods Study [87]	Canada	2022	Identify the benefits and challenges geriatric care professionals face when using telemedicine technologies with frail older patients, their caregivers, and their families and how to maximize the benefits of this method of providing care.	Mixed-method. Quantitative (Cross-sectional survey) Qualitative (Semi-structured interviews)	22 geriatricians 5 geriatric psychiatrist 3 geriatric nurse practitioners	Analysis of interview data identified 5 using the Consolidated Framework for Implementation Research (CFIR) contextual barriers (complexity, design quality and packaging, patient needs and resources, readiness for implementation, and culture) and 13 CFIR contextual facilitators (relative advantage, adaptability, tension for change, available resources, access to knowledge, networks and communications, compatibility, knowledge and beliefs, self-efficacy, champions, external agents, executing, and reflecting and evaluating).

Table A3. *Cont.*

N°	Title	Country	Year	Aim	Type of Research	Sample Size (n=)	Results
32	Barriers and facilitators to virtual care in a geriatric medicine clinic: a semi-structured interview study of patient, caregiver and healthcare provider perspectives [88]	Canada	2022	Describe barriers and facilitators experienced by people accessing and providing virtual care in a geriatric medicine clinic.	Qualitative. Semi-structured interviews	7 healthcare providers 7 OP 7 caregivers	Identified eight themes: impact of the COVID-19 pandemic on virtual care uptake, complexity of virtually caring for older adults, uncertain accuracy of virtual assessments, inequity in access to virtual care, importance of caring for the patient-caregiver dyad, assimilating technology into the lives of older adults, impact of technology-related factors on virtual care uptake and impact of clinic processes on integration of virtual care into outpatient care. Further, identified knowledge, skills, belief in capabilities, and environmental context and resources as key barriers and facilitators to uptake.
33	Determining the Factors that Impede or Facilitate the Utilization of Telemedicine (Video Visits) for Geriatric Patients [91]	USA	2022	Evaluate the barriers and facilitators of telemedicine utilization experienced by geriatric patients at the University of Iowa Family Medicine Clinic and selected Senior Living Communities in Iowa City, to inform recommendations for improving the telemedicine delivery process for older adults.	Mixed-method. Quantitative (Cross-sectional survey) Qualitative (Semi-structured interviews)	3 OP 4 caregivers 19 physicians 5 medical assistants 2 schedulers	Geriatric patients and their caregivers, as well as health and non-healthcare personnel experience barriers, including difficulty navigating technology, privacy concerns, and lack of technical support; and facilitators, such as customer service support and having protocols to guide patients on telemedicine use.
34	Enabling Rural Telehealth for Older Adults in Underserved Rural Communities: Focus Group Study [92]	New Zealand	2022	Investigate enablers for telehealth use in underserved rural populations to improve access to healthcare for rural older adults.	Qualitative. Focus group and Semi-structured interviews	98 OP	Those who had used telehealth reported positive experiences (time and cost savings) and were likely to use telehealth again. A total of 2 main themes were identified through an equity lens. The first theme was trust, with 3 subthemes—trust in the telehealth technology, trust in the user (consumer and health provider), and trust in the health system. Having access to reliable and affordable internet connectivity and digital devices was a key enabler for telehealth use. Most rural areas had intermittent and unreliable internet connectivity. Another key enabler is easy access to user support. Trust in the health system focused on waiting times, lack of and/or delayed communication and coordination, and cost. The second theme was choice, with 3 subthemes—health service access, consultation type, and telehealth deployment. Access to health services through telehealth needs to be culturally appropriate and enable access to currently limited or absent services such as mental health and specialist services. Accessing specialist care through telehealth was extremely popular, although some participants preferred to be seen in person. A major enabler for telehealth was telehealth deployment by a fixed community hub or on a mobile bus, with support available, particularly when combined with non-health-related services such as internet banking.

Table A3. *Cont.*

N°	Title	Country	Year	Aim	Type of Research	Sample Size (n=)	Results
35	Personalized Telehealth: Redesigning Complex Care Delivery for the 65+ During the COVID Pandemic: a Survey of Patients, Caregivers, and Health-care Providers [93]	USA	2023	Identify perceptions, barriers, and possible facilitators to telehealth use amongst elderly patients with comorbidities, their caregivers, and healthcare providers (HCPs).	Quantitative. Cross-sectional survey	40 OP with multiple comorbidities 39 healthcare providers 22 Caregivers	Most patients (90%), caregivers (82%), and healthcare providers (97%) had experienced telephone visits, but few were conducted via videoconference platforms. Patients and caregivers showed interest in pursuing some future telehealth visits (68%, 86%, respectively), but felt they lacked access to technology and skills, and some felt that telehealth visits may be inferior to in-person visits. Health-care providers showed interest in incorporating telehealth visits into practice, but identified challenges in lack of administrative support, lack of Health-care providers and patient technological skills, and limited infrastructure/internet access.
36	Barriers and challenges to telemedicine usage among the elderly population in Israel in light of the COVID-19 era: A qualitative study [94]	Israel	2024	Investigate the challenges and barriers (if any) experienced by the elderly population when using telemedicine services in Israel.	Qualitative. Semi-structured inter-views	14 OP	Most participants recognized the advantages of telehealth services, particularly for the elderly population during pandemics and normal times. Many participants were concerned that the quality of telemedicine sessions may not be good enough compared to in-person sessions, and expressed a lack of confidence in telemedicine services, and frustration from the absence of in-person interaction and communication. Many participants highlighted the technological challenges in the use of computers and applications in general and in the context of healthcare, in particular, in addition to physiological and literacy difficulties. Finally, the participants suggested several ways to increase the accessibility and usage of telemedicine solutions by elderly people.
37	Barriers to Telemedicine Video Visits for Older Adults in Independent Living Facilities: Mixed Methods Cross-sectional Needs Assessment [95]	USA	2022	Understand the barriers to telemedicine in community-dwelling older adults to improve the access to and experience of virtual visits.	Mixed-method. Quantitative (Cross-sectional survey) Qualitative (Semi-structured interviews)	249 OP	Regarding video visits, 36.5% of all participants felt comfortable connecting with their healthcare team through video visits. Regarding top barriers, participants at site A reported not knowing how to connect to the platform, not being familiar with the technology, and having difficulty hearing, whereas for site B, the top barriers were not being able to speak English well, lack of familiarity with technology and the internet, and lack of interest in seeing providers outside of the clinic. Three key themes emerged from the follow-up interviews: the perceived limitations of video visits, the overwhelming process of learning the technology for telemedicine, and the desire for in-person or on-demand help with telemedicine.
38	Awareness and attitudes of elderly Southeast Asian adults towards telehealth during the COVID-19 pandemic: a qualitative study [96]	Singapore	2025	Understand the awareness and attitudes of elderly Southeast Asians towards telehealth services during the coronavirus disease 2019 (COVID-19) pandemic.	Qualitative. Semi-structured inter-views	78 OP	Despite the advantages offered by telehealth services, participants preferred in-person consultations due to a perceived lack of human interaction and accuracy of diagnoses, poor digital literacy and a lack of access to telehealth-capable devices.

Table A3. *Cont.*

N°	Title	Country	Year	Aim	Type of Research	Sample Size (n=)	Results
39	Persisting Barriers to the Adoption of Telemedicine in Latin America After the COVID-19 Pandemic [41]	Argentina, Brazil, Chile, Colombia, Mexico	2023	Gives a broad-strokes update on the development of telemedicine after the COVID pandemic in Chile, Brazil, Mexico and Colombia—the four countries that made the greatest strides in the field of telemedicine and telehealth in Latin America, identifying which barriers still persist to its full integration into the health system.	Literature Review	12 documents were included	This gives a broad-strokes update on the development of telemedicine after the COVID pandemic in Chile, Brazil, Mexico and Colombia—the four countries that made the greatest strides in the field of telemedicine and telehealth in Latin America, identifying which barriers still persist to its full integration into the health system.
40	Implementation of telemedicine in the Americas: Barriers and facilitators [42]	Region of the Americas.	2021	To present an overview of the last twenty years of telemedicine, identifying its objectives, achievements, opportunities for improvement, lessons learned, and lessons learned during the COVID-19 pandemic. Academic aspects, public policy, regulations, hospital care, and knowledge networks from both the public and private sectors were covered, with a special emphasis on the Americas.	Literature Review	21 documents were included	The past 20 years have seen an increase in the availability of resources and technical capacity, improvements in digital education, empowerment of patients regarding their treatment, and increased public interest in this area. Successes have included the use of interdisciplinary teams, academic and professional networking, and virtual medical consultations. After reviewing the state of telemedicine in the Region of the Americas, the authors recommend the urgent adoption of measures aimed at implementing national telemedicine policies and programs, including a regulatory framework and adequate funding. Implementation of the measures should be integrated and interoperable and include the support of academic networks and the collaboration of specialized institutions. The policies should generate an enabling context that ensures sustainability of the progress achieved, bearing in mind the possible barriers mentioned.
41	Telerehabilitation for Geriatrics [9]	Not specified	2021	This article reviews the scope, need, and implementation of telehealth and telerehabilitation in the aging population from the perspective of both clinicians, patients, and caregivers.	Literature Review	82 articles were included	Telehealth use was accelerated by the coronavirus disease 2019 pandemic and became an essential part of the rehabilitation service. Telehealth has a great potential in alleviating social isolation as well as addressing the medical needs of older individuals. Challenges to effective and efficient implementation include willingness to adapt to the technology by older adults, reliable Internet connections, identifying the area where telehealth is most effective, and evaluating the patients and administrative outcomes of telehealth interventions. Telerehabilitation refers to rehabilitation services involving evaluation and treatment. It is an attractive option for older adults who may have multiple comorbidities. Limited access to in-person services and the concern about potential exposure to severe acute respiratory syndrome coronavirus-2 during this pandemic accelerated the implementation of telerehabilitation.

Table A3. *Cont.*

N°	Title	Country	Year	Aim	Type of Research	Sample Size (n=)	Results
42	Asynchronous Telehealth [20]	Not specified	2022	Discuss the use of asynchronous telehealth in the form of e-visits and e-consults.	Literature Review	28 articles were included	Asynchronous telehealth, which includes both e-visits and e-consults. The highest utility for e-visits is for lower acuity illness that does not require immediate evaluation and for which diagnosis does not require a physical examination. The potential benefits of asynchronous telehealth e-consultation between primary care and subspecialty care providers depend on the nature and framework of the local implementation, the breadth of available subspecialties, and the ability of the primary care physician to follow through on the recommendation provided by the subspecialist. Asynchronous virtual care is recognized for providing scale, value, and efficiency. Tracking volume, turnaround time, and quality variables involved in service delivery are critically important in ensuring patient satisfaction, programmatic success, and sustainability.
43	Telehealth Use in Geriatrics Care during the COVID-19 Pandemic-A Scoping Review and Evidence Synthesis [40]	USA, UK, Italy, Canada, Australia, France, Spain, Switzerland, Germany, Ireland, Israel, Japan, South Korea, Netherlands, New Zealand, Poland, Chile, Mexico, China, India	2021	Conducted a scoping review and evidence synthesis for telehealth use in geriatric care to summarize learning from these new data.	A Scoping Review and Evidence Synthesis	79 articles were in-cluded	The articles provide some evidence of effective provision of preventive, curative, and rehabilitative telehealth services for older people, but they highlight a greater focus on curative services and are mostly concentrated in high-income countries. We identified convenience and affordability as the strengths of telehealth use in geriatric care. Weaknesses identified include the inability of telehealth to cater to the needs of older people with specific physical and cognitive limitations. While the threats of increasing inequity and the lack of standardization in the provision of age-friendly telehealth services remain, identified opportunities for technologic advancements driven by simplicity and user-friendliness for older people.
44	Application and implementation of telehealth services designed for the elderly population during the COVID-19 pandemic: A systematic review [66]	Singapore, Poland, Italy, Tunisia, Turkey, Netherlands, USA, Ireland	2022	Explore the availability, application, and implementation of telehealth services during the COVID-19 era, designed for the aged population (age 65 and more).	Systematic review	11 articles were included	Among the telehealth services, there were services aimed for triage and control during the outbreak of the COVID-19 pandemic, remote monitoring and treatment, follow-ups online meetings for patients residing in health centers, and application of online services.

Table A3. *Cont.*

N°	Title	Country	Year	Aim	Type of Research	Sample Size (n=)	Results
45	Telemedicine in the primary care of older adults: a systematic mixed studies review [86]	Ireland, USA, Spain, UK, Netherlands, Poland, Portugal, Switzerland, China, Sweden, New Zealand, Scotland	2023	Explore the effects of TM and the determinants of its use in primary care for older adults.	Systematic mixed studies review	20 articles were included	They used either phone, videoconference or both. Among studies reporting positive outcomes in TM experience, 'user habit or preferences' was the most cited barrier and 'location and travel time' was the most cited facilitator. Only one study reported negative outcomes in TM experience and reported 'comfort with patient communication' and 'user interface, intended use or usability' as barriers, and 'technology skills and knowledge' and 'location and travel time' as facilitators. Among studies reporting positive outcomes in service use and usability, no barrier or facilitator was cited more than once. Only one study reported a positive outcome in health-related and behavioral outcomes
46	Facilitators and barriers to the adoption of telehealth in older adults: an integrative review [64] Comment: This scientific article is included because it provides a pre-pandemic comparison for the barriers and facilitators of telehealth in OP.	USA, UK, Germany, Netherlands, Austria, France, Denmark, Norway, Canada	2014	Identified the current telehealth technologies that are available to older adults with a discussion on the facilitators of and barriers to those technologies.	Integrative review	14 articles were in-cluded	50% of the studies did not specifically address facilitators of and barriers to adopting telehealth with older adults. Also, studies in this population did not address caregivers' perceptions on the facilitators of and barriers to telehealth.

References

1. Huenchuan, S. *Envejecimiento, Personas Mayores y Agenda 2030 Para el Desarrollo Sostenible: Perspectiva Regional y de Derechos Humanos*; CEPAL: Santiago, Chile, 2018; pp. 1–259. Available online: https://repositorio.cepal.org/server/api/core/bitstreams/431e4d95-46d9-4de6-a0a6-d41b1cb7d0b9/content (accessed on 1 September 2025).
2. Naciones Unidas. Se Acaba la Emergencia Por la Pandemia, Pero el COVID Continua. 2023. Available online: https://news.un.org/es/story/2023/05/1520732 (accessed on 1 September 2025).
3. Pinazo, S. Psychosocial Impact of COVID-19 on older people: Problems and challenges. *Rev. Esp. Geriatr. Gerontol.* **2020**, *55*, 249–252. [CrossRef]
4. Roschel, H.; Artioli, G.; Gualano, B. Risk of Increased Physical Inactivity During COVID-19 Outbreak in Older People: A Call for Actions. *J. Am. Geriatr. Soc.* **2020**, *68*, 1126–1128. [CrossRef]
5. McGarrigle, L.; Todd, C. Promotion of Physical Activity in Older People Using mHealth and eHealth Technologies: Rapid Review of Reviews. *J. Med. Internet Res.* **2020**, *22*, e22201. [CrossRef] [PubMed]
6. Mukhtar, S. Psychological impact of COVID-19 on older adults. *Curr. Med. Res. Pract.* **2020**, *10*, 201–202.
7. Manca, R.; De Marco, M.; Venneri, A. The Impact of COVID-19 Infection and Enforced Prolonged Social Isolation on Neuropsychiatric Symptoms in Older Adults With and Without Dementia: A Review. *Front. Psychiatry* **2020**, *11*, 585540. [CrossRef]
8. Damiot, A.; Pinto, A.; Turner, J.; Gualano, B. Immunological Implications of Physical Inactivity among Older Adults during the COVID-19 Pandemic. *Gerontology* **2020**, *66*, 431–438. [CrossRef]
9. Oh-Park, M.; Lew, H.; Raghavan, P. Telerehabilitation for Geriatrics. *Phys. Med. Rehabil. Clin. N. Am.* **2021**, *32*, 291–305. [CrossRef]
10. Broche, Y.; Fernández, E.; Reyes, D. Psychological consequences of quarantine and social isolation during COVID-19 pandemic. *Rev. Cuba. Salud Pública.* **2021**, *46*, 1–14.
11. Soto, M.; Ramos, M.; Camargo, L.; Calizaya, J.; Caldichoury, N.; López, N. The impact of SARS-CoV-2 on emotional state among older adults in Latin America. *Int. Psychogeriatr.* **2021**, *33*, 193–194. [CrossRef] [PubMed]
12. Brooks, S.; Webster, R.; Smith, L.; Woodland, L.; Wessely, S.; Greenberg, N.; Rubin, G. The psychological impact of quarantine and how to reduce it: Rapid review of the evidence. *Lancet* **2020**, *395*, 912–920. [CrossRef] [PubMed]
13. Murukesu, R.; Singh, D.; Shahar, S.; Subramaniam, P. Physical Activity Patterns, Psychosocial Well-Being and Coping Strategies Among Older Persons with Cognitive Frailty of the "WE-RISE" Trial Throughout the COVID-19 Movement Control Order. *Clin. Interv. Aging* **2021**, *16*, 415–429. [CrossRef]
14. United Nations. *Policy Brief: The Impact of COVID-19 on Older Persons*; United Nations: New York, NY, USA, 2020; pp. 1–16.
15. Hill, J.; Harrington, A.; Adeoye, P.; Campbell, N.; Holden, R. Going Remote-Demonstration and Evaluation of Remote Technology Delivery and Usability Assessment With Older Adults: Survey Study. *JMIR mHealth uHealth* **2021**, *9*, e26702. [CrossRef]
16. Nicol, G.; Piccirillo, J.; Mulsant, B.; Lenze, E. Action at a Distance: Geriatric Research during a Pandemic. *J. Am. Geriatr. Soc.* **2020**, *68*, 922–925. [CrossRef] [PubMed]
17. World Health Organization. *Mental Health and Psychosocial Considerations During the COVID-19 Outbreak*; WHO: Geneva, Switzerland, 2020; pp. 1–6. Available online: https://www.who.int/docs/default-source/coronaviruse/mental-health-considerations.pdf (accessed on 1 September 2025).
18. Dillon, J.; Wick, J. Telehealth: Moving Older People Along the Adoption Trajectory. *Sr. Care Pharm.* **2023**, *38*, 416–422. [CrossRef] [PubMed]
19. Ministerio de Salud de Chile. *Programa Nacional de Telesalud. En El Contexto de Redes Integradas de Servicios de Salud*; Ministerio de Salud: Santiago, Chile, 2018; pp. 1–76.
20. Stephens, J.; Greenberg, G. Asynchronous Telehealth. *Prim. Care Clin. Off. Pract.* **2022**, *49*, 531–541. [CrossRef]
21. Joughin, A.; Ibitoye, S.; Crees, A.; Shipway, D.; Braude, P. Developing a virtual geriatric perioperative medicine clinic: A mixed methods healthcare improvement study. *Age Ageing* **2021**, *50*, 1391–1396. [CrossRef] [PubMed]
22. Davoodi, N.; Chen, K.; Zou, M.; Li, M.; Jiménez, F.; Wetle, T.; Goldberg, E. Emergency physician perspectives on using telehealth with older adults during COVID-19: A qualitative study. *J. Am. Coll. Emerg. Physicians Open* **2021**, *2*, e12577. [CrossRef]
23. Khanassov, V.; Ilali, M.; Ruiz, A.; Rojas, L.; Sourial, R. Telemedicine in primary care of older adults: A qualitative study. *BMC Prim. Care* **2024**, *25*, 259. [CrossRef]
24. Quesada, M.; Carmona, A.; Chami, S.; Caballero, A.; Fernández, O.; Cañadas, G.; Romero, J. Telemedicine in Elderly Hypertensive and Patients with Chronic Diseases during the COVID-19 Pandemic: A Systematic Review and Meta-Analysis. *J. Clin. Med.* **2023**, *12*, 6160. [CrossRef]
25. Tan, S.; Lee, C.; Yong, C.; Ding, Y. Scoping review: Facilitators and barriers in the adoption of teledentistry among older adults. *Gerodontology* **2021**, *38*, 351–365. [CrossRef]
26. Lai, Y.; Chen, W.; Hsu, L.; Fu, C. The Effect of a Tele-Health Intervention Program on Home-Dwelling Persons with Dementia or MCI and on Their Primary Caregivers during the Stay-at-Home-Order Period in the COVID-19 Pandemic Outbreak: Evidence from Taiwan. *Healthcare* **2022**, *10*, 969. [CrossRef]

27. Banerjee, D.; Vajawat, B.; Varshney, P.; Rao, T. Perceptions, Experiences, and Challenges of Physicians Involved in Dementia Care During the COVID-19 Lockdown in India: A Qualitative Study. *Front. Psychiatry* **2021**, *11*, 615758. [CrossRef] [PubMed]
28. Quail, Z.; Bolton, L.; Massey, K. Digital delivery of non-pharmacological intervention programmes for people living with dementia during the COVID-19 pandemic. *BMJ Case Rep.* **2021**, *14*, e242550. [CrossRef]
29. Schwartz, H.; Har, I.; Wenhoda, T.; Halperin, I. Staying physically active during the COVID-19 quarantine: Exploring the feasibility of live, online, group training sessions among older adults. *Transl. Behav. Med.* **2021**, *11*, 314–322. [CrossRef]
30. Mukamal, R.; Dias, L.; Sarti, T.; Nunes, R.; Rego, G. The role of telemedicine in enhancing palliative care for older adults: Opportunities and challenges. *BMC Geriatr.* **2025**, *25*, 474. [CrossRef]
31. Rainsford, S.; Hall, S.; Phillips, C. Effectiveness of telehealth palliative care Needs Rounds in rural residential aged care during the COVID-19 pandemic: A hybrid effectiveness-implementation study. *Aust. J. Rural Health* **2021**, *30*, 108–114. [CrossRef]
32. Choi, N.; DiNitto, D.; Marti, C.; Choi, B. Telehealth Use Among Older Adults During COVID-19: Associations With Sociodemographic and Health Characteristics, Technology Device Ownership, and Technology Learning. *J. Appl. Gerontol.* **2022**, *41*, 600–609. [CrossRef]
33. Smith, K.; Torous, J.; Cipriani, A. Teaching Telepsychiatry Skills: Building on the Lessons of the COVID-19 Pandemic to Enhance Mental Health Care in the Future. *JMIR Ment. Health* **2022**, *9*, e37939. [CrossRef] [PubMed]
34. Chuen, V.; Dholakia, S.; Kalra, S.; Watt, J.; Wong, C.; Ho, J. Geriatric care physicians' perspectives on providing virtual care: A reflexive thematic synthesis of their online survey responses from Ontario. *Age Ageing* **2024**, *53*, afad231. [CrossRef] [PubMed]
35. Esfandiari, E.; Miller, W.; Ashe, M. The Effect of Telehealth Interventions on Function and Quality of Life for Older Adults with Pre-Frailty or Frailty: A Systematic Review and Meta-Analysis. *J. Appl. Gerontol.* **2021**, *40*, 1649–1658. [CrossRef]
36. Dong, M.; Steuwe, S.; Barry, L.; Siegel, C. The Use of Telemedicine in Older Patients with Gastrointestinal Diseases. *Curr. Treat. Options Gastroenterol.* **2022**, *20*, 594–604. [CrossRef]
37. Masterson, R.; Dodson, J.; Bidwell, J.; Breathett, K.; Lyles, C.; Harmon, C.; Ooi, S.; Yancy, C.; Kitsiou, S. Telehealth and Health Equity in Older Adults with Heart Failure: A Scientific Statement from the American Heart Association. *Circ. Cardiovasc. Qual. Outcomes* **2023**, *16*, E000123. [CrossRef]
38. Elbaz, S.; Cinalioglu, K.; Sekhon, K.; Gruber, J.; Rigas, C.; Bodenstein, K.; Naghi, K.; Lavin, P.; Greenway, K.; Vahia, I.; et al. A Systematic Review of Telemedicine for Older Adults With Dementia During COVID-19: An Alternative to In-person Health Services? *Front. Neurol.* **2021**, *12*, 761965. [CrossRef]
39. Dervan, K.; Mulkerrin, G.; McDonnell, T.; Mulkerrin, E. Technology and Specialist Care for Older Patients in the Post Covid-19 Era. *JAR Life* **2020**, *9*, 35–39. [CrossRef]
40. Doraiswamy, S.; Jithesh, A.; Mamtani, R.; Abraham, A.; Cheema, S. Telehealth Use in Geriatrics Care during the COVID-19 Pandemic—A Scoping Review and Evidence Synthesis. *Int. J. Environ. Res. Public Health* **2021**, *18*, 1755. [CrossRef]
41. Chueke, D. Persisting Barriers to the Adoption of Telemedicine in Latin America After the COVID-19 Pandemic. *Telehealth Med. Today* **2023**, *8*, 1–5. [CrossRef]
42. Garcia, S.; Marti, M.; Malek, V.; Pacheco, A.; Luna, D.; Plazzotta, F.; Nelson, J.; Tejerina, L.; Bagolle, A.; Savignano, M.; et al. Barriers and facilitators to the implementation of telemedicine in the Americas. *Rev. Panam. Salud Pública* **2021**, *45*, e131. [CrossRef]
43. Grant, M.; Booth, A. A typology of reviews: An analysis of 14 review types and associated methodologies. *Health Info. Libr. J.* **2009**, *26*, 91–108. [CrossRef] [PubMed]
44. Chigbu, U.; Atiku, S.; Du Plessis, C. The Science of Literature Reviews: Searching, Identifying, Selecting, and Synthesising. *Publications* **2023**, *11*, 2. [CrossRef]
45. Pizarro-Mena, R.; Rotarou, E.; Chavarro, D.; Wachholz, P.; López, M.; Perdomo, C.; Parra, S.; Barrientos, I.; Retamal, F.; Riveros, G. Comprehensive Gerontological Assessment: An Update on the Concept and Its Evaluation Tools in Latin America and the Caribbean—A Literature Review. *Int. J. Environ. Res. Public Health* **2024**, *21*, 1697. [CrossRef]
46. Colegio de Kinesiólogos de Chile. *Practical Telerehabilitation Guide for Physical Therapy*; Colegio de Kinesiólogos de Chile: Santiago, Chile, 2020; pp. 1–181.
47. Centro Nacional en Sistemas de Información en Salud. *Telemedicina Durante La Epidemia de COVID-19 En Chile. Guía de Buenas Prácticas y Recomendaciones*; Centro Nacional en Sistemas de Información en Salud: Santiago, Chile, 2020; pp. 1–19.
48. Organización Panamerican a de la Salud. *Marco de Implementación de Un Servicio de Telemedicina*; Organización Panamerican a de la Salud: Washington, DC, USA, 2016; pp. 1–82.
49. De Fátima, A.; Fernández, A. *Desarrollo de la Telesalud en América Latina. Aspectos Conceptuales y Estado Actual*; Naciones Unidas Comisión Económica para América Latina y el Caribe: Santiago, Chile, 2013; pp. 1–614.
50. Organización Panamericana de la Salud. *COVID-19: Salud Digital Facilitando la Telerehabilitación*; Organización Panamericana de la Salud: Washington, DC, USA, 2020; pp. 1–4.
51. Sixsmith, A. COVID-19 and AgeTech. *Qual. Ageing Older Adults* **2020**, *21*, 247–252. [CrossRef]

52. Ministerio de Salud de Chile. *Exempt Resolution N° 161. Program: More Self-Reliant Older Adults*; Ministerio de Salud de Chile: Santiago, Chile, 2021; pp. 1–26.
53. Mendoza, C.; Jiménez, R.; Montalvo, R.; Rodríguez, A. *Situación y Retos de la Gerontología en Latinoamérica*; Universidad Autónoma de Tlaxcala: Tlaxcala, México, 2023; ISBN 987-607-545-091-9.
54. Ministerio de Salud de Chile. *Actualización Manual de Geriatría Para Médicos*; Ministerio de Salud de Chile: Santiago, Chile, 2019; pp. 1–444.
55. Barrera, F.; Sarasola, A.; Sarasola, J. Telegerontologia, Robótica y entrevistas holográficas: Gerontologia y tecnologias emergentes. In *IDOSO 4.0. Envelhecer em Tempos de Futuro*; Carioca, V., Fernandes, A., Eds.; RVJ—Editores: Castelo Branco, Portugal, 2021; pp. 129–151. ISBN 978-989-53072-2-7.
56. Tieppo, A.; Wen, C.; Mukamal, R.; Júnior, R. Guia de Telegeriatría. *Soc. Bras. Geriatr. Gerontol.* **2023**, 1–84.
57. Boriani, G.; Maisano, A.; Bonini, N.; Albini, A.; Imberti, J.; Venturelli, A.; Menozzi, M.; Ziveri, V.; Morgante, V.; Camaioni, G.; et al. Digital literacy as a potential barrier to implementation of cardiology tele-visits after COVID-19 pandemic: The INFO-COVID survey. *J. Geriatr. Cardiol.* **2021**, *18*, 739–747. [CrossRef]
58. Programa Convive Digital de VTR, Criteria. Radiografía Digital Personas Mayores: Seniors Tech. 2021. Available online: https://www.vtr.com/radiografia-digital (accessed on 1 September 2025).
59. Qin, W. Technology Learning and the Adoption of Telehealth Among Community-Dwelling Older Adults During the COVID-19 Outbreak. *J. Appl. Gerontol.* **2022**, *41*, 165–1656. [CrossRef]
60. Lee, K.; Hyun, K.; Mitchell, J.; Saha, T.; Oran, N.; Krejci, C. Exploring Factors Enhancing Resilience Among Marginalized Older Adults During the COVID-19 Pandemic. *J. Appl. Gerontol.* **2022**, *41*, 610–618. [CrossRef] [PubMed]
61. Goldberg, E.; Lin, M.; Burke, L.; Jiménez, F.; Davoodi, N.; Merchant, R. Perspectives on Telehealth for older adults during the COVID-19 pandemic using the quadruple aim: Interviews with 48 physicians. *BMC Geriatr.* **2022**, *22*, 188. [CrossRef] [PubMed]
62. Kalicki, A.; Moody, K.; Franzosa, E.; Gliatto, P.; Ornstein, K. Barriers to telehealth access among homebound older adults. *J. Am. Geriatr. Soc.* **2021**, *69*, 2404–2411. [CrossRef] [PubMed]
63. Franzosa, E.; Gorbenko, K.; Brody, A.; Leff, B.; Ritchie, C.; Kinosian, B.; Sheehan, O.; Federman, A.; Ornstein, K. "There Is Something Very Personal About Seeing Someone's Face": Provider Perceptions of Video Visits in Home-Based Primary Care During COVID-19. *J. Appl. Gerontol.* **2021**, *40*, 1417–1424. [CrossRef]
64. Foster, M.; Sethares, K. Facilitators and barriers to the adoption of telehealth in older adults: An integrative review. *Comput. Inform. Nurs.* **2014**, *32*, 523–533. [CrossRef]
65. Weiss, E.; Malik, R.; Santos, T.; Ceide, M.; Cohen, J.; Verghese, J.; Zwerling, J. Telehealth for the cognitively impaired older adult and their caregivers: Lessons from a coordinated approach. *Neurodegener. Dis. Manag.* **2020**, *11*, 83–89. [CrossRef]
66. Haimi, M.; Gesser, A. Application and implementation of telehealth services designed for the elderly population during the COVID-19 pandemic: A systematic review. *Health Inform. J.* **2022**, *28*, 14604582221075560. [CrossRef]
67. Brodoehl, S.; Wagner, F.; Klingner, C.; Srowig, A.; Finke, K. Telemedicine Care of Dementia Patients During the COVID-19 Pandemic. *Fortschr. Neurol. Psychiatr.* **2023**, *91*, 444–454. [CrossRef]
68. Hajela, N.; Kwon, B.; Penson, K.; Lee, A. Telehealth Implementation and Teaching Strategies during COVID-19 and beyond in Gait, Balance, and Mobility Clinic for Community-Dwelling Older Adults. *Top. Geriatr. Rehabil.* **2023**, *39*, 240–252. [CrossRef]
69. Chen, K.; Davoodi, N.; Strauss, D.; Li, M.; Jiménez, F.; Guthrie, K.; Goldberg, E. Strategies to Ensure Continuity of Care Using Telemedicine with Older Adults during COVID-19: A Qualitative Study of Physicians in Primary Care and Geriatrics. *J. Appl. Gerontol.* **2022**, *41*, 2282–2295. [CrossRef]
70. Alexander, K.; Hamlin, P.; Tew, W.; Trevino, K.; Tin, A.; Shahrokni, A.; Meditz, E.; Boparai, M.; Amirnia, F.; Sun, S.; et al. Development and implementation of an interdisciplinary telemedicine clinic for older patients with cancer—Preliminary data. *J. Am. Geriatr. Soc.* **2023**, *71*, 1638–1649. [CrossRef] [PubMed]
71. Pizarro-Mena, R.; Duran, S.; Causa, M.; Rios, C.; Parra, S. Perceived Facilitators and Barriers, From the Perspective of Users, of a Multicomponent Intervention in Older People Using an Asynchronous Telehealth Modality During the COVID-19 Pandemic: A Qualitative Research. *J. Aging Res.* **2025**, *2025*, 6839569. [CrossRef] [PubMed]
72. Mann, D.; Chen, J.; Chunara, R.; Testa, P.; Nov, O. COVID-19 transforms health care through telemedicine: Evidence from the field. *J. Am. Med. Inform. Assoc.* **2020**, *27*, 1132–1135. [CrossRef]
73. Ufholz, K.; Sheon, A.; Bhargava, D.; Rao, G. Telemedicine Preparedness among Older Adults with Chronic Illness: Survey of Primary Care Patients. *JMIR Form. Res.* **2022**, *6*, e35028. [CrossRef]
74. Abdallah, L.; Stolee, P.; Lopez, K.; Whate, A.; Boger, J.; Tong, C. The Impact of COVID-19 on Older Adults' Perceptions of Virtual Care: Qualitative Study. *JMIR Aging* **2022**, *5*, e38546. [CrossRef]
75. Callisaya, M.; Lee, A.; Khushu, A. Rapid implementation of telehealth in geriatric outpatient clinics due to COVID-19. *Intern. Med. J.* **2021**, *51*, 1151–1155. [CrossRef] [PubMed]
76. Reyes, E.; Silvis, J.; Gandhi, M.; Shi, Y.; Greene, M. Telehealth access and experiences of older adults with HIV during the COVID-19 pandemic: Lessons for the future. *J. Am. Geriatr. Soc.* **2024**, *72*, 2816–2824. [CrossRef]

77. Barriga, F.; Ccami, F.; Alarcon, A.; Copa, J.; Yauri, J.; Oporto, B.; Quispe, C. Satisfaction of health personnel and patients with a telehealth service in a hospital in Peru. *Rev. Peru. Med. Exp. Salud Publica.* **2022**, *39*, 415–424. [CrossRef]
78. Romero-Albino, Z.; Tenorio-Mucha, J.; Cuba-Fuentes, M. Psychosocial telemonitoring and teleorientation for older adults in the Social Security (EsSalud) during the first six months of the COVID-19 pandemic in Peru. *Rev. del Cuerpo Médico Hosp. Nac. Almanzor Aguinaga Asenjo* **2022**, *15*, 392–396. [CrossRef]
79. Diniz, C.; Coelho, L.; De Almeida, S.; De Aguiar, V.; De Amorim, C.; Corrêa, M.; De Moraes, R.; Barbosa, P.; Gontijo, E.; Ribeiro, A.; et al. Understanding the Personal Barriers of Elderly Patients for Carrying out Teleconsultations During COVID-19 Pandemic: An Observational Study. *Telemed. J. E. Health* **2024**, *30*, 2712–2720. [CrossRef] [PubMed]
80. Hernández, C.; Jimenez, M.; Morales, A.; de la O-Murillo, A.; Soto, E. Providing geriatric oncology care using telemedicine for older patients with cancer during the COVID-19 pandemic in Mexico. *Ecancermedicalscience* **2023**, *17*, 1528. [CrossRef] [PubMed]
81. Beltrán, V.; Von Marttens, A.; Acuña, P.; Sanzana, C.; Rueda, S.; Alvarado, E.; Flores, M.; Cerda, A.; Venegas, B. Implementation of a Teledentistry Platform for Dental Emergencies for the Elderly in the Context of the COVID-19 Pandemic in Chile. *Biomed Res. Int.* **2022**, *2022*, 6889285. [CrossRef]
82. Caldichoury, N.; Soto, M.; Camargo, L.; Porto, M.; Herrera, J.; Shelach, S.; Rivera, C.; Ramos, M.; Gargiulo, P.; López, N. Clinical utility of Phototest via teleneuropsychology in Chilean rural older adults. *Dement. Neuropsychol.* **2022**, *16*, 316–323. [CrossRef]
83. Chávarri, Y.; Ramos, W.; Covarrubias, A.; Sánchez, S.; Quiroz, P.; Alcocer, N.; Del Pilar Milke, M.; Carrillo, M.; Morales, A.; Medina, M.; et al. Providing Supportive and Palliative Care Using Telemedicine for Patients with Advanced Cancer During the COVID-19 Pandemic in Mexico. *Oncologist* **2021**, *26*, e512–e515. [CrossRef] [PubMed]
84. Gutiérrez, M.; Mauro, J.; Asecio, J.; Acevedo, F.; Herrada, J.; Torres, C.; Delgado, C.; Fasce, G. Implementation of a virtual telehealth course for Chilean older adults and health students. *Rev. Med. Chil.* **2023**, *151*, 61–71. [CrossRef]
85. Brandão, L.; Bauer, M.; Haas, A.; Silveira, R.; Alves, C.; Souza, D.; Beber, B.; Oliveira, W. Playing remotely in times of crisis: A program to overcome social isolation. *Int. J. Geriatr. Psychiatry* **2022**, *37*, 1–12. [CrossRef]
86. Ilali, M.; Le Berre, M.; Vedel, I.; Khanassov, V. Telemedicine in the primary care of older adults: A systematic mixed studies review. *BMC Prim. Care* **2023**, *24*, 152. [CrossRef]
87. Chen, W.; Flanagan, A.; Nippak, P.; Nicin, M.; Sinha, S. Understanding the Experience of Geriatric Care Professionals in Using Telemedicine to Care for Older Patients in Response to the COVID-19 Pandemic: Mixed Methods Study. *JMIR Aging* **2022**, *5*, e34952. [CrossRef]
88. Watt, J.; Fahim, C.; Straus, S.; Goodarzi, Z. Barriers and facilitators to virtual care in a geriatric medicine clinic: A semi-structured interview study of patient, caregiver and healthcare provider perspectives. *Age Ageing* **2022**, *51*, afab218. [CrossRef] [PubMed]
89. Jarvis, M.; Padmanabhanunni, A.; Chipps, J. An Evaluation of a Low-Intensity Cognitive Behavioral Therapy mHealth-Supported Intervention to Reduce Loneliness in Older People. *Int. J. Environ. Res. Public Health* **2019**, *16*, 1305. [CrossRef] [PubMed]
90. Kharicha, K.; Manthorpe, J.; Iliffe, S.; Chew, C.; Cattan, M.; Goodman, C.; Kirby, M.; Whitehouse, J.; Walters, K. Managing loneliness: A qualitative study of older people's views. *Aging Ment. Health* **2021**, *25*, 1206–1213. [CrossRef]
91. Oche, O.; Dobyns, R.; Lin, C.; Kennelty, K.A. Determining the Factors that Impede or Facilitate the Utilization of Telemedicine (Video Visits) for Geriatric Patients. *Telemed. Rep.* **2022**, *3*, 156–165. [CrossRef]
92. Hunter, I.; Lockhart, C.; Rao, V.; Tootell, B.; Wong, S. Enabling Rural Telehealth for Older Adults in Underserved Rural Communities: Focus Group Study. *JMIR Form. Res.* **2022**, *6*, e35864. [CrossRef] [PubMed]
93. Nene, S.; Rauch, M.; Belanger, D.; Bennett, R.; Berry, G.; Saad, N.; Wall, M.; Morais, J.A.; Morin, S.N. Personalized Telehealth: Redesigning Complex Care Delivery for the 65+ During the COVID Pandemic: A Survey of Patients, Caregivers, and Health-care Providers. *Can. Geriatr. J.* **2023**, *26*, 150–175. [CrossRef]
94. Haimi, M.; Goren, U.; Grossman, Z. Barriers and challenges to telemedicine usage among the elderly population in Israel in light of the COVID-19 era: A qualitative study. *Digit. Health* **2024**, *10*, 20552076241240236. [CrossRef]
95. Mao, A.; Tam, L.; Xu, A.; Osborn, K.; Sheffrin, M.; Gould, C.; Schillinger, E.; Martin, M.; Mesias, M. Barriers to Telemedicine Video Visits for Older Adults in Independent Living Facilities: Mixed Methods Cross-sectional Needs Assessment. *JMIR Aging* **2022**, *5*, e34326. [CrossRef]
96. Man, R.; Ho, A.; Lee, E.; Fenwick, E.; Aravindhan, A.; Ho, K.; Wei Tan, G.; Wei Tan, D.; Wong, T.; Yeo, K.; et al. Awareness and attitudes of elderly Southeast Asian adults towards telehealth during the COVID-19 pandemic: A qualitative study. *Singap. Med. J.* **2023**, *66*, 256–264. [CrossRef]
97. Calvo, M.; Román, C.; Basualto, P.; Bannen, G.; Chamorro, M. Experience in the use of videos for the promotion of physical exercise at home in online mode in older adults in Chile during the COVID-19 pandemic. *Rev. Esp. Geriatr. Gerontol.* **2022**, *57*, 79–84. [CrossRef]
98. Wardlow, L.; Leff, B.; Biese, K.; Roberts, C.; Archbald, L.; Ritchie, C.; DeCherrie, L.; Sikka, N.; Gillespie, S. Development of telehealth principles and guidelines for older adults: A modified Delphi approach. *J. Am. Geriatr. Soc.* **2023**, *71*, 371–382. [CrossRef]

99. Hawley, H.; Boulton, E.; Hall, A.; Pfeiffer, K.; Todd, C. Older adults' perceptions of technologies aimed at falls prevention, detection or monitoring: A systematic review. *Int. J. Med. Inform.* **2014**, *83*, 416–426. [CrossRef]
100. Moretti, F.; Scazufca, M.; Nakamura, C.; Souza, C.; Seward, N.; Araya, R.; Moreno, D. Use of WhatsApp by older adults screened for depression in socioeconomically deprived areas of Guarulhos, São Paulo State, Brazil: Challenges and possibilities for telehealth. *Cad. Saude Publica.* **2023**, *38*, e00093422. [CrossRef] [PubMed]
101. De Luca, R.; Torrisi, M.; Bramanti, A.; Maggio, M.; Anchesi, S.; Andaloro, A.; Caliri, S.; De Cola, M.; Calabrò, R. A multidisciplinary Telehealth approach for community dwelling older adults. *Geriatr. Nurs.* **2021**, *42*, 635–642. [CrossRef] [PubMed]
102. Aslan, A.; Mold, F.; van Marwijk, H.; Armes, J. What are the determinants of older people adopting communicative e-health services: A meta-ethnography. *BMC Health Serv. Res.* **2024**, *24*, 60. [CrossRef]
103. Ali, M.; Alam, K.; Taylor, B.; Ashraf, M. Examining the determinants of eHealth usage among elderly people with disability: The moderating role of behavioural aspects. *Int. J. Med. Inform.* **2021**, *149*, 104411. [CrossRef] [PubMed]
104. Dykgraaf, S.; Desborough, J.; Sturgiss, E.; Parkinson, A.; Dut, G.; Kidd, M. Older people, the digital divide and use of telehealth during the COVID-19 pandemic. *Aust. J. Gen. Pract.* **2022**, *51*, 721–724. [CrossRef]
105. Dong, Q.; Liu, T.; Liu, R.; Yang, H.; Liu, C. Effectiveness of Digital Health Literacy Interventions in Older Adults: Single-Arm Meta-Analysis. *J. Med. Internet Res.* **2023**, *25*, e48166. [CrossRef]
106. Pichan, C.; Anderson, C.; Min, L.; Blazek, M. Geriatric Education on Telehealth (GET) Access: A medical student volunteer program to increase access to geriatric telehealth services at the onset of COVID-19. *J. Telemed. Telecare* **2023**, *29*, 816–824. [CrossRef]
107. Chung, G.; Ellimoottil, C.; Mccullough, J. The Role of Social Support in Telehealth Utilization Among Older Adults in the United States During the COVID-19 Pandemic. *Telemed. Rep.* **2021**, *2*, 273–276. [CrossRef]
108. Steinman, L.; Chavez, E.; Chadwick, K.; Mayotte, C.; Johnson, S.; Kohn, M.; Kelley, J.; Denison, P.; Montoc, C.; Spencer, L.; et al. Remote Evidence-Based Health Promotion Programs During COVID: A National Evaluation of Reach and Implementation for Older Adult Health Equity. *Health Promot. Pract.* **2024**, *25*, 475–491. [CrossRef] [PubMed]
109. Brownson, R.; Colditz, G.; Proctor, E. *Dissemination and Implementation Research in Health: Translating Science to Practice*, 2nd ed.; Oxford University Press: Oxford, UK, 2017.
110. Pinnock, H.; Barwick, M.; Carpenter, C.; Eldridge, S.; Grandes, G.; Griffiths, C.; Rycroft, J.; Meissner, P.; Murray, E.; Patel, A.; et al. Standards for Reporting Implementation Studies (StaRI) Statement. *BMJ* **2017**, *356*, i6795. [CrossRef]
111. Lee, K.; Jeong, G.; Yim, J. Consideration of the Psychological and Mental Health of the Elderly during COVID-19: A Theoretical Review. *Int. J. Environ. Res. Public Health* **2020**, *17*, 8098. [CrossRef]
112. Roque, N.; Boot, W. A New Tool for Assessing Mobile Device Proficiency in Older Adults: The Mobile Device Proficiency Questionnaire. *J. Appl. Gerontol.* **2018**, *37*, 131–156. [CrossRef] [PubMed]
113. Huang, Y.; Liu, L.; Goodarzi, Z.; Watt, J. Diagnostic accuracy of eHealth literacy measurement tools in older adults: A systematic review. *BMC Geriatr.* **2023**, *23*, 181. [CrossRef]
114. Verdugo, C.; Pizarro, R. Effects of physical exercise on quality of life in older people. Literature review. *Mem. Del Inst. Investig. En Cienc. La Salud* **2022**, *20*, 118–134. [CrossRef]
115. Gagnon, C.; Olmand, M.; Dupuy, E.; Besnier, F.; Vincent, T.; Grégoire, C.; Lévesque, M.; Payer, M.; Bérubé, B.; Breton, J.; et al. Videoconference version of the Montreal Cognitive Assessment: Normative data for Quebec-French people aged 50 years and older. *Aging Clin. Exp. Res.* **2022**, *34*, 1627–1633. [CrossRef]
116. Watt, J.; Lane, N.; Veroniki, A.; Vyas, M.; Williams, C.; Ramkissoon, N.; Thompson, Y.; Tricco, A.; Straus, S.; Goodarzi, Z. Diagnostic accuracy of virtual cognitive assessment and testing: Systematic review and meta-analysis. *J. Am. Geriatr. Soc.* **2021**, *69*, 1429–1440. [CrossRef]
117. Parra-Soto, S.; Duran-Aguero, S.; Vargas-Silva, F.; Vázquez-Morales, K.; Pizarro-Mena, R. Social Outbreak in Chile, and Its Association with the Effects Biological, Psychological, Social, and Quality of Life. *Int. J. Environ. Res. Public Health* **2023**, *20*, 7096. [CrossRef] [PubMed]
118. Hao, X.; Qin, Y.; Lv, M.; Zhao, X.; Wu, S.; Li, K. Effectiveness of telehealth interventions on psychological outcomes and quality of life in community adults during the COVID-19 pandemic: A systematic review and meta-analysis. *Int. J. Ment. Health Nurs.* **2023**, *32*, 979–1007. [CrossRef] [PubMed]
119. Mendoza, P.; Mendoza, J. Telemedicine: Expected challenges in Chile based on the experience in the United States during the pandemic. *Rev. Med. Chil.* **2021**, *149*, 1198–1204. [CrossRef]

MDPI AG
Grosspeteranlage 5
4052 Basel
Switzerland
Tel.: +41 61 683 77 34

Healthcare Editorial Office
E-mail: healthcare@mdpi.com
www.mdpi.com/journal/healthcare

www.ingramcontent.com/pod-product-compliance
Lightning Source LLC
Chambersburg PA
CBHW061519210926
51850CB00008B/1972
* 9 7 8 3 7 2 5 8 6 3 4 6 4 *